OPTIMAL DIGESTION

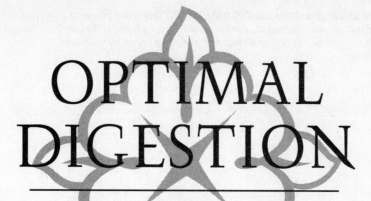

OPTIMAL DIGESTION

New Strategies for Achieving Digestive Health

EDITED BY

TRENT W. NICHOLS, M.D.

and NANCY FAASS, MSW, MPH

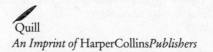

Quill
An Imprint of HarperCollins*Publishers*

The information contained in OPTIMAL DIGESTION is not intended to replace the care prescribed by your physician. Always consult your physician before beginning a new health regimen or altering any course of treatment set up by your doctor.

First WholeCare Edition published 1999.

Reprinted in Quill 2000.

Designed by Stanley S. Drate/Folio Graphics Co. Inc.

Library of Congress Cataloging in Publication Data:

Optimal digestion : new strategies for achieving digestive health /
    edited by Trent W. Nichols and Nancy Faass.
        p. cm.
    ISBN 0-030-80498-0
    "An Avon book."
    1. Digestive organs—Diseases—Popular works.   2. Digestion—Popular
works.   3. Digestive organs—Diseases—Alternative treatment.
    I. Nichols, Trent W.   II. Faass, Nancy.
RC801.0685   1999   99-29600
616.3—dc21   CIP

00 01 02 03 04 QBM 10 9 8 7 6 5 4 3 2

CONTENTS

❖

Preface   *ix*

PART I

HOW YOUR BODY WORKS

1 Redefining the Problem / JERRY STINE   *3*

2 How Digestion Works / JERRY STINE   *14*

3 Your Five Protective Barriers / SCOTT ANDERSON, M.D.   *26*

4 Immunity Against Invaders /
       MICHAEL ROSENBAUM, M.D.   *35*

5 Friendly Flora / NIGEL PLUMMER, PH.D.   *46*

6 Harmful Flora / LEN SAPUTO, M.D.   *54*

7 Leaky Gut Syndrome / LEN SAPUTO, M.D.   *62*

8 Effects of Food Allergies / MICHAEL ROSENBAUM, M.D.   *71*

9 Harm from Toxins / JEFFRY ANDERSON, M.D.   *80*

10 Stress and Digestion / MARTIN ROSSMAN, M.D.   *96*

11 Toxic Overload / JEFFREY BLAND, PH.D.   *105*

12 Damage from Free Radicals / JEFFREY BLAND, PH.D.   *115*

13 How Problems with Digestion Can Cause Illness
       Anywhere in the Body / JEFFRY ANDERSON, M.D.   *125*

PART II

NEW TOOLS TO EVALUATE
YOUR HEALTH

14 Testing to Rule Out Disease / TRENT NICHOLS, M.D.   *135*

Unraveling the Mystery of Digestive Illness /
ARISTO VOJDANI, PH.D., M.T.   *141*

15 Detecting Microbes / OMAR AMIN, PH.D.   *145*

16 Testing in Preventive Medicine / THE INSTITUTE FOR
FUNCTIONAL MEDICINE   *153*

Food Allergy Testing / SIDNEY MACDONALD
BAKER, M.D.   *156*

17 How to Find Out What's Working
and What Isn't / JOHN FURLONG, N.D.   *160*

18 Assessing Immunity and Inflammation /
WILLIAM TIMMINS, N.D.   *170*

PART III

NEW STRATEGIES FOR
INNER HEALTH

19 Remove, Replace, Restore, and Repair /
JEFFREY BLAND, PH.D.   *181*

20 Minimize Food Allergies / MICHAEL ROSENBAUM, M.D.   *183*

21 Clearing Bad Bugs / THE TEAM   *192*

22 The Problem of Viruses / RICHARD KUNIN, M.D.   *209*

23 Avoid Toxic Exposure / JEFFRY ANDERSON, M.D.   *214*

24 Replace Digestants and Restore Flora / THE TEAM   *230*

25 Repair the GI Tract / THE TEAM   *240*

26 Detoxing from Toxins / JEFFRY ANDERSON, M.D., AND
JERRY STINE   *252*

27 Detox from Damaging Habits / ELSON HAAS, M.D.   *262*

28 Rebalance Lifestyle / ELSON HAAS, M.D.   *271*

29 Renew Immunity: A Checklist /
MICHAEL ROSENBAUM, M.D.   *278*

30 The Basics / THE TEAM   *280*

31 The Ideal Diet / RICHARD KUNIN, M.D.   *293*

32 First Aid for Inflammation / PAUL LYNN, M.D.   *302*

33 Nutrients for Repair / RICHARD KUNIN, M.D.   *309*

34 The Role of Hormones in Healing / PAUL LYNN, M.D.   *324*

35 Drugs and Nutrition in Combination /
TRENT NICHOLS, M.D.   *332*

36 Drug Cautions / LEN SAPUTO, M.D.   *343*

37 Benefits of Herbal Therapies / TIMOTHY KUSS, PH.D.   *349*

38 Treating Allergies with EPD Immunotherapy /
W. A. SHRADER, JR., M.D.   *370*

39 Medicine for the Future: Bioelectromagnetic
Therapy / TRENT NICHOLS, M.D.   *379*

40 Chinese Medicine and Digestion /
EFREM KORNGOLD, O.M.D.   *384*

41 Homeopathic Remedies / MAESIMUND PANOS, M.D. AND
JANE HEIMLICH, M.S.   *402*

42 Ayurvedic Medicine / VASANT LAD, M.D.   *415*

43 Gentle Exercise / ROGER JAHNKE, O.M.D.   *422*

PART IV

THERAPIES FROM
MIND-BODY MEDICINE

44 Quality of Life / MICHAEL LERNER, PH.D.   *441*

45 Meditation: Spirit in Healing / JON KABAT-ZINN, PH.D.   *443*

46 Guided Imagery / MARTIN ROSSMAN, M.D.   *452*

47 Self-Care / Tom Ferguson, M.D.   463

48 Getting the Support You Need / Len Saputo, M.D., and
   Nancy Faass, M.S.W., M.P.H.   469

49 Support Groups / Rebecca McLean   482

50 Resources Online / Tom Ferguson, M.D.   491

51 The Healer Within / Roger Jahnke, O.M.D.   495

52 The Proactive Patient / Nancy Faass, M.S.W., M.P.H.   503

Part V

TREATMENT OPTIONS
FOR SPECIFIC CONDITIONS

Trent Nichols, M.D.

Cancer of the Colon / 511
Candida / 515
Celiac Disease (Sprue) / 519
Cirrhosis / 522
Constipation (Chronic) / 525
Diarrhea (Chronic) / 530
Diverticulosis and Diverticulitis /
   535
Dyspepsia—Without Ulcers / 538
Fissures / 541
Fistulas / 541
Food Allergies / 542
Gallstones / 543
Gastritis / 546
Hemorrhoids / 549
Hepatitis (Chronic) / 553

Inflammatory Bowel Disease (IBD)
   and Crohn's Disease / 555
Irritable Bowel Syndrome (IBS) /
   561
Lactose Intolerance / 566
Liver Disease / 567
Malabsorption / 571
Pancreatic Cancer / 574
Pancreatitis / 575
Pruritus Ani / 578
Reflux and Heartburn—GERD /
   579
Strictures and Structural
   Conditions / 585
Ulcers/Ulcer Disease / 588

Resources   591

Index   604

PREFACE

❖

This book offers new approaches to the treatment and healing of digestive illness. You'll find a wealth of resources here and a guide to navigating the new terrain. This is the perfect time to reevaluate your situation because now there is a new and different understanding of sickness and health—think of it as "the New Medicine."

You will want to seek the most skilled medical expertise available to you. This book is not offered as a prescription for self-treatment, because self-understanding alone will not replace expert medical care. However, as you may have found, medication alone does not always restore health. The greatest potential for recovery will evolve through your active participation in your own healing process, paired with the consistent efforts of a capable and compassionate healer.

The best strategy is to become highly educated about your condition, because in the long run, you are the one who has to live with your illness and you know firsthand how your body responds to various medications, treatments, and foods. It is also important to track your symptoms, because the way you respond to different therapies will provide vital clues to solve the mystery of your condition.

Use this book as a tool to evaluate your symptoms and create a personalized healing program. Take the questionnaires in Part I, explore the new testing in Part II, review the self-healing and alternative strategies in Parts II and IV, or jump to the treatment options for your particular condition in Part V. Another approach is to look over a chapter each week.

Whether you are a patient or a doctor, there may be information here that views health and illness from a new perspective. Give these ideas serious consideration. This knowledge is hard won: The driving force for the creation of this book has been the suffering of so many people with digestive disease. The hope is that doctors and patients together, using approaches such as these, can reduce needless suffering.

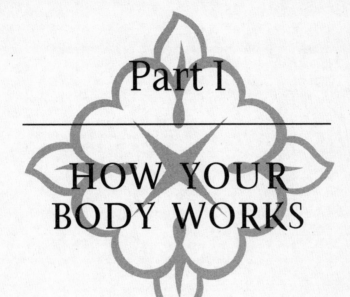

Part I

HOW YOUR BODY WORKS

1
Redefining the Problem

JERRY STINE
NUTRITIONAL CONSULTANT

❖

This book is about you. This book is written for you.

This book is drawn from the experience of people like you. It is based on your needs and the details of your situation. Your experience and responses hold the clues to solving the mystery of your situation. Individualizing the treatment to fit your unique symptoms and circumstances will enhance your opportunities for healing.

The New Medicine involves an understanding of the dynamics of disease, the complexity of the body's chemistry, and how illness is expressed differently in each of us. In this paradigm, each person's treatment is based on his or her unique makeup and responsiveness. Therapy involves skillfully manipulating the chemistry of the body through the use of diet, nutrients, medications, exercise, rest, and stress reduction. The promise of this approach is the freedom to lead a rich life, unencumbered by the pain and distress of illness.

The information in this book is not yet widely available through the existing health care system. But it is not just theory; it is the result of years of experience by both doctors and patients. The fruits of this knowledge are presented here as specific techniques and therapies. To those of us suffering from gastrointestinal illness, this information can be precious and critical.

NEW TOOLS FOR HEALING

We want to introduce you to three key areas of research and understanding:

- ◆ A focus on the unique physical chemistry of each individual, which is called *biochemical individuality*.

◆ An emphasis on intervening in the early stages of an illness by identifying problems through innovative new lab testing: *functional testing*.

◆ Using nutrition to adjust our body's chemistry and promote healing: *nutritional medicine*.

These approaches are part of the New Medicine that is now growing in acceptance and availability. The therapies are grouped under the term *integrative medicine*, which means using both mainstream and alternative treatments.

The new resources do not discard or discount mainstream Western medicine. We all take comfort in knowing that hospital emergency and surgical care is there when we need it. But the challenges of chronic illness sometimes require a different approach—the safe, effective treatments of the New Medicine complement mainstream treatments. Integrative medicine draws from the best of both worlds.

Applying the New Information to Address Chronic Illness

These resources offer hope for many difficult-to-resolve illnesses, from frustrating problems such as hidden food allergies to chronic illnesses such as Crohn's disease. This is not to say that all the answers are available yet, but in many cases, we can now make real advances toward health using the new information and resources. To the degree that we can heal, we can function better and improve our quality of life.

Determining Our Unique Makeup: Biochemical Individuality

An important first step in healing involves understanding the very individual nature of our physical makeup. Our uniqueness is described in nutritional medicine as *biochemical individuality*, a term coined by the Nobel Prize–winning Texas researcher Roger Williams. He was one of the first to define the wide range of variation in body chemistry that occurs from one person to the next—a uniqueness as individual as our fingerprints and our DNA.

We know intuitively that we're not all the same. We may function quite differently from those around us. We might experience strong reactions to foods that others can eat without any problem. We may have unusual symptoms of illness or alarming reactions to medication. Although our response is unusual, that doesn't discount its significance. By fully understanding the very individual nature of our responses, we can come to appreciate their importance.

Our physical and mental reactions reflect the status of our biochemistry, including our minute-to-minute reactions to the foods we eat and to the substances in our environment such as air pollution. Our biochemistry consists of the complex interaction between nutrients, hormones, brain and immune function, and all the other aspects of our body. Although we inherit some of these tendencies, other aspects evolve as we grow, influenced by our environment and lifestyle.

Our body's chemistry is fluid and ever-changing: If you miss a single meal, you may notice a series of dramatic differences in your mood and energy. This is your body's chemistry affecting how you function.

Another hallmark of the New Medicine is that it takes a more personal approach to treatment. In nutritional and functional medicine, treatment focuses on the individual rather than the illness. Describing the status of our body's chemistry is the starting point for a treatment plan. Once a therapeutic program has been developed, a skillful healer can shape the treatment by evaluating our ongoing reactions to foods, supplements, medications, and other remedies. As we monitor what actually works and doesn't work in our body, we can adjust the therapy and move toward healing, step by step.

Testing to Detect Problems Before They Become Serious: Functional Testing

The metabolism of food is a primary focus in the new functional and nutritional medicine and now has center stage. Food is now recognized as the primary source of the chemicals we require for life. Our responses to food are an excellent example of biochemical individuality, since food is also one of our primary chemical interactions with our environment. We are chemical beings. The way our body reacts to foods and processes them is a significant component of maintaining health or developing illness.

Our individual levels of vitamins, minerals, and amino acids can now be evaluated through basic, affordable lab testing. Tests are also available to evaluate our digestive flora, our immunity, and the presence of harmful microbes and markers for inflammation. Other assays can test the success or failure of our digestive processes and look for predictors of illness in the digestive tract and elsewhere in the body. These new tests can also define and measure how we respond to stress and other environmental factors. This testing is now available in affordable, easy-to-use, at-home kits, which can be requested from doctors. The information from these functional tests makes it possible to target treatment to our specific needs.

Healing Through Optimal Nutrients: Nutritional Medicine

Deficiencies of vitamins or minerals can be a significant cause of illness. It is well known that vitamin C can prevent scurvy, for example, but did you know that magnesium deficiency is implicated in muscle spasms of the esophagus and in diverticulosis? Extensive research has found a correlation between illness and nutrient depletion. When those crucial nutrients are supplied, the body can heal more rapidly.

In the early stages of an illness, the strategies of nutritional medicine are particularly valuable, before extensive tissue damage has occurred. Nutritional approaches are also useful in managing chronic illness on a day-to-day basis, to maximize functioning. The nutritional practitioner applies the same elements the body uses: foods, vitamins, minerals, amino acids, flora, fiber, and water. Nutrition offers the ongoing opportunity to strengthen the body by replenishing depleted resources. The new lab tests have improved the ability to detect deficiencies and monitor treatment more precisely.

A wide range of nutritional supplements are now available to you. These new products are more specific and better assimilated, and the nutrients are provided through enhanced delivery systems. Consequently, an unparalleled level of precision is now available in nutritional prescribing. The ultimate logic of nutritional medicine is being realized by addressing illness with the same elements used by the body.

REEVALUATING YOUR HEALTH

At this moment, the way you experience your life and your health is the result of thousands of interrelated factors. Different aspects of your life, your unique physical nature, and your lifestyle are interacting to produce the health you experience at this moment.

If you are currently dealing with chronic illness, this may be the ideal time to reassess your situation. The first step in a self-evaluation is to take a fresh look at your health. A reevaluation offers an opportunity to start over, to describe where you are right now, and to begin putting together a plan for healing.

Before you begin the evaluation, let's review some of the factors that influence overall health: our genetic heritage, our environment, and our habits.

Genetic Factors

Our genetic heritage is the basis for our uniqueness. We each have our own genetic makeup, encoded on the chromosomes of our DNA. However, genetic coding is only one of many influences. The health we each experience is the result of our genetic coding plus the thousands of influences from our environment from the moment of our conception.

Research has demonstrated that for most people, the strongest influences on health are environmental factors. For example, new evidence indicates that the quality of nutrition can actually change genetic expression (that is, our genetic makeup in adult life). We now know that although we were brought into the world with a certain genetic code, we can significantly influence our health through our nutrition and lifestyle. Genetics are *not* destiny.

Influences from Our Environment

The major environmental factors for most people include the quality of food, water, and air, hygiene, physical and emotional stresses, and exposure to toxic substances and to microbes.

Our first exposure to these environmental factors occurred while we were a developing fetus. The second phase began when we started making our own choices about foods and lifestyle. As we become more conscious of how environmental factors affect us, we are better able to maintain our health by consciously choosing habits that support us. This means educating ourselves about nutrition and water quality, becoming informed about environmental toxins and how to avoid them, making the effort to maintain good hygiene, and learning how to minimize the effects of stress in our lives.

The Importance of Lifestyle and Habits

Much of our life is composed of the habits that we have absorbed from our family and the social environment. But habits that work for one person may not work for another, and those that work in one situation may not work in another, due to individual body chemistry and personality type.

Our habits, even those that seem harmless, can aggravate illness. A habit may not cause an illness, but the continual stress on our system can lead to a loss of functioning and eventually to disease. Good habits increase and strengthen our vitality and make the load lighter. Profound influences on our health include:

◆ *What we eat and when we eat it.* Eating foods to which we are allergic can contribute to many gastrointestinal (GI) illnesses. Allergic responses may be delayed and therefore difficult to detect. Skipping meals, letting ourselves become too hungry, or eating too late at night can impose stresses that increase our vulnerability to digestive illness.

◆ *Whether we do or don't exercise.* Regular exercise activates balancing and cleansing activities in the body, improves immune function, regulates appetite, moderates the effects of emotional stress, and improves digestion and elimination. If you find it difficult to exercise, suggestions are included for getting started in Chapter 43.

◆ *The time we go to bed.* Keeping your rest in sync with normal day-night patterns can be a key to regulating many body systems. When you have an illness, it's important to get enough rest.

◆ *Our emotional and mental patterns.* These patterns influence the level of stress and how stress affects our physical health. Emotional tension caused by stresses such as unemployment or divorce has been found to trigger digestive illness, such as Crohn's disease.

◆ *The level of responsibility we take for our health.* Being actively involved in the treatment process can promote healing and reduce relapse.

The Effect of Innocent Habits

❖

A classic example of the impact of apparently innocent habits on health can be observed in people with an undiagnosed lactose intolerance who frequently eat dairy products. Their discomfort and reactions have become part of their daily experience. If they remain unaware of the possible connection, they may continue to suffer low-grade symptoms for years without ever realizing that their response could be due to a familiar food. We encourage you to think about your experiences in a new way and to develop new understandings out of your increased awareness.

SELF-EVALUATION

We have chosen the Health Profile because it's subtantiated by research and provides a reliable basis for self-appraisal. It has been used worldwide in more than 150,000 health assessments.

Approach the exercise as if you were evaluating someone else. Note and report everything, no matter how insignificant it seems. Even if a symptom has been with you for a long time, report it. Be honest with yourself and take your time.

Fill out the Profile with an innocent mind-set—with what the Buddhists refer to as "beginner's mind." Because an open mind offers the clearest possible perspective, we suggest that you suspend your ideas about your health and its potential. For the few minutes it takes to do this evaluation, leave behind any preconceptions. Forget about any assumptions that may be associated with your age or gender. A neutral mind-set is also important if you have a genetic predisposition or a diagnosis that has not led to healing.

You may want to give yourself two scores, one for good days and one for bad days. To do this, make two columns: one for your good time of day, month, or year; the other for times when you don't feel as well.

We encourage you to take yourself seriously; honor your intuitions and observations. Give yourself credit. You have lived within your body your whole life; no one knows it better than you.

Scoring the Health Profile

Once you've taken the test, let's review your scores. The Profile can be a useful screening tool and focusing device. The total score can indicate the overall severity of your symptoms, while the individual sections can serve to highlight the problem areas.

A high score of 50 or above may reflect increased intestinal permeability and suggest the need for further testing. There are many causes of hyperpermeability and many associated symptoms throughout the body. Permeability can be checked using a simple at-home test prescribed by your doctor.

A high score may also suggest the possibility of food allergies, which can pose a real threat to GI health. Unfortunately, food allergies are often difficult to diagnose. Some allergies can cause a direct response in the body, but others cause a delayed reaction and are there-

The Health Profile
by Immuno Laboratories, Fort Lauderdale, Florida

Rate each of the following symptoms based on your typical health profile for:

_____ INITIAL TEST: *the past 30 days* _____ RETEST: *the past 48 hours*

POINT SCALE: 0 = Never or almost never have the symptom
                1 = Occasionally have it, effect is not severe
                2 = Occasionally have it, effect is severe
                3 = Frequently have it, effect is not severe
                4 = Frequently have it, effect is severe

HEAD

_____ Headaches
_____ Faintness
_____ Dizziness
_____ Insomnia   Total _____

EYES

_____ Watery or itchy eyes
_____ Swollen, reddened, or sticky eyelids
_____ Bags or dark circles under eyes
_____ Blurred or tunnel vision
       (does not include near- or far-sightedness   Total _____

EARS

_____ Itchy ears
_____ Earaches, ear infections
_____ Drainage from ear
_____ Ringing in ears, hearing loss   Total _____

NOSE

_____ Stuffy nose
_____ Sinus problems
_____ Hay fever
_____ Sneezing attacks
_____ Excessive mucus   Total _____

MOUTH/THROAT

____ Chronic coughing

____ Gagging, frequent need to clear throat

____ Sore throat, hoarseness, loss of voice

____ Swollen or discolored tongue, gums, lips

____ Canker sores   Total _____

SKIN

____ Acne

____ Hives, rashes, dry skin

____ Hair loss

____ Flushing, hot flashes

____ Excessive sweating   Total _____

HEART

____ Irregular or skipped heartbeat

____ Rapid or pounding heartbeat

____ Chest pain   Total _____

LUNGS

____ Chest congestion

____ Asthma, bronchitis

____ Shortness of breath

____ Difficulty breathing   Total _____

DIGESTIVE TRACT

____ Nausea, vomiting

____ Diarrhea

____ Constipation

____ Bloated feeling

____ Heartburn

____ Intestinal/stomach pain   Total _____

JOINTS/MUSCLES

____ Pain or aches in joints

____ Arthritis

____ Stiffness or limitation of movement

____ Pain or aches in muscles

____ Feeling of weakness or tiredness   Total _____

WEIGHT

___ Binge eating/drinking
___ Craving certain foods
___ Excessive weight
___ Compulsive eating
___ Water retention
___ Underweight   Total _____

ENERGY/ACTIVITY

___ Fatigue, sluggishness
___ Apathy, lethargy
___ Hyperactivity
___ Restlessness   Total _____

MIND

___ Poor memory
___ Confusion, poor comprehension
___ Poor concentration
___ Poor physical coordination
___ Difficulty in making decisions
___ Stuttering or stammering
___ Slurred speech
___ Learning disabilities   Total _____

EMOTIONS

___ Mood swings
___ Anxiety, fear, nervousness
___ Anger, irritability, aggressiveness
___ Depression   Total _____

OTHER SYMPTOMS

___ Frequent or urgent urination
___ Genital itch or discharge
___ Frequent illness   Total _____

                                    TOTAL SCORE _____

fore harder to detect. See the testing section for additional information on allergies and allergy testing.

If you got a high score on the Profile, you will also want to take a look at the candida questionnaire and the parasite questionnaire, both in Chapter 2. Remember that all the symptoms on the test can result from any of a number of causes. To explore the interrelated nature of inner health, let's examine the complex world inside our body.

JERRY STINE is a nutritional consultant and the director of the Lifespan Institute for Functional Nutrition and Anti-Aging Medicine, which he founded in 1987 to develop advanced life-extension and performance-enhancement programs. He also founded and directed Health Evaluations, a non-profit research group with a nutritional consulting clinic and research lab. For the past eight years, he has been an independent nutritional counselor with an active private practice and serves as a consultant for several respected vitamin manufacturers.

The Lifespan Institute provides individual nutritional consultations by phone and access to a variety of the latest functional testing, including evaluations for allergies, GI health, parasites, adrenal function, oxidative stress, and general screening (415-479-3552).

2

How Digestion Works

JERRY STINE
NUTRITIONAL CONSULTANT

❖❖❖

OUR INTERNAL ECOSYSTEM

Let's think of the digestive tract as an entire ecosystem, a self-contained environment supporting a community of hundreds of species of bacteria. This ecology consists primarily of friendly bacteria at work, our digestive flora. Without these positive bacteria to ferment and digest our food, we can't have complete digestion or a healthy body. Our body is constructed from the products of our digestion—we literally are what we eat.

The bacteria in our GI tract number in the trillions. A healthy adult has five to fifteen pounds of living bacteria in their digestive tract, most of which are beneficial. These bacteria perform an essential part of our digestive function, and we are completely reliant on their activities. This huge engine of fermentation completes our digestive processes, producing the nutrients essential to our functioning.

Researchers have found that the lining of the gut is nourished primarily by the nutrients produced by the favorable bacteria. Previously it was thought that these cells were nourished by our blood supply. The beneficial bacteria acts as our primary source of short-chain fatty acids. A number of other important nutrients are also almost completely unavailable from external sources in our food.

Without the nutrients from the bacteria, there would be a loss of function in the lining of the gut. Cell damage can also occur. Consequently, the body devotes an enormous amount of energy to maintaining the proper balance in the digestive system.

WHEN THE BALANCE IS LOST

A number of influences can upset this elegant balance:

- ◆ Overgrowth of yeast, including candida
- ◆ Overgrowth of undesirable bacteria

Microecology Relationships

FOODS
Nutrients
Minerals
Vitamins
Fibers

GUT SECRETIONS
Electrolytes
Enzymes
Protein
Water
Fat

esophagus
stomach
mouth
small intestine

Digestion
Absorption
Immune Function
Detoxification
Hormone Production

colon

MICROFLORA
Bacteria
Viruses
Fungi
Parasites

© 1999 Great Smokies Diagnostic Laboratory

- Microscopic parasites, such as amoebas
- Parasites, such as worms
- Viral illnesses, including measles
- Poor hygiene
- Bad water
- A starchy diet
- Too many sweets
- Excessive alcohol intake
- Food allergies
- Certain medicines
- Frequent use of antibiotics
- Radiation
- Surgical complications
- Physical injury
- Stress
- Genetic tendencies
- Environmental toxins

OUR PROTECTIVE IMMUNITY

Our digestive immune system performs the tremendous task of distinguishing friend from foe in our internal world, playing traffic cop to more than 500 species of bacteria. Most of these are friendly, but even in a healthy digestive tract, small numbers of destructive microbes are always present. We also consume a wide range of bacterias, yeasts, and molds in our food and water; these microbes can be harmful if they survive and flourish. Consequently, the protective mechanisms of our GI tract are designed to neutralize these common organisms. A significant portion of our immune function is strategically located in the gut to keep a favorable balance between the helpful and destructive organisms. This immune function is so vital that 50 percent of the lymph tissue is located in the intestinal lining and 80 percent of all our protective immune globulins are produced there.

UNFRIENDLY FLORA

When the immune system is weakened, the destructive bacteria or yeast may not be held in check. Then colonies of the harmful organisms (pathogens) can establish themselves in numbers great enough to disturb the intestinal environment and harm the body. This imbalance in the microorganisms of the digestive tract is called *dysbiosis*.

If the friendly flora are compromised, the intestinal lining can become malnourished, because the supply of vital nutrients is diminished. What's worse, the destructive microbes produce toxic chemicals that can cause tissue damage in the GI tract and elsewhere in the body. The immune system may then become further impaired.

NUTRIENT ABSORPTION

The ultimate priority of the GI tract is to contain the substances that are toxic and to admit the nutrients our body requires. To accomplish this, the gut membrane acts as a selective barrier. This is the single most important activity of the digestive tract. These functions—containing toxins and absorbing nutrients—use an incredible amount of our energy. Digestive activities include regulating and accepting just the nutrients needed and rejecting everything else. And most of the material in the GI tract is rejected; very little is actually absorbed. You can see why the breakdown of these protective systems can cause a toxic condition in the body, a condition referred to as *leaky gut*; it can also create the potential for illness.

LOSS OF INTEGRITY IN THE GUT: HYPERPERMEABILITY

The leaking of the gut wall—also called *hyperpermeability*—may be triggered by a number of factors, including food allergies, certain medications, alcoholism, radiation, chemotherapy, infections including HIV, severe trauma such as burns, or hereditary tendencies. As the gut becomes excessively porous or permeable, the bloodstream begins receiving both nutrients and toxins. All this material is picked up by the blood vessels lining the gut wall, and the increased load must then be processed by the liver. Much of this inappropriately absorbed material is a source of metabolic stress and is potentially damaging to the body.

THE WORK OF THE LIVER: DETOXIFICATION

The liver has the job of making sense of all this material. If the substance is a nutrient, the liver processes it into an active form the body can use. If the material is toxic, the liver's job is to neutralize it. This process is essential because even a perfectly healthy gut will release some toxic matter.

Our liver is capable of neutralizing an amazing variety of substances in enormous quantities. However, if it is continually overloaded by toxins, detoxification may be incomplete. These toxins can suppress the immune system and compromise its ability to recognize and defend against infection. This excessive load can also directly damage the self-repair mechanisms within each cell. Detoxification stress occurs in a feedback loop: The more toxins are absorbed, the more the liver's capacity to detoxify is compromised. This depletion progressively reduces the ability to detoxify. At some point, real problems can begin to occur.

THE DEVELOPMENT OF ALLERGIES AND HYPERSENSITIVITIES

When permeability increases, unprocessed substances can be passed on to the liver completely intact. This means that the liver would have to process undigested food substances, bacteria, toxic chemicals, or whatever happens to be in the gut. The system could become overwhelmed and release these substances directly into the bloodstream. When this toxic material begins to circulate in the body, the immune system can become triggered, producing allergic responses to foods or other material released from the GI tract. An allergy or a hypersensitivity is typically an overreaction by the immune system that can cause symptoms anywhere in the body. The food or substance causing the reactions may be relatively innocent; it is actually the overactive response of our immune system that causes the damage.

This dynamic can work in more than one way. Eating an allergic food is also a common *cause* of hyperpermeability and can be such a powerful trigger that permeability can increase within a matter of hours. This is a vicious cycle: Hyperpermeability increases the absorption of more toxins and food fragments, which stimulates more allergic responses and amplifies the reactions in a snowball effect.

INNOCENT FOODS CAN PRODUCE DIRECTLY TOXIC EFFECTS

An overloaded liver can cause harm to the body in a number of ways. One is the hypersensitization of the immune system just described. Another is the damage to the body's tissues caused by the direct toxic effects of chemicals in food or digestive debris. For example, certain elements in milk or wheat can have direct toxic effects on the nervous or immune system. Specific sensitivities to proteins in wheat have been implicated in certain forms of schizophrenia.

AUTOIMMUNE DISORDERS

The chronic overstimulation of the immune system can also lead to an autoimmune disorder in which the immune system can mistake the tissues of the body for an invader. The white blood cells and T cells may actually attack the body, rather than the invasive bacteria or the offending substance. This can be a cause of chronic conditions such as rheumatoid arthritis, asthma, lupus, and multiple sclerosis.

With the development of chronic illness, an even greater toxic burden is placed on the liver. Under this increased stress, the liver may no longer be able to perform competently. This sets the stage for a whole new arena of possible problems.

CHALLENGES TO THE IMMUNE SYSTEM: FREE RADICALS

The chronic overwork of the liver's detoxification mechanisms caused by hyperpermeability sets in motion a series of stresses. The first of these is the increased production of toxic by-products called free radicals. We hear about free radicals in the media, because they have been identified as a major cause of cancer. The assault of free radicals, also referred to as oxidative stress, further overstimulates the liver, causing it to send out signals that can confuse the immune system. These signals may trigger inappropriate reactions in both the immune and neurological systems and cause inflammation. Such adverse effects can occur even in a liver that is still generally functional.

FREE RADICALS: WHY THEY ARE DANGEROUS

If the liver's detox mechanisms are held in constant operation, its functions may eventually become compromised. Increased stress on the liver can also be caused by even minor but frequent GI complaints, such as chronic constipation or an overgrowth of bacteria or yeast. Continual stress may ultimately lead to compromise of the liver's detoxification capacity. At the same time, free radicals (with the potential to cause cellular damage) could be generated in excessive amounts. Their effects are experienced throughout the body in cell membranes, connective tissue, and genetic material. This oxidative stress can lead to serious chronic illnesses such as Parkinson's disease, diabetes, irritable bowel syndrome (IBS), and Alzheimer's disease.

Oxidative stress from free radicals can also cause problems by consuming essential biochemicals that our body needs for normal energy production, immune function, the activity of our nervous system, and the production of hormones. It is directly connected to potentially fatal conditions such as heart disease and cancer, and has been identified as a primary cause of aging.

YEAST OVERGROWTH: MORE UNFRIENDLY FLORA

An overgrowth of *Candida albicans* is an example of the dynamic that can occur when the delicate balance in the GI tract is lost. Candida is an undesirable species of yeast that is normally found in the gut even when we are healthy, but usually in small numbers. However, when candida develops too large a population, it can overwhelm the positive digestive flora, like weeds taking over a garden. An overgrowth can also be caused by other bacteria or microbes in the gut. Imbalance in the flora has the potential to set in motion the entire sequence of harmful effects we have just described. Candida can cause illness and create symptoms anywhere in the body.

We have included a frequently used questionnaire developed by practitioners to assess the likelihood of a *Candida albicans* infection.

Scoring the Candida Questionnaire

A high score on the candida questionnaire suggests the possibility of an overgrowth of *Candida albicans* or other microbes. If your score is over 100, you have a number of symptoms often seen in people with a yeast overgrowth. Additional follow-up with your doctor and with relevant lab work could be very worthwhile. A score over 150 reflects the strong possibility of a problem caused by yeast.

If you find that you have candida, don't view that as the primary problem. An overgrowth typically occurs when the digestive tract is no longer able to protect itself. Other stresses may be causing a depressed immune function, allowing the candida to proliferate. Factors that promote the candida overgrowth include the frequent use of antibiotics, a highly sweet or starchy diet, low levels of stomach acid or digestive enzymes, chronic stress, exposure to toxic chemicals, or microscopic parasites.

It is quite possible to score high on more than one of these questionnaires. These problems are by no means separate from one another; frequently, they occur as overlapping conditions. If your scores are high on any of the tests, we encourage you to see your health care professional.

A QUESTIONNAIRE ABOUT MICROSCOPIC PARASITES

The next questionnaire is designed to assess the possibility of intestinal parasites, particularly the single-celled parasites. When we think of parasites, we often think of worms, but here in the U.S., most parasites are single-celled protozoa, so small they can only be seen by microscope. Research by the Centers for Disease Control has found that more than 90 percent of all parasites in 400,000 lab samples were microscopic protozoa. Microscopic parasites are a growing public health problem and are now viewed as one of the root causes in a number of serious illnesses, including chronic fatigue, arthritis, neurological disorders, and immune suppression.

The Possibility of a Yeast Overgrowth—Candida

A. MAJOR SYMPTOMS

Choose the score that fits your symptoms: Mild = 4   Moderate = 8
Severe = 12

Energy/Toxicity

4 8 12 ____ Fatigue or lethargy
4 8 12 ____ Irritability or discomfort when hungry
4 8 12 ____ Headache

Mental/Emotional Functioning

4 8 12 ____ Anxiety, sometimes without apparent cause
4 8 12 ____ Depression
4 8 12 ____ Feeling spacey, light-headed, or disoriented
4 8 12 ____ Poor memory
4 8 12 ____ Inability to make decisions and to concentrate

Digestive Symptoms

4 8 12 ____ Bloating or gas
4 8 12 ____ Chronic diarrhea
4 8 12 ____ Chronic constipation
4 8 12 ____ Abdominal pain

Reproductive System

4 8 12 ____ Loss of sexual interest or ability
4 8 12 ____ Troublesome vaginal burning, itching, or discharge
4 8 12 ____ Premenstrual tension or cramps

Muscles and Joints

4 8 12 ____ Muscle aches and weakness
4 8 12 ____ Cold hands or feet or physical chilliness
4 8 12 ____ Pain or swelling in joints

B. OTHER SYMPTOMS

Scoring: Mild = 3   Moderate = 6   Severe = 9

3 6 9 ____ Chronic eczema, rashes, or itching
3 6 9 ____ Body odor not relieved by washing or bad breath
3 6 9 ____ Chronic sore throat, laryngitis, cough, or tender glands
3 6 9 ____ Urinary frequency, burning, or urgency
3 6 9 ____ Pain or tightness in chest, wheezing, or shortness of breath
3 6 9 ____ Recurrent ear infections, fluid in ears, or nasal congestion
3 6 9 ____ Tendency to bruise easily
3 6 9 ____ Insomnia

3 6 9   ____ Lack of coordination, dizziness, or poor balance

3 6 9   ____ Food sensitivity or intolerance

          ____ **TOTAL—SECTIONS A AND B**

C. MAJOR INFLUENCES—PERSONAL HISTORY

Antibiotics and Drugs as Factors

35   ____ Have you taken tetracycline or other antibiotics for one month or longer?

35   ____ Taken frequent short courses of other broad-spectrum antibiotics?

15   ____ Taken prednisone or other cortisone-type drugs for one month or more?

10   ____ Taken birth control pills for more than a year?

Symptoms and Sensitivities

25   ____ Have you had persistent prostatitis, vaginitis, or other reproductive problems?

20   ____ Been frequently exposed to high mold environments? Are you sensitive to mold?

20   ____ Severe athlete's foot, nail or skin fungus, ringworm, or other chronic fungal infections?

20   ____ Have you been treated for internal parasites?

10   ____ Do perfumes, insecticides, or chemicals provoke strong symptoms?

10   ____ Does tobacco smoke *really* bother you?

Cravings. Enter the score if this describes how you feel.

10   ____ Do you crave or eat lots of starches such as pastas or breads?

10   ____ Do you crave or consume lots of sweets?

10   ____ Do you crave or consume alcoholic beverages?

          ____ **TOTAL—SECTION C**

          ____ **GRAND TOTAL—SECTIONS A, B, AND C**

Scores over 100 suggest the possibility of a candida overgrowth. Scores over 175 indicate a high probability of candida and suggest the value of seeing a health care professional.

Scoring the Questionnaire About Microscopic Parasites

The symptoms described in the questionnaires could be correlated with any of a number of illnesses. Consequently, the scores from the tests point to possibilities, but not a diagnosis.

A test score above 30 on this questionnaire suggests the possibility

Symptoms from Microscopic Parasites

SCORING: 0 = Never   1 = Sometimes   2 = Often   3 = All the time

	0	1	2	3
1. Increased appetite	0	1	2	3
2. Allergies, food sensitivities	0	1	2	3
3. Irritability	0	1	2	3
4. Chronic fatigue	0	1	2	3
5. A tendency to hyperactivity	0	1	2	3
6. Restless sleep	0	1	2	3
7. Grinding teeth while sleeping	0	1	2	3
8. Night sweats	0	1	2	3
9. Fevers of unknown origin	0	1	2	3
10. Loose stools or bowel urgency	0	1	2	3
11. Constipation	0	1	2	3
12. Diarrhea alternating with constipation	0	1	2	3
13. An itchy bottom	0	1	2	3
14. Bloating or gas	0	1	2	3
15. Abdominal pain	0	1	2	3
16. Stuffy nose	0	1	2	3
17. Wrinkles around the mouth	0	1	2	3
18. Dark circles under the eyes	0	1	2	3
19. Track lines in the soles of the feet	0	1	2	3
20. Swollen or achy joints	0	1	2	3

TOTALS: _____

GRAND TOTAL: _____

SOURCE: T. Kuss, Infinity Health Systems, Pleasant Hill, California

Scores over 30 suggest the possible presence of microscopic parasites. The most important next step is testing by a lab with special expertise in this field and treatment by a knowledgeable health care professional.

of infection by microscopic parasites. They are extremely difficult to detect and can be difficult to treat. The single-celled species include a wide variety of organisms, each with unique characteristics and a wide range of damaging effects. Microscopic parasites can actually suppress the immune system and they can also cause other illnesses almost anywhere in the body.

The incidence of microscopic parasites in the United States is increasing rapidly. If you have had long-term chronic digestive illness and have not been tested for parasites, this may be the next logical step. Even if you were previously tested, retesting is appropriate, since new advances in lab detection are improving doctors' ability to diagnose this troublesome problem. Undiagnosed infection can underlay many other illnesses. Note that the symptoms from these chronic parasitic infections may not necessarily occur in the digestive tract.

If you think you have a parasitic infection, you may be tempted to undertake self-treatment. It is vitally important not to self-treat if you do have parasites. Many of these parasites can only be eradicated by a specific drug or drug combination. Herbs can be very useful in combination with prescription drugs and may enhance the effectiveness of the eradication program. However, we advise against relying on the use of herbs alone.

We also want to emphasize that the questionnaires highlight only a few of the many aspects of digestive illness. The scores may indicate the value of lab testing for food allergies, hyperpermeability, candida, or parasites. These relatively simple conditions can play a role in maintaining the chronic nature of more serious digestive disease. We have included these health issues because they are often overlooked in traditional evaluations and treatments. The tests are also useful because low scores can help to rule out the presence of these problems. Your responses to the questionnaires will assist you in developing strategies to deal with digestive problems.

COPING WITH CHRONIC ILLNESS

Unresolved illness can be enormously confusing and frustrating. Consider viewing your situation as a complex puzzle. You may have two or more conditions that coexist. There could be a number of symptoms. A domino effect can occur—the original illness may cause other problems as well. And even your doctor may not be sure of exactly what is wrong.

If your illness is unresolved, you probably already consider it a mystery. View yourself as a detective. The clues are your symptoms, the results of your lab work, and your responses to treatment. Consider all evidence important, including information on what has been successful and what has not. Here are some leads you might find helpful:

◆ Work with the most informed and capable healers and labs available to you.

◆ Review your entire history. The questionnaires in this book can be part of this process.

◆ Develop and prioritize a list of possible causes.

◆ Work with your doctor to get tested and explore the suspected causes step-by-step.

◆ Integrate the results of the lab work with the clues from your individual history to develop the most complete understanding possible.

◆ Be involved in the development of a complete treatment strategy.

◆ Let your doctor know how you respond to therapy so that adjustments can be made. Your doctor needs to know what is *not* working as well as what *is*.

◆ If you are seeing more than one practitioner, keep all of them informed of what you are doing.

◆ Educate yourself about your illness. Ask questions and make sure you understand.

◆ If it is possible for you to obtain copies of your testing, do so.

◆ Keep a journal and a record of information whenever it comes to you. Create a list of what has helped and what hasn't. Record all the circumstances—when, where, how. Include everything: diet, supplements, drugs and herbs, exercise, stresses, liquid intake, time of day, and seasonal response.

◆ Review the literature at your bookstore, neighborhood library, and medical library.

◆ Share your observations with your doctor.

◆ Remember that a good doctor will want to involve you in the healing process.

◆ Continue to adjust and develop your program in response to your progress.

◆ Be good to yourself.

We wish you well.

3

Your Five Protective Barriers

SCOTT ANDERSON, M.D.

❖

INTELLIGENCE: THE FIRST PROTECTIVE BARRIER

Intelligence is the first and most important barrier that guards our health. Although we may think of our brain as the source of our intelligence, we can also define intelligence as the way we live, the way we run our entire life. It is reflected in our capacity to be proactive—to see positive options and to act on them.

We each have a sphere of influence where we can make choices about our lives. We can choose what we bring into our life—the people we spend time with, the thoughts we think, and the foods we eat. The more intelligent these choices, the better. Although we often take our diet for granted, it's important to be very conscious of what we eat,

---

Anatomy of the Mouth and Esophagus

❖

Why is it so important to chew our food well?

- Chewing well mixes our food with saliva to begin digestion and makes it easier to swallow.
- Chemicals in our saliva (enzymes) start breaking down the food. The better they're mixed into the food, the more thoroughly it will be digested.
- Our food is moved down the esophagus by waves of muscle contractions (peristalsis) that act as a conveyor belt to the stomach.

Doctors have noticed that people who bolt down their food have a greater tendency to gastrointestinal problems than those who chew thoroughly. Think of chewing as a time to really taste and savor your food.

because if we consume only what tempts us, we may not be very healthy. So we should exercise intelligence on behalf of our whole body.

Eating smart means making wise choices about when, how, and where we eat, and all those other little decisions we make when we buy, prepare, and consume food. This may mean planning ahead to bring a healthy snack to work for an energy boost in the afternoon. It should include eating in a relaxed way, perhaps sitting in the sun or a cozy café. Eating smart means paying attention to details such as chewing our food rather than just bolting it down. And it's wise to know the basics of nutrition.

OUR SECOND LINE OF DEFENSE: STOMACH ACID

Believe it or not, our stomach acid (hydrochloric acid, or HCl for short) is one of the most important self-protections our body provides; it destroys the "bad bugs"—microbes that are always trying to invade our system.

Most of us don't even think about our stomach acid, and when we do, we are more likely to think of it as a problem. But our body invests an enormous amount of energy to produce HCl. If we drew an energy map of the body, the energy used to create this acid would be comparable to Mount Everest. Although we're used to hearing about the dangers of stomach acid on television, these gastric juices are actually an essential and vital protection to our digestion. Here's how they work:

◆ *Stomach acid basically sterilizes our food.* It destroys microbes such as bacteria or yeast seeking to colonize the warm and nutrient-rich folds of the intestines. As our food is mixed with acid in the stomach, the germs are destroyed on contact by burning them with a solution strong enough to literally burn a hole in this book. Germs such as bacteria, microscopic parasites, viruses, and molds can contaminate anything we eat or drink.

◆ *Stomach acid begins the process of protein digestion.* Stomach juices contain acid and an enzyme called pepsin. This creates just the right chemical conditions for digesting protein.

◆ *In the acid mix of the stomach, minerals are processed for absorption.* Without enough stomach acid, we'd have poor absorption of minerals. In fact, malabsorption of minerals is one of the tip-offs to doctors that a patient may have chronically low stomach acid. The trace

OVERVIEW OF THE DIGESTIVE SYSTEM

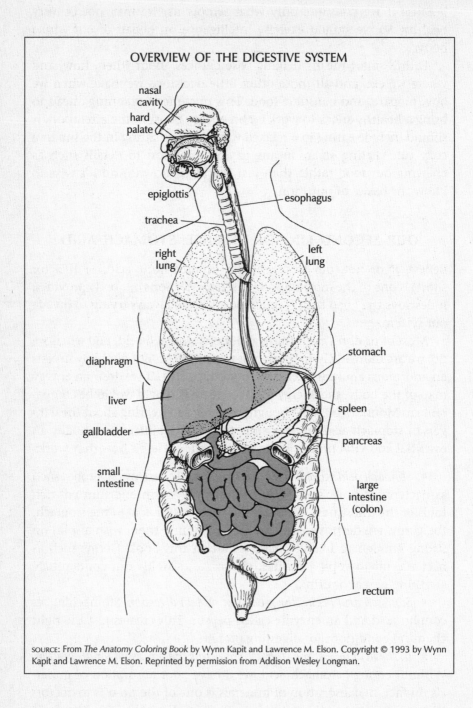

SOURCE: From *The Anatomy Coloring Book* by Wynn Kapit and Lawrence M. Elson. Copyright © 1993 by Wynn Kapit and Lawrence M. Elson. Reprinted by permission from Addison Wesley Longman.

mineral deficiencies that may result can be identified through simple lab tests such as hair analysis.

♦ *Stomach acid stimulates secretions from the pancreas that are essential to good digestion (enzymes and bicarbonate).* The acidity of the food coming out of the stomach signals the pancreas to pour out its juices. When the acid mix comes in contact with the gut wall, this stimulates the next phase of digestion. If the stomach's output is only mildly acidic, then the pancreas gets a weak signal and the whole digestive process is compromised.

Digestion: Our Food Furnace

After we've eaten, food stays in our stomach for a while. How long depends on the size and content of what we've just eaten and how well our digestive equipment is working. During that time (typically at least ninety minutes), food is confined in the stomach under very acid conditions. Here's what's happening when our food is digesting:

A Note from the Doctor

❖

As a doctor, when I identify patients who have frequent indigestion, one of the first things I have them try is an over-the-counter supplement of hydrochloric acid, betaine hydrochloride, which they can get from most any health food store. In some cases, just that addition will resolve their digestive problems. If not, the next step is to try adding over-the-counter pancreatic enzymes. So my first strategy is to support natural processes in the body that may be weakened, with supplements such as stomach acid and digestive enzymes.

♦ If you have any concerns or questions, be sure to talk about them with your doctor.
♦ When you begin a new supplement, make that the only addition to your diet for at least two weeks so you can more easily identify unwanted effects.
♦ Start by taking only one capsule a day for about four days—just as you start eating.
♦ If it agrees with you, then gradually increase the dose every two to four days until you are taking the recommended dose.
♦ Remember that we're all different—the nutritional requirements of a 100-pound woman are quite different than those of a growing child of 50 pounds or a man who weighs 200.

—*Scott Anderson, M.D.*

- The food is being churned in the stomach, grinding it to the consistency of cornmeal.
- This mixture is "cooking" in the stomach acid.
- Germs are being killed.
- Protein digestion is beginning.
- Minerals are being processed.

When this process has been competed, the food is ready for the next phase of digestion, which takes place in the small intestine. There nourishment from our food will be absorbed by the body, to actually become part of our tissues.

As the stomach sends the food into the small intestine, the food-acid mix needs to be neutralized. If this didn't occur, the mix would burn the delicate lining of the small gut. By adding bicarb into the mix, the tender lining of the gut (the epithelium) is protected from the chemical burn of digestive acid. This food mixture (called chyme) is about the consistency of liquid oatmeal and contains saliva, stomach acid, pepsin, bicarb, and enzymes.

The Pancreas Takes Center Stage

At this point, the pancreas also makes its contribution. This gland is located near our stomach, a long, thin organ about 4 to 6 inches long, shaped like a fleshy leaf. It produces a number of important secretions that help us digest. The major ones include:

- Digestive enzymes
- Bicarbonate
- Insulin

In this next phase of digestion, food is moved into the small gut by the action of the pylorus, a thick muscular ring that acts as the gate-keeper, separating the opening leading out of the stomach from the small gut which is called the duodenum. The pylorus releases the food mix little by little. If it were to open fully and stay open, the entire contents of the stomach would come flooding out all at once. Instead, the contents of the stomach are released in small squirts, every few seconds or every few minutes. At this point, the pancreas secretes more enzymes to continue the digestive process, including:

- Lipase to digest fats
- Protease for proteins

- Amylase for starches
- Other enzymes with specialized functions

The Small Intestine: The Cradle of Our Nourishment

The primary job of the small gut is to absorb nutrients from our food. The breakdown and absorption of proteins and fats and the final digestion and absorption of starches and sugars all occur there.

The small intestine is essentially a tube—25 feet long! Its inner surface is covered with tiny folds which provide the greatest possible surface area for absorption, so we can get the maximum nutrition from our food. If you could unroll and unwrinkle the folds and lay the surface of the tissue out flat, the small gut would be about 60 feet across—at a size of 60 feet wide and 25 feet long, the small intestine has roughly the surface area of a tennis court. The large intestine, in contrast, is only about 5 feet long with a surface area smaller than the top of a desk.

If you were to view the digestive tract through a videoscope, as gastroenterologists now do, the small intestine has a velvety appearance because its surface is made up of minute folds, which are covered with tiny finger-like structures called villi. The villi themselves are covered with other much smaller hairlike structures (microvilli), which can be seen only through a microscope. All these structures are exquisitely constructed to absorb nutrients. The villi and microvilli are covered with a layer of protective mucus. The large gut is also lined with mucus, but it has a smooth, glistening surface when seen through the videoscope.

In the small gut, the finger-like villi shrink when chronic irritation is present. As the absorptive area decreases, people usually have problems with malabsorption. In fact, the loss of the villi is one of the findings doctors use to diagnose irritations such as wheat/gluten intolerance (celiac disease, or sprue). If there is infection or irritation, absorption is compromised and the sufferer may lose weight or experience failure to thrive.

After the digested food moves into the colon or large intestine, water is absorbed from the spent food, preparing it to be discarded from the body as stool. Another major function of the colon may be its role as host to a huge population of bacteria, including the friendly flora. Some nutrients are also transferred to the blood here, but the vast majority of absorption has already taken place in the small gut.

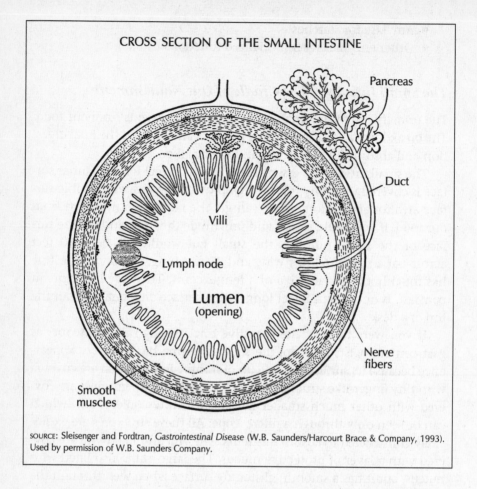

CROSS SECTION OF THE SMALL INTESTINE

Pancreas

Duct

Villi

Lymph node

Lumen
(opening)

Nerve
fibers

Smooth
muscles

SOURCE: Sleisenger and Fordtran, *Gastrointestinal Disease* (W.B. Saunders/Harcourt Brace & Company, 1993). Used by permission of W.B. Saunders Company.

THE THIRD BARRIER: OUR INNER DEFENSE SYSTEM

We have marvelous safeguards built into our digestive tract, there to destroy invaders from the outside world, microbes hiding in our food and coming in with our water, waiting to do us harm.

Our protections include microbe fighters (antibodies) concealed in the mucous lining of the gut. Antibodies target antigens, which are anything the body has identified as unknown or potentially harmful. A wide range of substances can be tagged as antigens, from allergenic foods to microbes.

Secretory immunoglobulin A is one of our foremost defenders (sometimes called SIgA). When invading antigens, such as microbes, try to work their way into the folds of the gut, our antibodies attack. Each SIgA molecule resembles a microscopic arrow tipped with a suction cup. Hundreds of these arrows may adhere to the surface of an invader, making it fuzzier and stickier so it will become trapped in the mucous layer.

THE FOURTH BARRIER: OUR HARD-WORKING LIVER

Our liver is the Grand Central Station of our metabolism, handling an enormous amount of molecular traffic. The liver is the site of a huge variety of processing, whose vital roles include:

- ◆ Breaking down nutrients
- ◆ Filtering out toxins that come in from the gut and breaking them down
- ◆ Synthesizing important blood components

There are extensive networks of tiny blood vessels around the gut that absorb nutrients from our food. This nutrient-rich blood all flows directly into the larger collecting veins of the portal system and is carried on to the liver. Another network of capillaries comprises the bulk of the liver and surrounds the liver cells. Guarding this system are specialized cells called macrophages, that destroy much of the bacteria that comes in from the GI tract.

All the nutrients and other substances that have been absorbed from our food are processed by the liver and then transported to the rest of the body. Nutrients will be broken down to provide energy and the raw materials from which our body will actually be constructed and maintained. These are the building blocks of muscle, skin, and bone.

The liver also functions somewhat like the oil filter on your car; its job is to protect the rest of the body from all the debris and gunk that could be harmful. Essentially all the material absorbed from the gut passes through the liver, carried by the bloodstream. The liver cleans the blood before it enters the heart, and before it's pumped throughout the body.

So the liver is the center for toxic cleanup in the body. The majority of the toxins are processed and transformed there. Some substances are exiled: If they don't measure up, they may get processed out of the body, in the urine or in stool. If the liver is required to process too many toxins, an overload may occur. Then the impaired capacity can limit its ability to monitor incoming traffic and filter out harmful substances, like a police force outnumbered by thugs who then get into general circulation.

THE FIFTH BARRIER: THE FRIENDLY FLORA

The friendly flora are bacteria that have beneficial effects in the body. They are important because they help keep our immune defenses well tuned and provide valuable nutrients such as vitamin K, folic acid, and the essential fatty acid butyrate. This barrier is so central to our well-being that Chapter 5 has been devoted to the subject. Read on to learn more about your inner ecology.

Our Incredible Digestive System

❖

- In a cubic millimeter of the mucosal lining (smaller than the size of a grain of rice), there are 6 to 9 feet of nerve cell fibers.
- "Gut reactions" are transmitted by nerve impulses that travel through the gut in a matter of seconds.
- There are ten times more bacterial cells within the gut than there are cells in our entire body.
- Human cells are hundreds of times bigger than bacterial cells.

Although bacteria are microscopic and their DNA is tiny, if we were to take many billions of them and place their DNA end to end, the total length can be huge. For example, there are approximately 75,000 miles of bacterial DNA in a teaspoon of yogurt. And these are the same friendly bacteria that thrive in a healthy gut.

SCOTT ANDERSON, M.D., is currently staff physician at two preventive medical practices in the San Francisco Bay Area. His education includes a degree in biology from Harvard University, a masters in genetics (his thesis focused on human gut bacteria), and an M.D. degree from the University of Connecticut. He has practiced medicine in a variety of clinical settings, including hospitals, outpatient clinics, and medical centers. Dr. Anderson specializes in preventive, health promotive, and anti-aging therapies. Dr. Anderson can be reached for telephone consultations at 415-472-2343 or 707-586-5555.

4

Immunity Against Invaders

MICHAEL ROSENBAUM, M.D.

❖

Your digestive tract is the largest immune system in your body! We usually think of the GI tract as the place where our food is digested and then discarded. But the gut is a very active immune center, containing more than 80 percent of the antibody-producing cells in our entire body.

This immunity in the gut is different from the immunity in the body in general, an entirely separate immune system that was not really appreciated until recently. It's considered the largest lymph organ in the body, larger than the thymus and all the other lymph nodes scattered throughout our system.

WHY THERE'S SUCH A LARGE IMMUNE SYSTEM IN THE GUT

♦ *The gut is constantly under siege.* We coexist with a vast population of microscopic armies, consisting of viruses, bacteria, yeast, and parasites that are literally trying to feed off us. The immune system is our major defense against this constant bombardment. To combat a never-ending horde of enemies, our immunity must be dynamic and ever-vigilant.

In the gut, material from the outside environment literally enters the interior of our body as our food and water. They can contain all manner of pathogens. Our trusty immune system is there in the gut to protect us from this outside world inside us.

♦ *Our protective barrier is fairly vulnerable.* To penetrate the inner gut lining and get into the blood vessels, invaders need only penetrate the mucous barrier and a layer of cells (the epithelium). This is quite different from the skin, for example, which has several protective layers of cells.

◆ *There is a lot of internal area to be protected.* Consider that the small intestine is on average 25 feet long—more than four times most people's height. And the large intestine is typically 5 feet long. So you have about 30 feet of gut.

◆ *Resident bacteria have to be kept under control.* In that 30 feet of intestine you have an enormous number of resident bacteria. They're supposed to be there—they're normal flora. And it turns out that the normal bacterial population in the human gut is about equal to the number of cells in our entire body.

In the small gut, there are millions of bacteria in each teaspoon of liquid (about a cubic centimeter). In the colon, there are probably at least a trillion. There's just an incredible amount of normal flora. People have no idea that they carry so much bacteria inside them. And if you take an antibiotic, in a sense you're probably wiping out almost half the cells in your body. In fact, some antibiotics literally wipe out all the bacteria, harmful and helpful, all at once.

When things are in balance, we have a symbiotic, harmonious relationship with these bacteria. We need the bacteria for so many reasons. They actually produce vitamins such as vitamin K, which helps our blood clot, and folic acid, which is essential to the female reproductive system. They also preserve and maintain a healthy lining of the gut and they tend to crowd out the bad bugs.

◆ *There's rapid turnover.* What's even more amazing is that the gut lining is completely replaced about every four days. These cells work very hard and then they die. If our body can't keep up with the effort of destroying and replacing them, we could end up with an impaired gut lining. Then we're subject to intestinal permeability, food allergies, or all kinds of other potential problems.

GUT DEFENSES

Your immune system is a vast military service fighting a never-ending war! The gut marshals several different kinds of defenses to protect us from the outside world that literally comes inside our bodies with food and water. Immune functions can be compared to munitions factories, artillery, hidden attackers, sentries, and even guardsmen that check I.D.

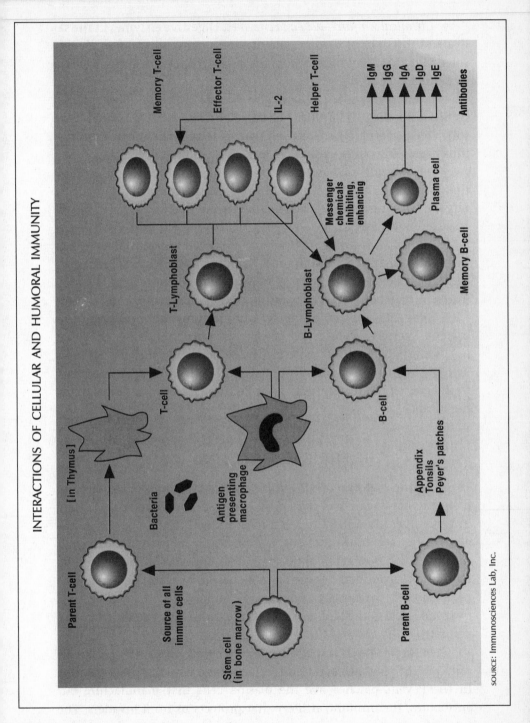

INTERACTIONS OF CELLULAR AND HUMORAL IMMUNITY

SOURCE: Immunosciences Lab, Inc.

◆ *Chemical warfare—acid and enzymes.* Digestive enzymes in the saliva and throughout the gut help us digest our food and literally dissolve invading "bad bugs." Stomach acid (HCl) also destroys bacteria and other pathogens.

◆ *The munitions factory—your lymph tissue.* The lymph tissue secretes antibodies, the artillery of our digestive immune system. Oral tolerance performs ID checks on invaders to separate friend from foe, thus protecting our friendly flora and digested food from attack.

◆ *Immune artillery—antibodies.* Antibodies are the immune artillery that target specific prey. The antibodies can be compared to ballistic missiles with a tracking device that seeks and finds and chases invaders—and never lets go.

◆ *The invaders—antigens.* The prey are called antigens; they trigger the antibodies' protective response. Antigens are any kind of invading agent perceived by the body as new, foreign, intrusive, or harmful. Antigens may be bacteria or parasites or even allergenic foods.

◆ *Killer cells—cellular immunity.* Our immunity also includes components such as T cells called killer cells and natural killer cells that police our body, targeted to destroy bacteria, viruses, and even tumors by releasing toxic enzymes. Note that there is little cellular immunity in the gut, so the secretory IgA, our immune artillery, are of supreme importance.

THE MUNITIONS FACTORY: GALT

The immune response of the gut is generated by a specialized kind of lymph tissue researchers call GALT (gut-associated lymphoid tissue). In general, the lymph system is a network within the body that provides certain immune functions. Lymph is a clear liquid that circulates through a series of interconnected spaces and vessels, including the lymph nodes, located between the tissues and organs. The lymph is responsible for removing bacteria and supplying white blood cells (lymphocytes) to the blood, as well as the transport of certain proteins and fats.

The GALT consist of specialized colonies of cells in the gut lining called Peyer's patches and also the lymphatic tissue in the appendix. In the Peyer's patches live the plasma cells that manufacture our antibodies, the immune artillery that protects us from invaders. The antibodies in the gut are primarily the secreted (or secretory) immuno-

YOUR AMAZING IMMUNE DEFENSES

Immunity in the Gut

Type of protector	Where it's made and lives	Its role in our defense
B cells (live for years)	Made in bone marrow and mature in spleen and lymph nodes	Mature into plasma cells
Plasma cells (live about four days)	Reside in Peyer's patches in the lower small intestine	Make all the antibodies: IgA, SIgA, IgE, IgG, IgM
Memory cells (may live as long as twenty years)	Originate in bone marrow, migrate to the thymus where they mature; live hidden away in the spleen and in Peyer's patches	Attack specific microbes encountered in the past

Immunity Throughout the Body

T cells—T helpers, T suppressors, killer and natural killer cells, T cytotoxic cells	Made in bone marrow Mature in the thymus	Roam the body to protect us; some stimulate immunity, others calm it

globulin A (SIgA), our first line of immune defense in the digestive tract.

Most of the gut lymph tissue is located at the juncture of the large and small appendix and also near the last part of the large intestine (the descending colon). This strategic concentration of lymph tissue appears to play an important role in protecting the small intestine against the migration of bacteria or parasites back up into the gut from the colon, where there's a much greater concentration of microbes.

It's probably no coincidence that most inflammation in the gut occurs at this juncture. There is a greater potential for infection here, and that's probably why there is so much lymphatic tissue. This is the area where Crohn's disease, for example, is most likely to occur (in the ileum). Appendix infections are well known. However, removing the appendix or a section of the ileum through surgery can be both a blessing and a curse, because while it can decrease inflammation, a lot of immune tissue is removed in the process. In most cases this seems to decrease immune defenses, and unfortunately, in some conditions such as Crohn's disease, the inflammation may reappear in other parts of the digestive tract. Research has found that people who have their appendix removed more often get Hodgkin's or Crohn's disease.

CAPTURING INVADERS

In the barrier lining there are specialized cells that function like guards on duty, called M cells. The M cells can't move, so they're like guardsmen who can't leave their post. They have the ability to bind onto anything considered dangerous—any kind of pathogen or oversized food particle. When an invader approaches them, they latch onto it and pull it underneath the surface to the lymphocytes below in the Peyer's patches. There in the trenches, white blood cells (lymphocytes) screen invaders to determine if they're friend or foe and produce the SIgA antibodies that line the entire tract and act against invasion. Macrophages are there to digest and process the invading microbes and alert T helper cells to the identity of the invader for future reference. Throughout the gut, the secretory IgA bombards any and all invaders in a generalized response. When a problem is detected, SIgA secretion tends to increase throughout the gut to bolster our defenses.

The antibodies are tiny little arrow-shaped molecules that are part of our mucous defense barrier. Their role is to attack and detain. If they perceive bacteria, for example, which are typically hundreds of times larger than the antibody, they cover its surface, until it resembles an orange stuck with cloves. Several hundred SIgA molecules may adhere to the surface of a single invading bacteria. The purpose is to create a rough or uneven surface that will catch the microbe in the mucous layer that covers the gut lining. The mucous acts like a slow conveyor belt, gradually sliding the food through the gut and also moving microbes and large food particles out of the gut. The bacteria can then simply be discarded with the spent food in the stool. If you decrease the body's secretions, you decrease immune defenses. Aspirin, for example, decreases the mucous lining, one reason it can cause intestinal bleeding.

Our First Line of Defense: SIgA

In the digestive tract, the secretory IgA is our first line of immune defense. The SIgA are produced in the lining of the gut in the specialized cells called Peyer's patches. These cells secrete the SIgA into the mucous barrier, so they're called *secretory* immune globulins (SIgA for short). SIgA is also an important part of the defense system found in the saliva, and lives in the mucous membranes of the nose and the lungs.

Fortunately, the entire digestive tract is loaded with SIgA, because there are very few of our protective roving scavenger T cells there. The SIgA is targeted against anything potentially harmful—bacteria, microscopic parasites, even large food particles that might cause inflammation. Note that other kinds of antibodies (IgE, IgG, and IgM) specifically target one subspecies of invader, such as a particular strain of flu or an allergenic food, but they won't attack any others. For example, if I caught the flu this year, I won't catch it again later this year, because I have built up antibodies against it. However, when a new strain of flu comes around next year, I will have no protective immunity against it. My antibodies are so specific, they recognize only illnesses to which I've already been exposed, but ignore all others. But our faithful SIgA offers *nonspecific immunity*—it will attack anything it perceives as potentially harmful.

Peacekeeping Roles: SIgA

SIgA is ingeniously programmed to be tolerant of our friendly flora. Although it will attack anything offensive, it's somehow able to recognize what belongs there and what doesn't—no friendly fire. SIgA targets only microorganisms that don't have the right identifier and binds to them—metaphorically speaking, only those without the right ID or badge. Macrophages in the GALT attach to the invader, consume it, and display its identity. T cells scan the ID to see if the immune system has been in combat with this invader before. The memory cells are checked (they function as a huge database documenting past offenders). If the scan matches the identity of an old enemy, the memory cells begin to rapidly replicate in a cloning-like activity which generates a huge immune response. In addition, SIgA has the ability to bind to particles that aren't fully digested or dissolved, typically large food particles, to minimize the wear and tear on the gut and the potential for problems such as the leaky gut syndrome. Basically, SIgA targets both pathogens and food.

In the gut, secretory IgA acts as a kind of peacemaker through an anti-inflammatory effect. Immunoglobulin A (IgA) in general prevents inflammation. It can reduce the biochemical panic response that can occur when the metabolic alarm system goes off in the body. This warning system includes immune messenger chemicals (the cytokines) that function like sirens sounding the call to respond when a threat is perceived. If the cytokines stimulate too heavy an attack, major inflammation can occur as a protective mechanism. By toning down the metabolic panic and the inflammation that could follow, SIgA maintains the integrity of the lining cells of the gut barrier.

There are some things that promote our body's arsenal of SIgA and others that deplete it. Some people are just born with less ability to make it. SIgA is reduced in people who have allergies in general, and in children born of parents who are allergic. And as a result, such children may be more prone to food allergy and to gluten/wheat intolerance. This is an important response to monitor, because gluten has the unique ability to inflame the lining of the small intestine, which can cause you to become allergic to everything else.

Vitamin A can significantly increase our ability to produce SIgA. If you are suddenly exposed to bacteria, the secretory IgA production usually goes up, particularly in response to bacteroides and nonpathogenic forms of *E. coli*. The level of SIgA in our body at any given time can now be measured through a simple mail-in lab test. One test is performed on saliva, the other on stools, and there are labs that do both. People with low levels of SIgA in saliva or stool tend to be much more prone to infection and to food allergy.

OTHER IMMUNE DEFENSES

IgM is also found in the gut, although it's not as important as SIgA. It's produced whenever there is a definite infection in the gut. Anything from botulism to salmonella will induce an IgM response.

Lysosomes are another kind of "chemical warfare"—specialized enzymes. They're a very primitive form of immune defense that's present in saliva, tears, and in gut secretions. Lysosomes are also capable of killing pathogens in the gut, essentially by digesting them, just as the enzymes in meat tenderizer break down meat tissue.

TELLING FRIEND FROM FOE: ORAL TOLERANCE

The second major immune defense of the GALT is oral tolerance. Oral tolerance is extremely important because it's the mechanism by which

OUR IMMUNE ARTILLERY—THE ANTIBODIES

Type and location	Source	Task	Effect
B cells become plasma cells and memory cells	Develop and mature in bone marrow	Plasma cells produce antibodies; memory cells direct them	Antibodies (immunoglobulins, or Ig) are our immune artillery
SIgA secreted into the mucous lining	Peyer's patches (GALT): lymph tissue in small gut, appendix, elsewhere in the gut	Targets any invader (nonspecific immunity)	First line of defense; tones down inflammation
IgA in saliva and mucus of nose, lungs	From B cells including lymph tissue in nose and tonsils	Targets any invader	Tones down inflammation
IgE made by plasma cells	Produced by B cells throughout the body	Targets specific invaders	Immediate response
IgG in bloodstream—80% of blood immunity	All immunoglobulins are made by plasma cells (mature B cells)	Highly specific (work through a lock-and-key mechanism)	Delayed response that can cause inflammation
IgM—secreted into gut mucus lining	Peyer's patches	Fights any specific infection	Immediate response

your gut immune system tells friend from foe and it deals with both food and microbes.

Our oral tolerance system has learned to distinguish what we can tolerate and what we can't. As adults, we consume about a ton of food a year. If the immune system attacked everything that came into the gut, it would attack all the food we eat, since it's actually all foreign to our body. But fortunately it doesn't. Food that's undigested, in large particles, or allergenic can be attacked by both SIgA and IgM antibodies. Sometimes our oral tolerance doesn't work. When it doesn't, we are more prone to food sensitivities.

Oral tolerance has the job of identifying the friendly bacteria—again, no small task. There are also ten trillion bacteria in an adult gut. Without oral tolerance, our immune system would attack all of the zillions of bacteria in the gut, even those that belong there. Fortunately, this system has learned to distinguish between what should be there and what shouldn't. It identifies normal flora and signals the body not to attack. So the gut immune response attacks only pathogenic organisms.

SUPPORTING YOUR IMMUNITY AND YOUR ANTIBODIES

Any kind of infection, even a flu, can lower our stores of antibodies (our precious SIgA). An infection anywhere in the body, even a tooth abscess, can affect the gut by increasing stress and reducing the secretory IgA.

Stress reduces secretory IgA. Any kind of stress can do this. Two German studies indicate that mental relaxation procedures, such as meditation or biofeedback, can lead to increased secretion of SIgA. To promote this positive effect, stress reduction, moderate exercise such as yoga, tai chi, or Qigong, meditation, or any kind of mental relaxation are very important for a healthy digestive tract.

Poor diet and low nutrient levels generally also lower SIgA. It's been shown that kids in third world countries who have protein calorie malnutrition (PCM) have lower SIgA levels and therefore frequently get diarrhea because they're lacking the SIgA to protect them against it. Once you get diarrhea, you lose even more lining in the gut and it becomes a vicious cycle.

SIgA decreases with age. It seems that there are many more things that reduce secretory IgA than easily increase it, so you really have to be on guard.

The key influences on your immune system are (1) genetics, (2) inherited allergies, (3) nutrition, (4) stress, (5) lack of breast feeding,

IMMUNE DEFENSES IN THE GUT

Type	Primary Task	Role with microbes	Role with food
Size of the job	Must differentiate friend from foe	Ten trillion microbes in a normal adult GI tract	One ton of food is eaten yearly by a normal adult
Secretory IgA	On the attack—"up-regulates" immunity	Attacks pathogens: yeast, bacteria, parasites	Attaches to larger undigested food particles and allergens
Oral tolerance	Calms the system— "down-regulates" it	Identifies and protects normal flora	Assures the passage of digested, dissolved foods

(6) age, (7) the integrity of the gut lining, (8) the health of the microflora, and (9) the presence of infection in the gut or anywhere in the body. Research has found that nutrition can actually affect the way your genetic makeup is expressed. Good nutrition can tip the balance toward health.

Vitamin A in particular is critical in replenishing the lining of the gut and maintaining the integrity of the mucosa. Unfortunately, lack of vitamin A happens to be the most common vitamin deficiency in the entire world. Other nutrients that increase SIgA include zinc taken with vitamin A, colostrum (for people who are not dairy intolerant), and probably L-glutamine.

MICHAEL ROSENBAUM, M.D., of Corte Madera, California, has had an active private practice since 1977 focused on immunology, clinical nutrition, and allergy. He is a graduate of the Albert Einstein College of Medicine in New York City and holds an M.S. in clinical biochemistry from the Hebrew University in Jerusalem. He is the author of *SuperSupplements* (Viking Penguin and Signet), *Solving the Puzzle of Chronic Fatigue Syndrome* (Life Science Press), and numerous articles on nutrition. He has been a frequent lecturer to professional medical groups and has participated in numerous television and radio talk shows on the topics of chronic fatigue syndrome, nutrition, and immunity.

Dr. Rosenbaum is available for consultations on nutritional therapy, allergy treatment, and anti-aging medicine, which can be arranged by calling his office at 415-927-9450.

5

Friendly Flora

NIGEL PLUMMER, Ph.D.

❖

You often hear about ecology, the relationship between organisms and their environment. As you read in Chapter 2, within your body there is an entire miniature ecosystem, a microecology, which has a major influence on your health. This inner ecology is made up of the microflora, more than 400 species of microscopic living bacteria, creating an internal environment that is diverse, complex, interrelated, and ever-changing. This population, although minute, is so enormous that the number of microbial cells in our body at any one time is greater than the number of our own cells.

The microflora are essential to our well-being. These bacteria provide very real beneficial effects. They limit the populations of harmful bacteria. They assist in the process of digestion. And they even manufacture some essential nutrients, like butyrate, an essential fatty acid, a primary fuel for the gut lining. So when our gut ecology is in balance, we thrive.

THE BENEFICIAL EFFECTS OF FLORA

◆ *Crowding out the harmful microbes.* It appears that the beneficial flora may actually interfere with the ability of some pathogens to adhere to the gut lining by covering all available surfaces, which is reported to limit the colonization of microbes such as *E. coli*, candida, and giardia.

◆ *Producing natural antibiotic effects.* Lactobacilli are believed to produce substances that suppress the growth of potentially harmful organisms.

◆ *Slowing the growth of pathogens.* Many pathogenic microbes re-

---

The Benefits of Good Flora

❖

Joel had suffered from inflammatory bowel disease for more than ten years, when he was first diagnosed and treated with standard drug therapy (5-ASA drugs and steroids, the treatment of choice at that time). Following his first episode, he had many periods of relapse, most often in the spring and fall. The colonoscopic exam showed nothing unusual, but a comprehensive lab analysis of his stool indicated that he had severe dysbiosis with an overgrowth of *E. coli* bacteria that may have become pathogenic.

Although it was necessary to put him back on steroids, Joel also began a program of nutritional support that included probiotics, a friendly flora product with bifidus and acidophilus. He also began taking vitamins and minerals and replaced one meal a day with liquid nutrition to rest his digestive tract. He was gradually able to taper off the steroids, but continued with the nutritional program. Joel's job took him to another state, but when he returned two years later, he told us that he'd never been in such good health before in his life. He's had no relapses and no longer has to take steroids every spring and fall. He continues to use one medication in low doses, the rice powder supplement, extra glutamine, and the flora products. We are delighted to know he's been "feeling great!"

—*Trent W. Nichols, M.D.*

---

quire iron in order to be highly active and destructive. Our bodies have a mechanism to minimize microbe growth by ensuring that very little free iron remains in the bloodstream. In the gut, bifidobacteria appear to aid in binding iron, making it unavailable to microbes by concentrating it up to a thousand times the normal content.

◆ *Discouraging destructive organisms.* Most gut pathogens stop growing in highly acid environments, so creating a more acidic environment in the mucous lining (with a low pH, below 5) potentially stops colonization by pathogenic types.

◆ *Improving digestion.* Digestive absorption can be enhanced in people who lack the enzyme to digest dairy products (lactose). In some cases, the consumption of fermented milk products or the addition of *L. acidophilus* to dairy products can be quite helpful. The fermenting process reduces the level of lactose and makes it more easily absorbed. Lactose digestion is greatly enhanced by the addition of *L. acidophilus*, whether the milk is fermented or not.

◆ *Reducing the harmful effects of cholesterol.* Researchers have noticed repeatedly that eating yogurt-like foods is beneficial for health.

A study of the Masai peoples of Africa found a very low incidence of heart disease, despite a diet high in animal fat. Diets high in animal fat normally tend to raise cholesterol levels and increase clogging of the heart arteries (atherosclerosis). In another study, a 5 to 10 percent decrease in cholesterol was seen in subjects after they had been eating yogurt for just seven days! This effect was also found to be true in studies of animals and even poultry. So yogurt can be a great addition to your diet if you're not dairy intolerant. When this is the case, use a good acidophilus/bifidus supplement.

◆ *Increasing the efficiency of the body.* Bile salts can inhibit harmful flora, the bad guys. By recycling bile salts, the helpful flora maximize the levels of bile in the system. This conservation saves the body precious energy and increases the protection of the gut.

◆ *Regulating the immune system.* Yogurt has been found to significantly enhance the production of B-interferon in the human immune system. This effect was observed when cultures of *L. bulgaricus* and *Streptococcus thermophilus* were introduced.

◆ *Protecting against cancer.* Supplementing the diet with *L. acidophilus,* researchers found that levels of potentially harmful enzymes in the gut were reduced. These included the enzymes that convert nitrates into much more harmful nitrosamines, documented to cause cancer in children and adults. They also included enzymes that convert azo-compounds, found in food colors, into potentially toxic products.

◆ *Suppressing tumors.* Animal studies have found that it took twice as long for cancer to form when fermented milk was part of the diet. *L. bulgaricus* was observed consistently to be more effective than *Streptococcus thermophilus*. A number of studies also found that yogurt had the capacity to suppress tumors or halt tumor growth.

FACTS ABOUT FLORA

There are half a dozen types of bacteria present in the gut in large numbers. Of these, *Lactobacillus acidophilus* (in the small gut) and bifidobacteria (in the large gut) are two of the primary strains. Although researchers have identified more than 400 species of microflora that can live in the gut environment, most of them are transient, occur in low numbers, and contribute little to our overall functioning. Friendly flora are:

◆ Present in children once they begin eating solid food and in normal healthy adults
◆ Predictably found in specific areas of the GI tract

♦ Often associated with the lining of the gut
♦ Mostly live without air; in ratio, there are 1,000 anaerobes for each of the aerobic bacteria

THE ORIGIN OF OUR FLORA

Just before birth, a human infant has a sterile GI tract, with no flora whatsoever. The development of the flora of a newborn depends on whether the child is breast or bottle fed. In breast-fed children, the flora of the GI tract quickly becomes dominated by a species of friendly flora called bifidobacteria and a few other types of bacteria. If left undisturbed, this community of flora remains stable until the child is weaned, when the changeover to solid food marks the development of typical adult flora.

In bottle-fed babies, a different microflora develops in early infancy. The population is mainly lactobacilli, with a much lower incidence of bifidobacteria. There is a large body of evidence to suggest that this difference in the makeup of the flora is connected with the greater susceptibility of bottle-fed infants to infection by harmful microbes which typically cause mild to severe diarrhea.

Once a child begins solid food, distinct changes occur in the flora of the gut, due to the changes in diet. By mid-childhood, the commu-

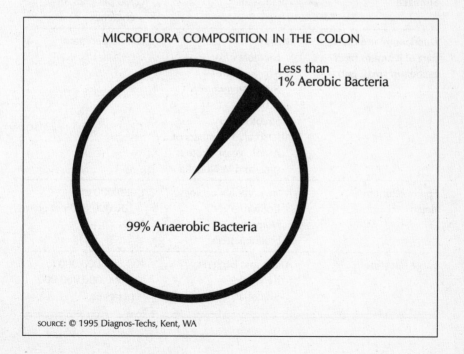

MICROFLORA COMPOSITION IN THE COLON

Less than
1% Aerobic Bacteria

99% Anaerobic Bacteria

SOURCE: © 1995 Diagnos-Techs, Kent, WA

nity of microflora that has developed should remain stable through-out most of adult life, under normal conditions. However, this delicate balance can be significantly disrupted by antibiotic treatment, mi-crobial infection (such as traveler's diarrhea), or periods of stress, sometimes leading to overgrowth by other potentially harmful micro-organisms.

IMPORTANCE OF THE FLORA TO THE GUT

Since the turn of the century, there have been recurring reports from researchers worldwide that supplementing the diet with viable bacte-ria, mainly lactobacilli, has beneficial effects on health that range from reestablishing flora to preventing cancer. Elie Metchnikoff is often quoted as the first researcher to identify the benefits of lactic acid bac-teria. He suggested that yogurt and fermented milk products in the diet of the Bulgarian people contributed to their longevity. He sug-gested that the lactobacilli in these foods prevented the overgrowth of harmful bacteria in the gut flora.

Part of the GI Tract	Kind of Flora	Task of the Flora
Stomach	Lactobacilli	1,000 per gram of contents
Duodenum and first part of jejunum (first section of small gut)	Mainly: *Lactobacillus acidophilus* *Bifidobacterium bifidus* Streptococci Also smaller numbers of *E. coli*, yeast, Proteus spp., and Veillonella	10,000 per gram
End of jejunum Ileum	More complex ecology Coliforms Numerous bifidobacteria	1,000,000 to 100,000,000 per gram
Large intestine	Anaerobic bacteria Bacteroides Bifidobacteria	100,000,000,000 to 1,000,000,000,000 per gram

INFLUENCES ON THE BALANCE OF FLORA

Our inner ecology can experience distress, just as any other ecosystem can. And like the environment, our internal ecosystem may seem to be intact, but the biodynamics may be stressed and the system out of tune.

What causes imbalances in the microflora? Research has found that stress, a poor diet, or antibiotic therapy can destroy many of the helpful bacteria. The use of certain drugs or the chronic use of processed laxatives can also have a negative effect. When the friendly flora decrease in number, our inner environment is open to invasion and colonization by destructive microbes—harmful bacteria such as *E. coli* and salmonella, parasites including giardia and cryptosporidium, or yeasts such as candida.

♦ *Stress.* When the mind or body are under stress, the changes in the makeup of the mucous lining can create an environment less favorable to the friendly flora. In addition, motility in the gut (peristalsis) may slow down, and then the food may be colonized by different and possibly harmful microbes, no longer held in check by the lactobacilli and bifidobacteria. *E. coli*, bacteroides, and candida can increase significantly at these times.

♦ *Your choice of food.* Diet has an extremely important influence on the quality and quantity of the flora. Researchers have found that a diet of wheat meal greatly favored the growth of lactobacilli and decreased the levels of potentially harmful bacteria (such as strep, *E. coli*, and clostridium). In contrast, rats fed a diet of pork developed microflora low in lactobacilli and high in *E. coli*. A diet of easily digested milk protein (casein) produced a decrease in all bacteria types, with the exception of streptococci. This research suggests that a diet high in meat and milk products could depress the levels of favorable flora.

♦ *Antibiotics.* The widespread use of antibiotics by their very nature induces a dramatic and destructive effect on the microflora in the GI tract. Unfortunately, the action of most antibiotics is not specific, so the harmful (pathogenic) organisms and the beneficial ones are often destroyed together. This is especially true of the lactobacilli and bifidobacteria, which are particularly sensitive to a wide variety of antibiotics and whose numbers fall dramatically following therapy.

STRESSORS THAT ARE DESTRUCTIVE TO FLORA

Effects	How They Can Be Harmful	Potential Invaders
Stress	Decrease in mucous secretions; causes changes in composition of the gut lining; flora may be unable to cling to the gut lining and can be washed away	*E. coli*, bacteroides, and candida
Diet	Meat-based diet suspended beneficial bacteria Milk-based diet suspended most bacterial growth	Meat: *E. coli* and clostridium Milk: Strep
Antibiotics	Eradicates both helpful and harmful bacteria; leaves the gut open to invasion by harmful microbes	*E. coli*, staph, strep, yeasts, especially candida

This reduction of the beneficial flora leaves the intestine open to invasion by opportunistic pathogens or overgrowth by less desirable components that the normal flora usually keep in check (including *E. coli*, staph such as *S. aureus*, strep, and yeasts, especially candida). It is worth noting that this situation is made worse when the undesirable microbes have developed drug resistance. In that case, they survive treatment, but ironically the beneficial flora are killed off—exactly the opposite of what the body requires. Then the "bad bugs" are left to thrive unopposed—like a lawless Western town with no sheriff. In fact, the imbalance that results can allow the overgrowth of normally harmless bacteria such as strep; if their number increase sufficiently, they can become so invasive as to cause severe problems such as inflammation of the heart lining (endocarditis). Yeast are also quite resistant to antibiotics, so an overgrowth of candida in the GI tract following antibiotics is a likely occurrence.

The results of any of these stressors—physical or mental stress, poor diet, or antibiotic therapy—is that the microflora can become unbalanced to such an extent that health is harmed. Symptoms of minor imbalance may include intestinal discomfort, indigestion, gas, and bloating. A major or prolonged imbalance can lead to severe diarrhea or even a bacterial infection in the bloodstream (septicemia).

The most effective way to reestablish the normal microflora is by taking flora supplements of lactobacilli and bifidobacteria, available from many health food stores. (See the Appendix for mail-order sources for supplements such as probiotics.)

Dr. Nigel Plummer is a British scientist who does collaborative research in conjunction with the American lab, Diagnos-Techs. Diagnos-Techs, Inc., USA, was established in 1987 in Kent, Washington, and in 1989 introduced salivary-based testing for evaluating stress and assessing hormone levels. These tests are considered the gold standard nationwide for salivary testing.

Their lab testing for digestive function includes panels to evaluate digestive efficiency; screening for GI infection due to candida, parasites, or bacteria; testing for markers that reflect GI inflammation and levels of secretory IgA; as well as tests that evaluate male and female hormone levels, measure adrenal hormones, and detect markers for adrenal stress.

Diagnos-Techs works directly with physicians and health care professionals, so patients should have their practitioner contact the lab: Diagnos-Techs, Inc., 6620 S. 192nd Place, Suite J-104, Kent, WA 98032; 800-878-3787, fax 425-251-9520

6

Harmful Flora

LEN SAPUTO, M.D.

❖

The balance that exists among our microflora is an example of nature's incredible perfection. When the microflora coexist in harmony, a healthy state of symbiosis results and we thrive. When they live not in symbiosis, but in dysbiosis, this disturbed ecology often results in a sense of unwellness or even disease.

Our GI flora have been equated to an entire system within itself. There are more than 500 different species of bacteria, which collectively produce more metabolic activity than any other organ system in our body. You've read about the many essential functions these flora provide. We don't often think about the flora, and their importance is often underestimated. But research shows that even in conditions as serious as AIDS, good flora can enhance health and prolong life.

WHEN OUR INNER BALANCE IS LOST

If the beneficial flora decline, due to heavy antibiotic use or consumption of the wrong foods, the harmful flora can overgrow. These include yeast and numerous kinds of bacteria. Abnormal flora in the GI tract can result in a number of harmful effects. They can:

- ◆ Allow infection by microbes
- ◆ Deplete vitamin B_{12} and some amino acids
- ◆ Short-circuit digestive enzymes
- ◆ Transform essential fatty acids into damaging saturated fats
- ◆ Encourage conditions such as inflammatory bowel disease
- ◆ Interfere with breakdown of bile acids and estrogens, setting up the potential for cancer

How Things Go Wrong

◈

Before Carol entered college, she hardly had a sick day in her life. That first semester at college was really tough. She was up late studying, she gulped down fast foods, and when she partied, she partied! When the cold season hit just before finals, Carol was one of the first to catch a cold, a cold that just wouldn't go away. She saw her doctor, who prescribed several courses of antibiotics because "she just couldn't afford to be sick," and after about three months, the cold went away.

But Carol was never the same again. She began to have recurring vaginal yeast infections, and finally what was called a spastic colon. Her yeast infections were controlled with anti-yeast suppositories, but the spastic colon would respond only to muscle relaxants and tranquilizers, and even then she never really felt well. She was finally told to see a psychiatrist, under the assumption that her gastrointestinal problems were probably related to her nerves. I saw Carol a full ten years later, when out of desperation she wanted to try an alternative approach. "There just has to be a better way." By that time, she'd had every test in the book, including X-rays of her GI tract, stool exams for parasites, blood work, and even a colonoscopy, but everything appeared to be "normal."

Carol was beginning to believe that she really was a "head case"! I requested lab tests to analyze her digestive capacity (the CDSA) and found she had a major imbalance of intestinal microflora—a severe overgrowth of yeast and a deficiency of normal beneficial bacteria. We devised a program of nutritional support for the intestinal tract, including mild anti-yeast herbs, a very low-sugar diet, antioxidant nutrients, and a rich source of friendly bacteria. Within ten days, Carol's symptoms cleared up, and she has remained free of symptoms ever since. We have been checking her flora levels about every four to six months now for two years, and she's slowly developing a healthy intestinal microflora. Carol has discontinued psychotherapy and is beginning to feel like her old healthy self.

The causes of flora imbalance—dysbiosis—occur far more often than we generally appreciate. Many doctors don't really focus on gut ecology. Basically, any situation that can alter the physical integrity or the chemical balance of the GI tract can result in changes in the makeup of the microflora by decreasing friendly flora and allowing harmful microbes to take over or overgrow. But the harmful microflora alone are rarely the single cause of dysbiosis. The essential questions to ask are: What is happening that enables some of these organisms to overgrow and upset the balanced ecology that previously existed? What makes an organism that is normally not destructive become pathogenic?

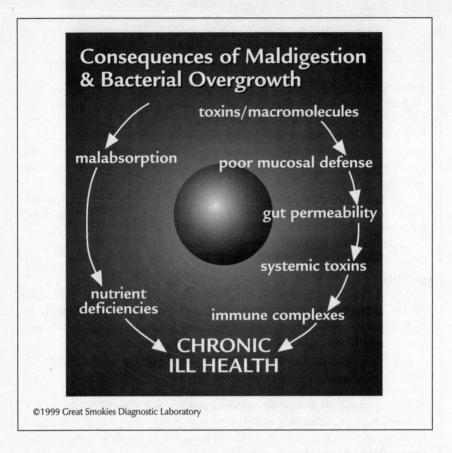

Consequences of Maldigestion & Bacterial Overgrowth

toxins/macromolecules

malabsorption

poor mucosal defense

gut permeability

systemic toxins

nutrient deficiencies

immune complexes

CHRONIC ILL HEALTH

©1999 Great Smokies Diagnostic Laboratory

Two primary factors determine just how pathogenic an organism can become. First is its ability to overgrow and produce toxins that can injure us. The second factor, our resistance or the strength of our immune defenses, is one that modern medicine acknowledges. But we don't always address it, especially in short-term illness. In fact, it is widely believed that invading organisms are the primary cause of illness and that removing them is the solution. But all the organisms inhabiting the intestinal tract (including friendly bacteria such as acidophilus) can cause serious illness, such as blood poisoning and even death, under certain circumstances.

The treatment goal in combating dysbiosis is often to aggressively kill all the pathogenic microbes in a war between man and germs. We need strategies that also strengthen our own defenses and restore the balance in our inner ecology. In a catastrophic illness such as AIDS, modern medicine honors the fact that host defenses have been weakened. Researchers predict that our increased understanding of immunity will lead to new therapies to strengthen our immunity.

WHY GOOD FLORA GO BAD

Overgrowth of flora and dysbiosis are clear signals that something's gone wrong in the GI tract and requires attention. There are at least nine pathways that can lead to dysbiosis. They include:

- Eating too much sweet and starchy food
- Overuse of antibiotics
- Stress
- Poor digestion
- Exposure to toxins
- Inflammation
- Infection
- Lowered immune defenses
- Unknown causes

THE EFFECTS OF POOR FOOD AND POOR DIGESTION

What we eat creates the chemical environment in our GI tract. This presents a growth advantage for certain organisms—the microflora have to eat too. Each species of bacteria has specific nutritional needs. If the right food is provided, that species will enjoy accelerated growth. The beneficial bacteria that inhabit the gut survive on high fiber diets. If we eat adequate amounts of fiber from vegetables and whole grains, these bacteria will have the nutrition they need to flourish.

Meals that are high in fat and meat and low in fiber tend to lead to what's called putrefactive dysbiosis. In this situation, a normal bacteria in the gut called bacteroides overgrows. Its toxic by-products results in the overproduction of ammonia. When this occurs, the stool in the large intestine becomes more alkaline and the production of essential gut fuel (butyrate) falls. As a result, nutritional shortages occur throughout the digestive tract. Increased levels of bile acids build, raising the risk of colon cancer; levels of estrogen also go up, which can increase the risk of breast cancer.

Certain illnesses such as Crohn's disease or infections from invading microbes can disrupt the GI lining and cause a loss of normal defenses. Then harmful microorganisms can take advantage of this change in the GI environment and result in a shift in the microflora. When the destructive flora overgrow, their concentration becomes toxic to the gut and can cause other negative conditions, creating a vicious cycle that will be self-perpetuating.

Other factors come into play. Digestion may be poor because there's not enough hydrochloric acid. This can allow more undigested food to reach the lower small intestine and colon, where the microflora typically overgrow. The overgrowth of bacteria can lead to the overproduction of certain enzymes (proteases), resulting in poor digestion. This type of dysbiosis has been called fermentation dysbiosis.

THE UNINTENDED SIDE EFFECTS OF ANTIBIOTIC THERAPY

The use and abuse of antibiotic therapy may be the single most frequent cause of dysbiosis today. When antibiotics are taken, profound changes can occur in the microflora of the GI tract and elsewhere in the body where there are flora (such as the mouth, the vagina, the lungs, skin). If your defenses are adequate and the flora balance is not too deeply disturbed, normal flora are often able to return to their original positive state.

However, repeated or prolonged antibiotic treatment can cause severe and ongoing dysbiosis, especially if our immune defenses are down. This can result in disease. When the beneficial flora have been substantially reduced, the condition is termed deficiency dysbiosis.

STRESS CAN CAUSE DYSBIOSIS

Stress can have profound effects on our immune defenses. It tends to affect all the systems of our digestive tract—psycho-neuro-endocrine-immune function. This usually has a compromising effect on our immunity.

In addition, stress can interfere with our digestion by slowing down the time it takes our food to move through the gut (constipation) or speeding it up (diarrhea). The movement of food through the GI tract (the transit time) affects the completeness of digestion. When these things happen, harmful microorganisms shift the ecological balance of the intestinal tract.

NOT ENOUGH FIBER TO FEED OUR FLORA

Lack of adequate fiber in our diets can also allow deficiency dysbiosis to develop. Fiber is the major source of nutrition for the normal, health-promoting flora. One of the most dreaded diseases that can develop in this situation is infection due to *Clostridium difficile*, the over-growth of a gut bacteria that can actually be a life-threatening complication of antibiotic use.

It is ironic that the standard treatment for this condition is to use more antibiotic therapy aimed at stopping the overgrowth of the *C. difficile*. Although this approach is successful at times, we are better assured of healing if we also address the underlying process in the ecology of the microflora and our immune defenses.

I have treated a number of cases of deficiency dysbiosis for patients who've had recurring colitis even though they underwent very aggressive antibiotic treatment for the overgrowth. An alternative approach is to give a short pulse of antibiotic therapy for a few days and then quickly begin replacing the friendly bacteria and the fiber. This can stimulate and stabilize immune function in the intestinal tract. As the flora rebuilds, it provides some of the nutritional support so the GI mucosal surface can repair itself. This has worked within a few days in every case I have managed.

TOXIC WASTE AND YOUR DIGESTION

Environmental exposures are increasing at an alarming rate in this era of widespread synthetic chemical production. Many of these toxins find their way into the intestinal tract through food, water, and products, including toothpastes, mouthwashes, and dental amalgams. These substances can damage the cells of our intestinal tract and lower our resistance. Toxins can also damage the microflora, setting the stage for dysbiosis. A wide variety of drugs are known to have profound effects on the balance of the gut microflora, including steroids, birth control pills, NSAIDs (nonsteroidal anti-inflammatory drugs), antacids, H2 blockers, and some chemotherapy medications.

THE BEST-KEPT SECRET: GUT IMMUNITY

One of the best-kept secrets in health care is that the gastrointestinal tract is the largest immune organ in our body. The intestinal lining has a huge surface area that separates the outer world from the internal milieu of our body. This is a strategic location for our body's defense system. Here is the very site of entry for potentially dangerous organisms or chemicals. It doesn't take a rocket scientist to see that when this large, strategically placed immune system isn't working well, our defenses are lowered. Once our barriers are down, it may not be possible to keep the ecology of the intestinal tract in balance. And it becomes more difficult to defend against invaders.

WHAT IF OUR IMMUNE DEFENSE IS DOWN?

Our immune system can malfunction in at least three ways. First, it can be weakened so that it can't fight off common illness. This occurs with cancer and AIDS, but can also result from everyday stress. It's called immune suppression. Second, it can overreact and become hyperresponsive to normal stimuli; this occurs in asthma, migraine, and food allergies. These hyperreactions can use up immune reserves of the body, but may also cause defensive immune responses that actually injure the tissue. Third, a malfunctioning immune system can cause autoimmune reactions—antibodies become targeted against our own tissues, as in rheumatoid arthritis or lupus. In any of these mechanisms, the end result is the same: Abnormal body defenses can lead to dysbiosis.

FINDING THE PROBLEM

The diagnosis of dysbiosis centers around three approaches:

- ◆ A careful history and physical exam
- ◆ A specific test called a comprehensive diagnostic stool analysis (CDSA)
- ◆ Testing for yeast, bacteria, and parasites

Keep in mind that dysbiosis is not a disease per se. As a matter of fact, dysbiosis is frequently found in patients who have no specific symptoms, though they often have a vague sense of not feeling well. The presence of disturbed gut ecology is clearly an abnormal situation. It serves as a warning for the potential of detectable disease. When dysbiosis is present, other related illnesses often develop as well. Since the primary causes of dysbiosis relate to almost everyone, it is the opinion of the author that a CDSA is a reasonable and cost-effective screening that should be done whenever there is unresolved illness.

RESTORING INNER HEALTH

Treating dysbiosis depends on the strength of one's immunity, the quality of support, and the severity of the infection or overgrowth.

In the management of dysbiosis, treat the underlying cause whenever possible. This means carefully evaluating all the possible causes and then finding ways to eliminate them.

The goals in managing dysbiosis are to restore the normal microflora, provide nutrients that will heal the intestinal mucosa, reduce toxic exposures, and increase antibodies in the GI tract (SIgA).

The health of the mucosal lining of the gut is important in maintaining our immune resistance, and this resistance is a powerful determinant that controls which microflora can survive. It is easy to understand that nutritional support for the gut mucosal cells is necessary to maintain our most effective defense mechanisms.

- ◆ Use a variety of vitamins (A, Bs, C and E), especially vitamin A
- ◆ Use minerals and nutrients (such as L-glutamine and phosphatidyl choline)
- ◆ Remember essential fatty acids and bioflavonoids (like quercitin)
- ◆ Support with antioxidants (coenzyme Q10, lipoic acid, glutathione, and ginkgo biloba)
- ◆ Consume organic food and juice whenever possible
- ◆ Minimize toxic exposures

THE WRONG FLORA AND LEAKY GUT SYNDROME

Dysbiosis and leaky gut are often intimately related. They can occur together or exist independently. Or they may be caused by each other, and often coexist. In Chapter 7 these interrelationships will be explored more fully.

LEN SAPUTO, M.D., has great enthusiasm for public education on alternative therapies. He is founder and president of the Health-Medicine Forum and the Health-Medicine Network, an organization of more than 300 members that provides weekly panels, monthly workshops, conferences, and cybercasting. The forum offers information on complementary and alternative medicine for both health care professionals and a broad public audience.

Dr. Saputo received his medical education at Duke University and his undergraduate degree at the University of California at Berkeley. He has been in private practice in internal medicine since 1971, with a therapeutic focus in the use of nutrition in preventive care and wellness. An avid tennis player, he was a world singles champion in 1995. Dr. Saputo can be reached for phone consultations at his Walnut Creek, California, office: 925-937-9550.

7

Leaky Gut Syndrome

LEN SAPUTO, M.D.

❖

Leaky gut is a surprisingly common problem. Basically, it's a condition that occurs whenever there is inflammation and the "pores" in the gut lining remain open too long. Then toxic by-products in the digestive tract can be absorbed into the bloodstream, transported on to the liver. The molecules of food and toxins "leaked" through the GI lining may eventually affect systems throughout the body by aggravating inflammation in the joints, expressing toxins in skin disorders, triggering food sensitivities, and causing "brain fog" or hyperactivity.

Managing hyperpermeability is definitely preventive medicine. Reducing this toxic load on the liver and the body can prevent illness or improve its outcome. Like dysbiosis, leaky gut is an example of a process that can lead to disease, rather than a specific disease. This condition is far more typical than many practitioners realize and is often overlooked in designing treatment. Resolving hyperpermeability can produce very real benefits.

Leaky gut (or hyperpermeability) is associated with a wide range of general symptoms, such as fatigue, fevers of unknown origin, abdominal pain or bloating, diarrhea, feelings of toxicity, memory problems and difficulty with concentration, and poor tolerance of exercise.

Hyperpermeability can cause:

- Attention deficit disorders
- Symptoms resembling autism
- Chronic and rheumatoid arthritis
- Chronic fatigue syndrome
- Eczema
- Food allergies and intolerances
- Inflammatory bowel disease
- Irritable bowel syndrome
- Joint and collagen problems
- Compromised liver function
- Malnutrition
- Multiple chemical sensitivities

- Psoriasis
- Symptoms like schizophrenia

- Skin disorders ranging from urticaria to acne and dermatitis

Hyperpermeability can also be *caused by* any number of different conditions. Any substance or condition that causes inflammation (such as GI infection), severe trauma (such as burns or surgery), or mechanical overstimulation (such as certain medications or NSAIDs)—anything that overstimulates the pores and keeps them open too long—is said to cause leaky gut, known as hyperpermeability.

The following conditions sometimes cause hyperpermeability:

- The aging process
- AIDS with diarrhea
- Alcoholism
- Burns
- Cancer
- Celiac disease
- Chemotherapy
- Crohn's disease
- Cystic fibrosis

- Certain drugs
- Giardia and other parasites
- Chronic hepatitis
- Intensive illnesses
- HIV
- Malnutrition
- NSAIDs
- Pancreatitis

- Psoriasis
- Radiation therapy
- Rheumatoid arthritis
- Shock or anaphylaxis
- Toxic shock syndrome
- Ulcerative colitis
- Trauma

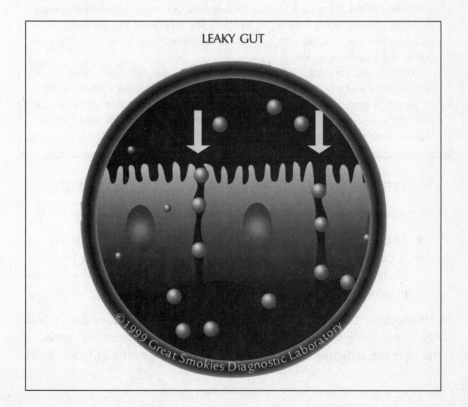

LEAKY GUT

©1999 Great Smokies Diagnostic Laboratory

When the Tests Come Out Normal, But . . .

❖

Debbie had complained of stomachaches since she was a child. Sometimes she would double over with crampy and dull, aching abdominal pains so severe she couldn't do anything but lie in bed for hours. Her symptoms seemed to come on a few minutes after eating. She had several thorough medical workups that were all normal. Her doctor prescribed muscle relaxants and tranquilizers, which seemed to help most of the time, and she got along reasonably well until she was in her mid-forties.

Out of the blue, at a time when Debbie was under enormous stress, she began having repeated attacks so severe they caused intense abdominal pain, explosive diarrhea, vomiting, hives, and a shock-like state in which her blood pressure would drop to almost undetectable levels. She was seen by many doctors and again had extensive testing that all came out normal. This time she was put on steroids, antihistamines, and Tagamet. Since the attacks were potentially life threatening, they had to be stopped.

When Debbie first saw me, she was developing additional problems from the steroids. Her physicians tried to taper her off the steroids, but whenever the doses were decreased, her attacks recurred. Her symptoms were consistent with a severe form of food allergies. A workup for intestinal permeability provided striking evidence of leaky gut syndrome. In addition, she was found to have severe dysbiosis that was associated with both yeast overgrowth and a parasitic infection due to *Blastocystis hominis*.

Debbie was successfully treated with nutrients and diet. She's been off all pharmaceuticals for five years now, and has not had a single attack. Her Cushing's syndrome is gone, and she has only an occasional episode of mild abdominal pain. Follow-up testing for leaky gut syndrome has been normal, and her dysbiosis is continuing to gradually clear.

WHY IT'S CALLED THE LEAKY GUT SYNDROME

The intestinal lining has two opposing functions:

- ◆ The absorption of nutrients from food in the digestive tract
- ◆ A barrier function, to contain microbes or large food particles (potential allergens) so they don't go beyond the gut environment (translocate) and get into our bloodstream

Our digestive tract has tiny porous openings between the cells (called tight junctions) so that nutrients can be absorbed from our food. If the porelike structures open too wide, toxins from the gut can flood into the bloodstream, overwhelming the liver and causing allergies or any of dozens of other ailments.

This is known as hyperpermeability because the lining has become too permeable (porous). It's also called leaky gut syndrome because the gut begins leaking larger food particles and toxins from the gut. It's not an illness but rather a natural process gone wrong. Normally, all these pores in the gut lining open and close whenever nutrients are absorbed from our food. It's only when the pores open too wide that leaky gut is said to occur.

HOW LEAKY GUT HAPPENS

Here's a blow-by-blow account of how leaky gut occurs. Let's use the example of someone who has an allergy. Suppose Sarah has a dairy allergy and unknowingly eats cheese; this can trigger a reaction in her body. If she has an immediate food allergy, her immune system may begin reacting right away. If she has delayed allergies, the reaction may not occur for as long as three hours, but it could take as long as forty-eight hours to occur.

What is amazing is that no matter when it occurs, Sarah may not even be aware that it's happening. She may have a vague feeling of discomfort that could include a mild stomachache, a headache, even joint or muscle aches. Although she may not notice anything more than vague discomfort at the time, later she may have a flare-up of some chronic problem such as allergies, asthma, or arthritis. And she probably won't link it to this microscopic process going on in her digestive tract as the lining becomes too "porous" and begins leaking tiny particles.

On the other hand, she may have noticed that if she cheats on her allergy diet and has milk for breakfast, sometime that day or the next her joints may be achy and exercise will become a major effort.

The response of Sarah's body to the offending food also activates her immune system. To alert the system that an invader is present (the dairy food she just ate), her immune system sounds the alarm through chemical messengers, the cytokines. They act like buglers calling out the cavalry, and their job is to bring in the infection fighters (the antibodies). This sets the immune system in motion. While we always have cytokines as an essential part of our system, when there are too many cytokines and other immune chemicals circulating in the bloodstream, the gut will start leaking.

WHEN THINGS ARE WORKING RIGHT

When Sarah's system is working properly, absorption is occurring through tiny structures in the lining of the small intestine. All this is happening on a microscopic level. Nutrients are being absorbed through three structures:

◆ Directly through the cells of the gut lining, called transcellular absorption
◆ Between the cells, in paracellular absorption
◆ In the crypts, tiny crevices in the lining of the gut

Each structure is programmed to absorb nutrient molecules of a particular size and electromagnetic charge. Between the finger-like villi that line the gut are the crypts, crevices at the base of each villi, like the webbing between your fingers. Because of their larger size, the crypts absorb bigger molecules, such as the disaccharides, which are complex sugars.

Between every cell in the gut lining is a tiny pore-like structure called a tight junction. These tiny pores are also active during digestion. They expand and contract just as other muscles do, opening and closing to release nutrients from the gut into the bloodstream or contain the food mix as it passes through the gut.

WHAT HAPPENS WHEN THERE'S INFLAMMATION

Too many immune chemicals can cause the pores to open too wide, causing too much permeability. When there's inflammation or any kind of crisis in the body, if too many of the immune signaling chemicals are circulating in the bloodstream, they can overstimulate the tight junctions, causing the pores to open too wide. This process can be compared to a house with doors wired to a fire alarm system. If the alarm system malfunctions, it may keep all the doors in the house open and won't let them close. Clearly other problems can result. Intruders could easily enter the house.

Leaky gut can increase the body's vulnerability to intruders, such as bacteria, yeast, or large food particles that would normally remain in the gut. Again, when the pores open too wide, material is inappropriately released into the bloodstream. In Sarah's case, if her immune system detects large food particles in the bloodstream (perhaps other innocent foods, released through the leaky gut), it will assume they're allergens and launch a second attack, flooding her system with more cytokines. Then the whole dynamic just gets worse.

THE IMPORTANCE OF THE LEAKY GUT SYNDROME

If leaky gut occurs frequently, it can cause chronic conditions. The importance of this increase in the permeability of the small intestine is not to be taken lightly, because two additional serious problems usually develop: liver overload and autoimmune conditions.

♦ *Stress on the liver.* Leaky gut places an increased toxic load on the liver, producing harmful chemical by-products as the liver attempts to clean up the overload. The free radicals that result form toxic bile, which can directly injure the gut lining. Contamination may also be a factor, caused by bacteria invading the system through dysbiosis. In the short term, this worsens leaky gut, creating a vicious cycle. Over time, these toxic by-products can cause gallstones or eventually even cancer. In order to break the cycle, it's important to control the underlying problem that has caused the leaky gut syndrome in the first place.

The liver is the major detoxifying organ of the human body. All products absorbed across the intestinal barrier must pass through the liver before entering the general circulation. There must be a balance between the size of the toxic load presented to the liver and the liver's capacity to metabolize this load. Unless the liver's detoxification system has enough reserve capacity to adjust to an increased toxic load, serious consequences can and often do result.

♦ *Autoimmune conditions.* Hyperpermeability sets the stage for possible autoimmune complications. When the total load of foreign material (antigens) is increased for a prolonged period, the immune system can become hyperactive, and a hyperimmune state can follow. As the immune system becomes overstimulated, "immune soldiers"— the antibodies—actually begin to attack the cells of the body as if *they* were the invaders. If one of the invading molecules resembles tissue within the body, the antibody produced to attack the foreign molecule will be unable to distinguish friend from foe, attacking both the original invader and the body's own tissue. This is known as the innocentbystander phenomenon. In the gut, these conditions include Crohn's disease, food allergies, and celiac disease. Elsewhere in the body, conditions such as asthma or rheumatoid arthritis can result.

THE VICIOUS CYCLE OF THE LEAKY GUT

Certain conditions trigger leaky gut and then are made worse as oversized molecules seep into the bloodstream and circulate throughout the body. These include:

♦ *Allergies*. Food sensitivity can induce leaky gut. The offending food stimulates an allergic reaction in the gut lining that increases permeability. The leaky gut then allows the passage of additional oversized macromolecules that the immune system perceives as invaders (since they are larger than usual) and therefore tagged as "different" or "antigen." This further stimulates the immune system to form antibody complexes that attack the tissue, causing additional aggravation of the leak in the gut lining and further allergic responses. Unless the vicious cycle is interrupted by avoiding the offending food or blocking the allergic reaction, the process will continue to tax the reserves and the functions of the liver, the immune system, and GI tract.

♦ *Overgrowth (dysbiosis)*. When potentially harmful flora take over, leaky gut can occur, allowing bacteria and bacterial fragments across the small intestinal lining (translocation). This can overstimulate the immune system and aggravate intestinal permeability, leading to additional overreaction and further aggravating the leak! Clearing the dysbiosis can break the cycle by removing the bacteria that are translocating across the gut lining. It's also important to increase the beneficial flora, stopping the immune reaction.

♦ *Malabsorption and malnutrition*. When the gut is starved for nourishment, whatever the cause, within days, hyperpermeability can occur. If malabsorption or malnutrition trigger the syndrome, a lack of nutritional supply to the lining of the gut can further limit the vital supply of blood or nutrients. Depriving the lining tissue of nourishment can cause shrinking, deterioration, and increased permeability. This increase in permeability tends to aggravate malabsorption and results in more atrophy and leaky gut syndrome. The cycle can be interrupted by carefully restoring proper nutrition to the cells of the small intestinal lining.

♦ *Inflammation*. The immune reactions (antibody responses)

within the gut wall, although intended to be protective, can create inflammation, further aggravating the leak in the gut, setting the stage for a vicious cycle.

OTHER LINKS TO LEAKY GUT

♦ *Genetics*. There appear to be genetic patterns of permeability. For example, Crohn's patients frequently have gut permeability; even their relatives with no symptoms also often have increased gut permeability. Although closely related individuals appear to have the same physical structures, some develop the symptoms characteristic of Crohn's disease and others do not. Relatives without symptoms also tend to have small areas of inflammation, not as extensive as fully developed Crohn's disease. These observations imply a genetic predisposition to leaky gut.

♦ *Mental disorders*. A number of mental conditions have been linked to increased permeability. The elevated toxins that leak into the system from hyperpermeability can produce symptoms that range from spaciness and brain fog to attention deficit disorder. We now know that many children with ADHD have increased gut permeability. In the most extreme form, hyperpermeability can cause disorientation resembling autism or schizophrenia. In some cases, these disorders are also linked to specific food sensitivities such as gluten intolerance. And a number of stresses can be affecting the body at once: toxic load on the system appears to affect neurotransmitter production and specific allergies may directly affect the nervous system as well. Recent research links some allergic responses with brain chemistry and reactions in the receptor sites (see Chapter 8).

Clearly, the presence of leaky gut syndrome, with its impact on the liver and the immune system, always extracts a metabolic price from the human body. This process is particularly important in patients with existing disease, but even in the absence of specific symptoms, it will tax wellness reserves and can eventually lead to serious consequences.

The widespread frequency and critical importance of the leaky gut syndrome has been largely underrated. In one study that tested for leaky gut syndrome in an intensive care unit, all patients studied had leaky gut syndrome, regardless of the condition that originally brought them to intensive care. Because of the incredibly high incidence of chronic diseases today and the high frequency of leaky gut syndrome in patients with chronic diseases, testing for intestinal permeability is worthwhile whenever associated conditions are present. Skillful management of this syndrome will help alleviate the primary illness, regardless of its nature.

8

Effects of Food Allergies

MICHAEL ROSENBAUM, M.D.

Allergies can cause digestive problems. It's that simple. For people who don't have allergies, this is not an issue. For those who do, it's a big deal.

In addition, some people have delayed responses that doctors now call food sensitivities. These are even more difficult to detect, because the response could occur even forty-eight hours after the triggering event. Some people go through their entire lives with an allergy, unaware that it's causing them chronic problems.

WHAT TO DO WHEN YOU SUSPECT ALLERGIES

If you have a digestive condition that hasn't gone away, explore the possibility of allergies, food intolerance, and sensitivity. Some aspect of these reactions could be an important component of your illness. Research shows that allergies are linked to Crohn's disease, colitis, irritable bowel syndrome, chronic constipation, malabsorption, and many other conditions.

It's also important to have a sense of what doctors mean by food allergy and food sensitivity. Although a doctor may find that you don't have an allergy, you may have a *food sensitivity,* and that can cause problems as well.

What is traditionally thought of as *allergy* is typically a strong reaction: immediate, obvious, and sometimes life-threatening. But this type of allergy accounts for only about 10 percent of allergic events.

In contrast, about 90 percent of the reactions to food seem to be delayed—and these are considered either *sensitivities* or *delayed food allergies.* Although the reaction can be observed, the mechanism isn't

---

How Allergies Can Affect Digestion

✥

At 37, David had a twenty-year history of abdominal pain, nausea, bloating, and diarrhea. During those years, he was seen by many doctors and specialists who diagnosed him as having irritable bowel syndrome. He was treated with a variety of medications, but his symptoms never really improved. David's life also involved a tremendous amount of stress. He was recently divorced and had sole custody of his two children, and he was both breadwinner and a full-time single parent. He often resorted to fast foods as the main staple for the family's diet (which probably didn't help his digestion).

When David's symptoms worsened, he consulted a surgeon and his gallbladder was removed. Unfortunately, he continued to experience nausea, bloating, and frequent diarrhea. When David was seen for a GI consult in a preventive medicine practice, he appeared to be chronically ill and fatigued. In addition to standard blood tests, stool testing for parasites was ordered and a gastro-colonoscopy was performed (scoping the stomach, esophagus, and upper small intestine—the duodenum). The lab studies were normal, but the scope revealed a hiatal hernia and an abnormally smooth texture to the duodenum. Biopsies showed evidence of celiac disease, an allergy to wheat gluten.

Blood tests found antibodies against wheat (anti-gliadin antibodies), which further confirmed the diagnosis of celiac disease. A low-allergenic and gluten-free diet was prescribed, which David has adhered to faithfully. Within a month, his diarrhea and bloating were gone for the first time in more than twenty years! He's being seen monthly for follow-up, and he continues to feel better, look better, and improve.

—Paul Thomas, D.O.

---

always known. Delayed reactions may occur from four to forty-eight hours after the offending food is eaten.

CLASSIC FOOD ALLERGIES—IMMEDIATE REACTIONS

Dr. Alan Levin's book *The Type 1 and 2 Allergy Relief Program* (Merla Zellerbach, 1986) was one of the first to describe classic immediate allergies as Type 1 allergies and delayed food allergies as Type 2.

With immediate Type 1 allergies, the same type of antibody that causes hay fever also causes allergies to specific foods. This is a relatively uncommon condition. Type 1 food allergies are *immediate* reactions that can often be life-threatening. People who have this condition typically carry adrenaline with them in case of emergency. (So when you think of Type 1 allergies, think of the IgE antibody—E for emergency.) The foods that usually cause these reactions are shellfish (such as crab, lobster, or shrimp) or nuts. Cinnamon (used as a spice) and peanuts can also be trigger foods.

People with Type 1 allergies have instant reactions and they know it. Their responses tend to be strong and clear-cut. Type 1 allergies (IgE-associated) tend to be hereditary. There is a genetic link, but people don't necessarily inherit an allergy to any specific food. Rather, they inherit a general tendency toward strong, specific allergic reactions. When someone tells me he is allergic to shellfish and he has had this problem since childhood, I have a strong suspicion of a Type 1 allergy.

Periodically there are stories in the newspapers about someone suddenly passing out in a restaurant, unable to breathe and having to be taken to a hospital immediately because of something he or she ate. The cause could be as innocent as a trace of peanuts in a sauce! The result can be a sudden, extreme reaction.

DELAYED FOOD ALLERGIES

Type 2 allergies are typically delayed reactions. Alan Levin suggests that Type 2 reactions are associated with the IgG antibody (think of G for gradual), but there may also be several other mechanisms involved. There may even be nonantibody mechanisms involved. These re-

Type Response	Type 1 Allergy	Type 2 Allergy	Sensitivity
Response time	Immediate	Delayed	Immediate and delayed
Frequency	10% of allergies	About 90% of allergic responses are delayed	
Associated antibody	IgE (remember E for emergency)	IgG (remember G for gradual)	May not trigger immunoglobulins
Severity	May be life-threatening	Mild to severe	Mild to severe
Origin	Allergic tendency is inherited	May be inherited or not	Genetic aspect unknown
Cause or trigger	Specific trigger food (antigen)	Food trigger that is difficult to identify because of the delay	A variety of causes including binding to opiate and serotonin receptors

sponses tend to be much more complicated. The reactions are typically delayed. Foods such as wheat, for example, have been found to cause responses with long delays—as long as two days after the food has been eaten.

In fact, because of the delay, it's much more difficult to diagnose delayed reactions to food, which constitute perhaps 90 percent of the responses reported to allergists. These are cases in which there is no obvious immediate cause and effect. There may or may not be a genetic link.

FOOD SENSITIVITIES

Another category of response is sensitivity to both foods and chemicals, including food additives and coloring, pesticides, and pollutants. With sensitivities, you see the response and the symptoms, but you don't know the cause. And research indicates that a number of different possible causes and mechanisms are associated with food sensitivities. Some of these processes may not be triggered by antibodies at all. One of the possible causes, for example, is intestinal permeability, the leaky gut syndrome (see Chapter 7). The intensity of the response is influenced by the degree of leaky gut and the levels of protective antibodies (secretory IgA). There's still a lot to be learned about the mechanisms that cause these frequently seen sensitivities.

Possible causes of delayed food sensitivities include:

◆ Stimulation of the nervous system
—Binding to opiate and serotonin receptor sites in the central nervous system
—Direct toxicity to nerve cells
◆ Foods and substances may have direct hormone-like activity or neurotransmitter-like activity
—Triggered by specific proteins (peptides)

THE LEAKY GUT CAN CAUSE ALLERGIES

Food allergies and sensitivities can be made worse by the leaky gut syndrome (high intestinal permeability). Many factors can trigger hyperpermeability: GI infection, an overgrowth of yeast or bacteria, viral illness, poor absorption, or genetic factors. In the leaky gut syndrome, oversized food particles begin sneaking in between the cells. These particles, which are not fully broken down, enter the blood-

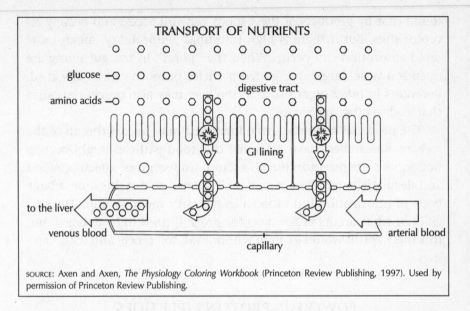

TRANSPORT OF NUTRIENTS

SOURCE: Axen and Axen, *The Physiology Coloring Workbook* (Princeton Review Publishing, 1997). Used by permission of Princeton Review Publishing.

stream, and the immune system identifies them as foreign material. At that point, the body mounts an immune response that creates a whole series of symptoms, a symptom complex. This dynamic is believed to be one of the causes of delayed food allergies and sensitivities.

ALLERGIES CAN GET ON YOUR NERVES

Research suggests that food particles which manage to sneak through the leaky gut into circulation can eventually occupy receptor sites in the brain and possibly in other organs. Fascinating research has shown that particles of foods such as milk and grains such as corn and wheat can occupy morphine or opiate receptor sites in the brain. This may trigger a variety of neurological responses. It can create problems with cognition, mood, or even pain, through responses in the brain described as cerebral reactions.

This receptor mechanism may explain why food allergies tend to obey the laws of addiction. Food particles that occupy morphine and opiate receptors create a craving for the allergenic food. When you don't have the food, you go into withdrawal. Then you crave it. And when you eat it, you may feel better.

Receptor stimulation does not necessarily depend on having high intestinal permeability. Even with normal permeability, research has found that by-products of these foods can still access and occupy receptor sites. But if there is high intestinal permeability, much more rapid absorption can occur. When the "pores" in the gut lining are open too wide, larger undigested particles of foods can be absorbed. Receptors in other organs such as the liver may also trigger responses that lead to other problems.

The processes that have been identified may be just the tip of the iceberg. Researchers have suggested that food particles might occupy not only opiate receptors but also serotonin receptors, affecting mood and sleep. Although there is no definitive evidence at this time, a large body of information links food allergies with mood swings. The specifics of what occurs at the receptor site still need to be detailed, but this mechanism would explain withdrawal, tolerance, and food cravings.

POWERFUL PROTEINS (PEPTIDES)
THAT TRIGGER ALLERGY

Clusters of protein molecules called peptides can stimulate hormone activity. These tiny peptides can be extremely powerful. Some of the hormone activity mediated by peptides occurs in the gut. For example, the intestine releases a powerful peptide called VIP. This potent hormone or transmitter affects gut motility (a vital issue to anyone suffering from chronic constipation or chronic diarrhea). The same peptide is found in certain foods and is now being used in the healing of GI illness. It is included in a product called Sea Cure, which contains peptides that seem to relax the gut and prevent spasm. Doctors report that such peptides (made from predigested whitefish) can be very useful in treating conditions such as irritable bowel syndrome.

Peptides can also act as neurotransmitters in the brain. Other peptides that control appetite are produced in the intestine and released in the stomach. They appear to control the amount of digestive enzymes that the body makes. They also may control the speed at which food is propelled through the gut. And they may control whether the GI tract is in spasm or not. They are extraordinarily potent in very minute levels.

Researchers have identified CCK (cholecystokinin), a polypeptide hormone that affects the gallbladder by causing the release of bile. As a neurotransmitter in the brain, it appears to shut off appetite. Researchers have been trying to isolate CCK for use in weight-loss programs.

Some peptides may have adverse effects. Fragments of peptides from undigested food may also have transmitter activity that can cause inflammation or mimic the activity of VIP and cause spasms. These peptides have direct hormonal effects on the gut wall. This is a third mechanism that can cause allergy, but it doesn't appear to be an immune mechanism.

YOU MAY BE SENSITIVE TO FOOD ADDITIVES AND PESTICIDES

The diet of the average American often contains food colors and food additives that can cause pharmacological actions. Some additives such as MSG have been found in lab experiments to affect the brain, and there are other additives that also act as excito-toxins—brain stimulants. So a lot of food sensitivities may be caused by food additives. Pesticides and heavy metals are also known to have adverse effects on the nervous system and may also stimulate inflammation in the gut. Since the food and water of most industrial nations contain pesticides, industrial chemicals, and heavy metals, these pollutants must also be considered when you're evaluating food sensitivity.

ANTIBODIES (SIgA) HELP FIGHT ALLERGIES

People with low levels of secretory IgA tend to be much more prone to infection and to food allergies. Sudden gastrointestinal infection or exposure to bacteria can cause secretory IgA production to increase rapidly. Some people are just born with less ability to make antibodies. SIgA tends to be reduced in people who have allergies and also in children born of parents who are allergic. As a result, they're more prone to food allergies and may be more prone to gluten/wheat intolerance. And gluten has the unique ability to inflame the entire lining of the gut, which can cause you to be allergic to everything else.

MINIMIZING FOOD ALLERGIES

Here are some suggestions about how to minimize allergies and sensitivities, digest your food better, and maintain the integrity of your digestive tract.

The Connection Between Infection and Allergies

❖

As an allergist, I've noticed that there's a connection between having a virus and being more allergic in general. People tell me their food allergies get worse when they have a flu. The interesting connection is that viral infection causes the blood levels of vitamin A to plummet. And when the level of vitamin A drops, the secretory IgA level in the gut goes down as well, so the defenses against allergy are down.

Lack of vitamin A is the major vitamin deficiency that causes a drop in secretory IgA. Before we had the modern vitamin industry, healthy kids took cod-liver oil. Of course now we can get vitamin A palmitate as a supplement. You have to maintain a balance by keeping up your levels of vitamin A without taking toxic doses. If you have very low nutrient stores in your liver, you can use them up by having a virus, and then it's important to replenish vitamin A.

◆ *Do everything you can to prevent dysbiosis and high intestinal permeability.* Then you are well on your way to preventing many food sensitivities.

◆ *Digest your food well.* When food is thoroughly digested, it's less allergenic. It's important that your digestive processes all work smoothly. Is your pancreas functioning properly? Is there enough bicarbonate for the intestine so the pancreatic enzymes can work? Are you eating in a hurry, with no time to really chew your food? Are you eating standing up? Eating under tremendous stress?

◆ *Do you have enough pancreatic enzymes?* The Chymex Test (from Meridian Labs) can actually test pancreatic enzyme levels in the body. This test and other useful lab work can be ordered by your doctor (see Resources for information on Meridian Laboratories).

◆ *Eat smaller, more frequent meals.* We tend to eat huge meals. Smaller meals usually encourage more thorough digestion.

◆ *Cook your food if you have a tendency toward sensitivities.* As a general principle, raw food is more allergenic than cooked food. So one way to prevent these allergies is to cook as much of your food as you can, because cooking changes its structure. That explains why apple sauce is less allergenic than raw apples. The same is true for tomato sauce as opposed to fresh tomatoes.

◆ *Use the rotation diet in planning your meals.* Be creative, so meals are still interesting and pleasurable.

◆ *Experiment with food combining.* Food-combining theory is based on not mixing grains and meat at the same meal (or at least not mixing large quantities of both). In this system, the main course of grain *or* protein is combined with vegetables. The idea is to encourage more complete digestion. Minimizing the amount of undigested food moving through the GI tract will decrease the allergic (antigenic) load on the system. Some people report that simpler meals, designed around food combining, are easier to digest.

◆ *Relax when you eat.* Make mealtime a time of quiet, relaxed pleasure, a refuge from the hectic nature of your day. Do this even if your meal is brief and simple.

◆ *Keep your immune system strong.* It has been proposed that food allergies are worse in the winter, in cold weather, and better in the summer. Keep your stores of secretory IgA up by taking a moderate amount of vitamin A.

◆ *Minimize stress.* The concept of stress reduction is important because stress will affect the amount of digestive enzymes you have and the degree of intestinal permeability. Stress is an underappreciated factor in digestion and in allergies and sensitivities. Few of us realize the degree to which stress impairs the lining of the gut.

9

Harm from Toxins

JEFFRY ANDERSON, M.D.

❖

Toxic chemicals can directly injure the lining of the GI tract and interfere with your digestion. Symptoms can result from minimal low-level exposures, as well as from intense or long-term exposures. Man-made chemicals, products of our high-tech industrial world, are released into the environment in staggering amounts—thousands of metric tons per year in the U.S. alone. Reports of toxic spills and new chemical pollutant threats are frequently reported in the media. We may feel a sense of concern when we hear about these pollutants, but few people with digestive illness connect their symptoms with toxic exposure.

TOXINS FROM CHEMICALS AND HEAVY METALS

Pollutants can trigger inflammation and interfere with the function of the GI tract. These toxins include pesticides such as everyday household bug sprays; solvents in paint thinner; petroleum products such as gasoline; industrial chemicals and by-products including dioxin and PCBs; and heavy metals like mercury and lead.

COMMON SOURCES OF LOW-LEVEL EXPOSURE

We may be sensitive to chemicals in water such as fluoride and chlorine. In agricultural areas, water often contains pesticides, herbicides, and inorganic fertilizer chemicals. In industrial or military areas, water may contain heavy metals, petrochemical derivatives, PCBs, and radioactive compounds, as well as other toxins.

The water supply to many urban/suburban areas contain some of these pollutants from distant runoff contamination, originating in agricultural and industrial areas. This is because water, as well as air, moves over great distances, carrying contaminants with it. In addition, chlorine in municipal waters can create new toxins such as THMs by interacting with organic pollutants. THMs have been linked to high rates of miscarriage. Many of these chemicals (particularly pesticides, PCBs, and dioxins) persist for long periods of time in our environment and break down slowly.

◆ *Pesticides and other chemicals in our food can trigger digestive symptoms.* Fruits, vegetables, and grains may be contaminated by any of the 800 pesticides currently in use. Meat, dairy products, and poultry often contain residues of hormones, antibiotics, tranquilizers, steroids, or other drugs, as well as pesticide residues from feed. Fish and shellfish commonly contain low levels of heavy metals, particularly mercury, as well as lead, arsenic, cadmium, chromium, and chemicals such as dioxins and PCBs.

◆ *Low level chronic exposure to toxins in the home and garden can actually affect our digestion.* Toxic chemicals in everyday home use include solvents such as turpentine, paint and paint thinner, paint and wax

---

Digestive Problems Can Be Caused by Toxins in Food

❖

Testing by the Food and Drug Administration (FDA) shows that about half our foods contain some level of pesticides, although legal, while perhaps 5 percent of our foods contain illegal residues (FDA data reported by the Environmental Working Group, 1994). Many toxic chemicals persist in our environment for a long period of time, and are said to have a long half-life (period of time before they begin breaking down). They accumulate in our food sources, and because we are the higher on the food chain, we get more concentrated amounts of pesticides in our food, particularly from the livestock and poultry we eat and the chemicals they have also been exposed to. The chemicals remain in our tissues and systems, stored in fats and bound to proteins. Researchers suggest that probably every person on earth has some residues of the pesticide DDT in his or her body, despite the fact that it was banned more than thirty years ago.

When one's nutritional status is compromised from poor absorption and poor digestion, combined with the effects of toxins present in the body, then subsequent damage to other tissues is likely, which can result in further illness.

SOURCE: M. Moses. *Designer Poisons.* San Francisco: Pesticide Education Center (1995).

strippers, spot removers, degreasers, and gasoline. Pesticides that are found in the home and garden include bug sprays, pet sprays, flea collars, and pest strips.

♦ *Other unknown low level chronic exposures include fluoride in toothpaste and chemicals in food and cosmetic products.* Fluoride, for example, is contained in most toothpastes. Researchers have linked conditions such as irritable bowel syndrome (IBS) to toothpaste—fluoride or carrageenan could be the irritant, or both. Recent studies have found toxic effects from common cosmetic and toothpaste additives such as propylene glycol (a major constituent of antifreeze!), sodium lauryl sulfate, DEA (di-ethanolamine), and other similar chemicals.

♦ *The effects of mercury amalgams.* Mercury (along with silver and tin) has been the material of choice for dental fillings (mercury-silver amalgams) in American dentistry and has been used extensively for over a century. Many scientific studies have documented the toxic effects of mercury on the brain, nervous system, kidney, liver, and GI tract. Tin is also known to cause these effects, especially in the brain, although to a lesser degree.

Toxic processes include the creation of antibiotic-resistant gut bacteria, which contributes to harmful overgrowth (dysbiois). The antibiotic-resistant bacteria may even become predominant residents in the GI tract. Recent research indicates that some species (Klebsiella, citrobacter, and Proteus) may play a role in perpetuating ulcerative colitis and Crohn's disease. They can also be communicable to immuno-compromised individuals.

Mercury is released from dental fillings continuously in very small amounts, but over a period of fifteen to twenty years can accumulate in the body in dangerous amounts, since most people have multiple fillings by midadolescence. Mercury-silver amalgams have been outlawed in Europe and Scandinavia for several decades, but continue to be widely used by American dentistry.

POSSIBLE SOURCES OF LONG-TERM OR HIGH INTENSITY EXPOSURE

♦ *Indoor exposure from tight or sick building syndrome.* Toxins inhaled or absorbed through the skin can circulate widely in the bloodstream, throughout the body and the GI tract, where they can cause specific damage.

Sick building syndrome can occur in commercial or public build-

---

Insight from Environmental Medicine

❖

Susan had a five-year history of chronic illness with what seemed like overwhelming problems—severe fatigue, repeated colds, bladder and GI infections, asthma, chronic constipation with frequent bouts of diarrhea with gas, bloating and cramps, mental fogginess and difficulty with memory, as well as generalized pains in her muscles and joints. Routine medical evaluations had found nothing abnormal, and she was told she was depressed.

An environmental medicine consultation revealed three significant aspects of her history: a long-standing hobby of silk screen printing that involved the use of numerous solvents; extensive fillings of mercury-silver amalgam present since adolescence; and several episodes of foreign travel prior to her illness. Lab tests revealed a number of significant abnormalities. Stool testing was positive for parasites and yeast overgrowth, as well as high levels of pathogenic bacteria and unusually low levels of normal flora. It also suggested increased hyperpermeability (leaky gut syndrome); abnormally low secretory IgA in saliva; suppression of her immune response (both antibody and white blood count); and major elevations of several toxic solvents in blood specimens (N-hexane, pentane, toluene, and benzene, all used in her silk screening hobby); and abnormally high levels of mercury in the urine analysis. Additional tests also demonstrated an autoimmune condition involving the thyroid gland and many allergic reactions, particularly to a number of foods.

Susan has improved significantly after three years of intensive treatment that involved avoiding the use of solvents; clearing her GI system of microscopic parasites, pathogenic yeast, and bacteria; and restoring normal flora. She has also benefited from the removal of her mercury amalgams (by a dentist with special expertise who performed the work in stages, over a period of months, taking great care not to reintroduce the mercury back into her body). Removal of the amalgams was followed by medically monitored sauna detox therapy and mercury chelation. Susan has experienced a major improvement in most of her symptoms and marked improvement in her daily functioning and general quality of life.

---

ings including schools and hospitals, as well as in residential buildings characterized by poor ventilation and a high level of synthetic materials. Toxic building materials and commercial chemicals include certain paints, most synthetic carpets and underpadding, adhesives, formaldehyde, sealers, waxes, disinfectants, cleaning agents, photocopier solution and toner, pesticide applications, and PCBs (from older electrical equipment such as fluorescent light transformers). These materials can build up in significantly high concentrations in buildings that lack adequate ventilation and outdoor air exchange.

◆ *Outdoor and industrial sources.* Occupational exposures have been associated with the use of pesticides (agricultural and pest control workers and landscapers), solvents (building trades), PCBs, dioxins, and hundreds of thousands of other chemicals (heavy industry, chemical manufacturing), and petroleum and its by-products (the petrochemical industry).

◆ *Acute, intense exposure from a single incident, an industrial accident, or spill.* This can involve solvents, pesticide spills, agricultural activities such as crop dusting and aerial spraying, petroleum spills, and other sources of exposure.

SYMPTOMS IN THE GI TRACT

Any condition that includes inflammation, poor digestion, or poor absorption could be caused partly by environmental toxins or be aggravated by them. Such illnesses include irritable bowel syndrome, peptic ulcer disease, Crohn's disease, ulcerative colitis, celiac disease, and colon cancer.

This can lead to a wide variety of distressing GI symptoms, such as abdominal pain, indigestion, bloating or distention, gas (flatulence), nausea, diarrhea, constipation, and leaky gut syndrome. If the problem in the digestive tract is not cleared up, it can lead to damage and dysfunction elsewhere in the body, which can translate into major illness, chronic illness, or degenerative disease.

GENERAL SYMPTOMS

This concern can affect anyone to some degree, but people who have greater exposure may also have a more serious problem. On the other hand, people who are highly sensitive, have a genetic tendency to GI problems, or have an infection may react more strongly to toxins. Any of a number of symptoms can occur.

They can occur singly or in combination, and may be constant or intermittent: fatigue, weakness, weight loss, headache, joint and muscle pain/fibromyalgia, and allergic responses. Repeated infections have been linked to immune system dysfunction, such as frequent colds, coughs, flu, bronchitis, or sinus infections. Other immune system disorders include many types of allergic responses and even autoimmune diseases, such as lupus, Lou Gehrig's disease, or MS (multiple sclerosis). A wide variety of neurological symptoms are frequently seen: migraine; impaired short memory or attention span; difficulty concentrating, brain fog or spaciness; tingling, numbness, and muscle tics; depression, irritability, and panic attacks.

THE MAJOR FACTORS

- These toxins can be the primary cause of illness.
- Most often they coexist with other problems and eventually cause a cascade of chronic illness.
- Other factors can play a significant role, such as genetic makeup, lifestyle, and nutritional status.
- In some cases, a second condition can develop or be made worse by this exposure. These include GI infections from yeast, bacteria, microscopic parasites, or viruses.

WHEN DO YOU SUSPECT EXPOSURE?

In an industrial society, almost no one is immune—most everyone has some degree of exposure through the air, water, and food. If you live in the average city or suburb, drink city water, and buy your food at the local supermarket, you are frequently exposed to toxic chemicals. If you live in an area of industry or agriculture, you are probably heavily exposed. Even those of us who live in pristine environments still have some amount of uncontrollable exposure to toxic chemicals. Such chemicals are universally present because they are carried via wind and water, which circulate around the planet.

Although most substances in nature break down and return to the earth, heavy metals and many man-made chemicals do not. Consequently, these toxins remain for long periods of time in our environment and in our bodies and break down slowly. Some, such as heavy metals, don't break down at all.

Many of us receive specific exposures at home or at work, in addition to the unavoidable exposure to pollution of the air we breathe, over which we have little control. This may occur frequently, such as the monthly spraying by the exterminator, dusting the garden, using pest strips, starting the barbecue with lighter fluid, or keeping flea collars on our pets. Everyone has some vulnerability.

It's important to know about intentional use, because some exposures can be controlled. We can monitor our health. If we find that we are sensitive to chemicals, we can effectively minimize our exposure by eating organic food, drinking purified water, and using non-toxic pesticides and building materials in our home. (See Chapter 23 on cutting toxic exposure for further solutions and strategies.)

When we are exposed to toxins, they are absorbed through the skin and mucous membranes of the gut and the lungs and can circulate throughout the body. They can cause damage to almost any cell or organ. Some tissues are more vulnerable than others, due to their unique structure and function:

- ◆ Cells that have rapid turnover and repair—gut lining, skin, liver, the respiratory tract, and the immune system
- ◆ Those with exceptionally slow growth, as well as reproductive cells—the brain, eggs, and sperm.

Connective tissues such as muscles, tendons, cartilage, and fat cells are relatively less vulnerable.

When digestive problem result from chemical exposure, it can be extremely difficult to discover the actual cause. However, it's important to find the source of the problem in order to eliminate the exposure. Many chronic health problems begin with compromised digestive function.

TOXINS CAN HARM GI STRUCTURE AND FUNCTION

Chemicals and heavy metals can harm the structure and functioning of the GI tract in a number of ways. The gut lining is the focal area where the external environment meets the interior of the body. For this reason, the GI tract is one of the most vulnerable organs of the body, where some of the most significant damage can occur. Toxins can directly injure the lining of the digestive tract.

The cells lining the gut have the complex and essential role of defending the GI tract against invading microbes that may enter the body, primarily through ingested materials in food and water. The mucosal cells provide a barrier against microbes by secreting mucus that contains protective secretory IgA antibodies (SIgA). At the same time, they provide a barrier against the introduction of large molecules of toxins and allergens from food. The lining cells also have a critical role in the selective transport of essential nutrients into the body.

Some of the most important functions of the gastrointestinal tract depend on the integrity of the gut lining and the health of each individual cell. Essential processes include:

♦ *Communication.* Sending and receiving information occurs through molecules and receptors that coordinate different components and organs in the GI tract to orchestrate digestion.

♦ *Defense.* Recognizing invading, foreign, or threatening microbes or materials and mounting an immune response.

♦ *Nutrition.* Identifying and preparing key nutrients for transport and assimilation into the body.

MECHANISMS OF DAMAGE

Damage to the Cells of the GI Lining

♦ Direct damage by chemicals and heavy metals to the structure of the cell wall, distorting the three-dimensional shape of protein and

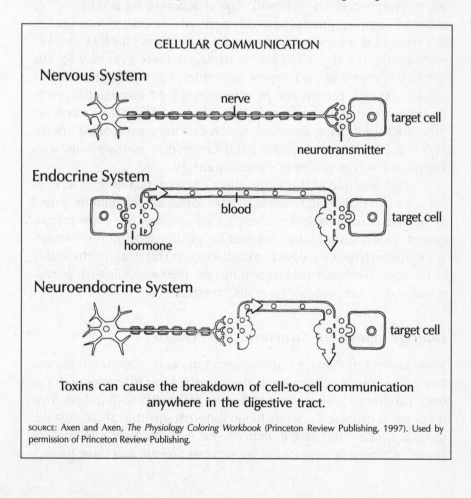

CELLULAR COMMUNICATION

Nervous System

nerve · target cell · neurotransmitter

Endocrine System

blood · hormone · target cell

Neuroendocrine System

target cell

Toxins can cause the breakdown of cell-to-cell communication anywhere in the digestive tract.

SOURCE: Axen and Axen, *The Physiology Coloring Workbook* (Princeton Review Publishing, 1997). Used by permission of Princeton Review Publishing.

fatty structures (receptor sites). (This is like distorting a lock so the key no longer fits and the lock no longer works.)

♦ Free radical or oxidative by-products that cause damage, making essential fatty structures of the cell wall more brittle and rigid. (This is comparable to the prolonged effects of sunlight and air on rubber or plastic materials—they become oxidized, stiff, and brittle.)

♦ Direct effects of certain chemicals, particularly solvents and related toxins, on the cell wall, through destruction of the fatty portions of the cell membrane. (This is similar to the action of solvents on grease.)

Interference with the Body's Ability to Absorb Nutrients

One of the ways nutrients are transported into our body is by attaching to receptors in the cell wall. The attachment signals the cell to initiate a complex process in which nutrients are carried into the cell in a series of specific steps. The receptor works through a lock-and-key mechanism, and if the receptor is damaged, there's no way for the nutrient to attach to the receptor and initiate the transport process. A second way this process can be interrupted is by damage to specific enzymes essential to the process. In either case, essential nutrients are prevented from being absorbed, which can have widespread effects. This is a form of malabsorption and can lead to malnutrition, with symptoms such as weight loss and low energy.

A good example of this is the effect of heavy metals such as mercury (from dental amalgam fillings) or colloidal silver (commonly used as an alternative antibiotic). These metals can bind up a key protein enzyme called glutathione, essential for the transport of trace minerals, so the enzyme no longer works effectively. This disrupts the ability of the body to obtain vital trace minerals. Heavy metals such as cadmium and nickel probably have similar effects.

Damage to Immune Structures and Processes

Some toxins can damage immune structures and processes in the gut lining (the mucosa). Damage to the mucosal layer interferes with the body's ability to produce SIgA and other antibodies such as IgM. Toxins can also damage the white blood cells living within and below the mucosa. These cells come in many forms with multiple roles and include lymphocytes (responsible for sentinel defense and surveillance), macrophages (scavenger cells), and others, which make up our cellular immune defense.

Compromise of immune function can increase our susceptibility to infections—both infections localized in the gut, such as GI viral infections and dysentery, and illness throughout the rest of the body, like colds, flu, bronchitis, and sinus infections. Toxic damage to immune functions can also increase the incidence of allergies, chronic fatigue syndrome, and autoimmune diseases.

Toxins can compromise the gut's barrier and defense functions against microbes—bacteria, parasites, yeast, viruses, and other pathogens. Reductions in SIgA antibodies also diminish protection against the undesirable absorption of oversized macromolecules of toxins and food.

Overstimulation of the Immune Response

Heavy metals such as cadmium and nickel and certain toxic chemical compounds can increase allergic and autoimmune responses. Overstimulation of the immune response can occur in localized areas where tissue is damaged, or generally throughout the GI tract. This can trigger sensitivity to other unrelated substances such as foods, molds, or even bacteria.

This process can also cause autoimmune conditions to develop—for example, ulcerative colitis or Crohn's disease in the GI tract, or general autoimmune disorders such as lupus or rheumatoid arthritis.

DISTURBING THE FLORA

Destruction of Beneficial Microflora

Damage can occur to normal beneficial gut flora, leaving the body vulnerable to infection. Unfortunately, these flora are often more vulnerable to toxins than the pathogenic bacteria. Beneficial microflora have an essential role in maintaining both normal GI health and general health. For example, maintenance of beneficial bacteria has been found to correlate with keeping the AIDS virus in remission. The flora produce antibiotic-like molecules and enzymes that inhibit the invasion of unfriendly microbes. They also synthesize and process essential nutrients, particularly key vitamins such as B_{12} and essential fatty acids such as butyrate.

In the absence of friendly flora, an overgrowth of harmful microbes can take place, particularly yeast and bacteria. This can result in secondary damage to the integrity of the gut wall, increased fermentation, putrefaction, and toxins.

◆ *The toxic metabolic by-products of putrefaction* can result in the common symptoms of gas and bloating.

◆ *Inflammation in the gut can be generated by the toxins.* White blood cells are then mobilized in response to the inflammation, bombarding the tissue with free radicals that produce further inflammation.

◆ *Carcinogenic by-products can result* from the interaction of free radicals with bacterial toxins and normally nontoxic substances such as nitrates and nitrites, which are transformed into potentially cancer-causing nitrosamines.

◆ *Chemical toxins and heavy metals bound in the stool for disposal can be released back into the body* when abnormal bacteria flora result in undesirable levels of an enzyme that unbinds toxins (beta-glucaronidase). This allows the toxins to be reabsorbed in a revolving door process.

◆ *Certain yeast and pathogenic bacteria produce neurotoxic substances,* which are then absorbed and go to the brain. These toxins are linked to conditions such as attention deficit disorders (ADD/ADHD), autism, panic disorders, chronic depression, and possibly schizophrenia.

Activation of Dormant Viruses

For unknown reasons, chemical damage to the gut lining can result in the activation of viruses such as measles or herpes which may remain dormant in the cells for years, but which then replicate and spread. The compromise of immune integrity, lowering levels of defending antibodies and white blood cells, can create an opportunity for viruses to more easily flourish. This can lead to either localized inflammation or infection anywhere in the body.

The activation of viruses in the gut may be associated with conditions like chronic fatigue syndrome and irritable bowel syndrome (IBS). Viral activation has also been associated with the mechanism of autoimmunity, both in the gut itself in diseases such as Crohn's and elsewhere in the body.

Induction of Antibiotic-Resistant Bacteria

Recent research has established that mercury, released from amalgam dental fillings, can encourage the development of bacteria that are resistant to antibiotics, particularly varieties of streptococcus. This can occur within two weeks of the amalgam placement. As it turns out, resistance to mercury and antibiotics are encoded on the bacteria's DNA on adjacent sites. Mercury exposure activates the DNA genetic expression for mercury resistance to protect the bacteria from toxic damage, but also induces the expression for antibiotic resistance. This resistance can be passed on to other bacteria of the same or other species. The effect can also be caused by other heavy metals. The implications are profound, considering the major problem that currently exists with antibiotic-resistant pathogens.

THE BREAKDOWN OF COMMUNICATION THROUGHOUT THE DIGESTIVE TRACT

All the organs of digestion must talk with one another: the stomach, all the parts of the lengthy small intestine—the duodenum, the ileum, the jejunum—as well as the pancreas, gallbladder, and large intestine. They all have to communicate in order for food to make it through the GI tract and get totally processed: all the nutrients extracted, all the toxins eliminated, all the enzymes and digestive juices secreted at the right time and place, and so forth. If that process doesn't occur, food won't be thoroughly digested and toxins won't be thoroughly eliminated. It means there's a much greater likelihood of leaky gut and dysbiosis.

The wrong signals can affect motility, causing diarrhea or constipation. If coordinated communication doesn't take place, it could mean that everything goes through the GI tract so quickly that diarrhea occurs, eventually causing malnutrition. Or it could mean that things move too slowly and there is stasis, excessive fermentation, and putrefaction, encouraging the overgrowth of yeast and bad bacteria. When constipation occurs, toxins may actually be reabsorbed back into the body.

Normally, the GI tract is elegantly coordinated by molecules of protein called peptides. They're secreted by specialized cells in the gut lining and released at the cell wall. Signals from the gut and from other distant organs are received by receptors in the cell wall that specialize in identifying these molecules and binding them through a lock-and-key mechanism.

The cell wall has literally thousands of receptors in order to communicate with a wide variety of signaling molecules. Once the molecule binds to the receptor, the cell is instructed to carry out a specific function, such as the production of a particular enzyme. This happens millions of times a day all over our body.

Toxins can damage the structure of receptors and the ability of cells to produce and release signaling peptides. This damage can block communication to such a degree that the digestive tract becomes nonfunctional. Or it can be overstimulated by too many molecules released too soon, so that they flood the system. Just as when too many people try to dial into the Internet at the same time, the system shuts down because of too much input. In the gut, communication can also be misread if the wrong molecule is released at the wrong time or goes to the wrong place. When any of these miscommunications occur, the digestive tract no longer functions properly.

Besides communicating within itself, the most critical digestive communication is with the brain. The GI tract is also regulated by peptides secreted by the brain that signal the gut when to move, when to become active. So just as localized miscommunication can cause diarrhea or constipation, so impaired communication with the brain can affect motility. There may be too much communication, like noise. Or there can be too little communication, resulting in lethargy, weakness, and chronic fatigue.

Some peptides have dual roles. For example, cholecystokinin signals the gallbladder to digest fats and perform other functions. It also controls appetite by notifying the brain that you're no longer hungry, so that you suddenly feel full.

Many of the peptides secreted in the GI tract have a major influence on brain function. Both physical, neurological, and even psychological symptoms can result, including irritability, spaciness, or anxiety. So damage to the gut doesn't affect only the digestive tract because the brain and GI tract have a profound synergistic role in communication and regulation. What happens in the gut doesn't just stay in the gut. When you have stomachache, you may also have a headache. Everything is interconnected.

In the GI tract, miscommunication can cause numerous symptoms—hypermotility, hyperperistalsis, diarrhea, cramping, spasms, reverse peristalsis, ulcers, pain, nausea, excessive appetite, regurgitation, heartburn, and other derangements. Impaired functioning can result in poor digestion, malabsorption, and poor assimilation, mild or severe.

There is also two-way communication throughout the digestive tract between the gallbladder and the liver, the GI tract and the pancreas, and many other locations. If that communication is interrupted, it can lead directly to digestive problems and the malfunction of other organs in the system.

Toxins can damage the regulation of the GI tract by the autonomic nervous system, which runs your body's functions automatically. This can interfere with functions that should happen as a matter of habit, such as motility and the secretion of digestive juices. Since many pollutants are neurotoxic, they can cause these disruptions by damaging junctions between muscles and nerves or damaging the brain centers that control these functions.

Toxins can also inhibit the function of key enzymes within the cell by inhibiting the production of energy in the "engine of the cell," the mitochondria. This can short-circuit the efforts of the cell to defend or repair itself. Certain pesticides that inhibit ATPase can severely inhibit energy-dependent functions. They inhibit mitochondrial ATPase. When these toxins infiltrate the gut lining, they damage the mitochondrial membrane and the cell wall membrane of the lining cells, the epithelium. As a result, all the functions of the gut lining that are dependent on energy production through ATP will be impaired.

Toxins and the Liver

Toxins can directly damage the liver in two ways. Toxic buildup can overwhelm the liver's ability to detoxify, leading to a bottleneck and the storage of toxins throughout the body. It can also directly impair the liver's ability to regulate metabolism. This includes the synthesis and breakdown of fats, sugars, and starches and to some degree proteins. Deranged metabolism of carbohydrates can lead to abnormalities in blood sugar levels. This can cause a tendency toward low blood sugar, resulting in fatigue, mood swings, or depression. Impaired fat metabolism can lead to elevated cholesterol and bad cholesterol (LDL), which has been found to increase the risk for heart disease. Damage to protein metabolism can lead to abnormal protein by-products, including the buildup of ammonia in the body that can produce mental impairment.

Toxins and Cancer

Many chemical pollutants have been documented as carcinogens, especially organo-chlorine pesticides, aromatic and chlorinated solvents, and chemicals such as dioxins and PCBs . Some carcinogens are produced by overcooking food, particularly meats done on the barbecue, producing what's called PAHs (polycyclic aromatic hydrocarbons). All these toxins can cause damage to cellular DNA, which can initiate or promote cancerous changes in cells. Cancers of the colon, stomach, esophagus, and pancreas have all been linked with exposure to these chemicals. Of course these toxins can also circulate throughout the body and cause cancers in other organs and tissues.

Leaky Gut Syndrome and Food Allergies

The gut lining membrane functions as a selective gate or barrier, allowing the passage and transport of small and medium-size molecules of essential nutrients and communication peptides. At the same time, the membrane bars the passage of larger molecules, including many toxins and allergenic substances. The cells of the gut lining play an essential role in this process. Their cell walls are made up of double-layered fatty and protein structures that act as semipermeable membranes, selectively allowing some substances through and barring others.

When nutrients are absorbed, small molecules are actively transported *through the cell* into the blood vessels beneath (transcellular transport) and other medium-size molecules are allowed to pass *between the cells* (paracellular transport). The passage of nutrients *between* the cells is regulated by specialized structures called tight junctions. Essentially, tight junctions are protein structures linking one cell wall to the next in a pore-like structure that can open or close selectively to allow nutrients to pass through. The tight junctions are crucial in preventing the passage of large undesirable molecules such as toxins and allergens, as well as whole bacteria.

Toxins can damage or disrupt the tight junctions and their functions. If the tight junctions open too wide, material from the gut can enter the bloodstream directly. This invasive material includes toxins and allergenic molecules, as well as microbes. The malfunction is called leaky gut, and can actually occur within a matter of minutes. Leaky gut can cause infection, allergies, direct toxic damage, or malabsorption and malnutrition. This syndrome can be caused by direct damage from toxins ingested in food and water, but also by toxins produced internally in the gut through fermentation, putrefaction, and inflammation.

This chapter has discussed the various ways in which toxins can damage the gastrointestinal lining and function, leading to a wide variety of diseases. It should be remembered that these mechanisms, although discussed individually, often occur simultaneously or concurrently. Sometimes all of them occur at once to produce a complex chronic condition.

Although our discussion is predominantly about environmental toxins, with dysbiosis, a large toxic load is created from within the gut itself by fermentation, putrefaction, and the toxin production of normal flora. These toxins can have an impact that is just as harmful as environmental toxins, if not more damaging. When both conditions coexist, the internally generated toxins, in combination with high intake of environmental toxins, can lead to the most serious conditions.

JEFFRY ANDERSON, M.D., is a physician in environmental medicine. His practice has included the treatment of hundreds of patients with environmental exposures and he has served as consultant on a number of major environmental spills. He received his medical degree from Indiana University, following study at Purdue. Dr. Anderson has provided medical care in a variety of hospital and clinical settings and has been in private practice in Marin County, California, since 1973. He also specializes in allergy-immunology and applied medical nutrition, using an integral approach to the diagnosis and treatment of chronic disease.

10

Stress and Digestion

MARTIN ROSSMAN, M.D.

❖

There is probably no system in the body that's more responsive to mind-body influences than the digestive tract. When we get sick, we tend to focus on the physical level, but our emotions and stress can affect digestion fairly profoundly. Problems are often initiated in the mind, as well as the body. Illness typically includes both physical and stress-related aspects.

Health issues can be challenging to sort out. Some conditions (like an overgrowth of yeast or bacteria) have mainly emotional symptoms when they're really a physical problem. On the other hand, research indicates that stress can have a negative effect on our flora and decrease antibody production, both factors in any overgrowth. So stress can directly affect our immune response.

No matter what the diagnosis, stress seems to make everything worse. Stress tends to interfere with digestion, whereas relaxation tends to promote good digestion. In some cases, digestive symptoms are simply a response to stress. And doctors report that with conditions such as Crohn's disease, flare-ups and relapses tend to correlate with stressful life events. This doesn't mean the cause is psychological or emotional, but that stress can amplify the level of illness.

We now know that positive emotional factors can promote healing. This has been demonstrated in the work of Dean Ornish on community support and love, Herbert Benson on the relaxation response, Norman Cousins on laughter, and Larry Dossey on prayer.

INSIGHT INTO DIGESTION

Some of the first modern research on the connection between stress and digestion grew out of the work of Dr. William Beaumont, a fa-

---

The Powerful Effects of Stress on Digestion

Beverly's situation is an interesting example of the powerful effects of stress on health. Her experience also demonstrates that coping with stress can improve health. I first saw Beverly ten years ago when she was diagnosed with Crohn's disease at the young age of 23. Over the years, whenever she was under extreme stress at home due to a rocky marriage, she would be seen for symptoms of abdominal cramping, diarrhea, rectal bleeding, and weight loss. These relapses would occur about every other year. Otherwise, she was generally well and free of symptoms, with the periodic support of medication.

For about five years, I saw her very occasionally, primarily to renew prescriptions. Then one day Beverly reappeared, about forty pounds underweight, anemic, and extremely emaciated. She confided that she had recently gotten a divorce and felt her whole life was falling apart. She was overwhelmed by the challenges of dealing with lawyers, an intense child custody battle, unemployment, and a lack of job skills. Her condition was extreme enough to require tube feeding, as well as medication.

Before long, we were able to get her back on solid food and supplements, while gradually decreasing the medication. On a program that included vitamin supplements, L-glutamine, and minerals with additional magnesium, she began regaining her weight. Once she developed some work skills and got a job, she was able to piece her life back together. As the stress decreased, she no longer needed most of the medications. At this point, her Crohn's disease has been in remission for several years. Although we haven't seen her as a patient, she comes in once a year to let us know how she's doing. She is a perfect example of what stress can do to you—and the health benefits of coping.

—*Trent Nichols, M.D.*

---

mous nineteenth-century physician and pioneer in American surgery. One of his patients, Alexis St. Martin, had been shot in the abdomen, resulting in a wound that healed but couldn't be closed. St. Martin's open wound provided a view directly into his stomach through the abdominal wall.

Alexis St. Martin became a guest in the Beaumont household, where he resided for many years. This provided Beaumont the opportunity to do a lot of observation. In 1833, Beaumont published a monograph, *Experiments and Observations on the Gastric Juices and the Biology of Digestion,* in which he detailed 238 experiments that suggested the presence of what we now know to be hydrochloric acids and enzymes such as pepsin. His book marks the beginning of modern study of the digestive system.

Beaumont's experiments included feeding St. Martin foods directly through the opening in his abdomen and then watching the process of digestion and timing how long it took. He noticed that if St. Martin became angry, his stomach lining became extremely red; there was a tremendous increase in blood supply and secretions in the stomach that were quite visible. If St. Martin became frightened, the stomach wall would blanch, as the blood flow left the stomach lining. So Beaumont was able to see the direct effects of stress and emotions on digestion.

THE STRESS RESPONSE

Research on stress in the 1930s provided additional insight into the interaction between stress and digestion. Studies by Hans Selye, who first named and defined the stress response, found that animals placed under prolonged stress developed physical conditions. Most often, the problems occurred in three primary areas:

- ◆ They developed multiple stomach ulcers.
- ◆ Their adrenal glands became enlarged—four or five times greater than normal—from the effort of producing the tremendous amounts of adrenaline to cope with the stress.
- ◆ The immune system atrophied; lymph nodes and lymph tissue in the gut became tremendously shrunken.

Selye noticed that those same three conditions occurred in both animals and humans whenever continuous stress was present. He decided they were characteristic of a prolonged stress response. Each of these dynamics is relevant to how well the digestive tract is functioning.

"FIGHT OR FLIGHT"

We now know that stress causes other changes in the body as well. During intense stress, the blood supply is shunted away from the digestive organs and into the large muscles, so you can fight or run for your life. This is usually termed the fight-or-flight response. Scientists suggest that this protective reaction evolved long ago among prehistoric people in response to the kind of intense life-threatening events hunters must have faced.

Imagine walking out of a cave and running into a saber-toothed tiger! An immediate response is triggered—fight or flight. The senses get very sharp, the heart rate and blood pressure go up, and blood goes into the large muscles so you can either fight for your life or run. This effort is orchestrated by your sympathetic nervous system. As part of this process, the blood flow is shunted away from the digestive tract, typically causing digestion and absorption to be less efficient until the stress response is over.

Half an hour later the event is over. After this supercharged period and intense response, you go into a relaxation phase, the opposite kind of response. Your muscles relax, your blood pressure comes down, and your heart rate decreases. All this happens through the action of the *para*sympathetic nervous system. The focus of the blood flow shifts from the muscles to the internal and digestive organs. This is a time when the body replenishes itself, rebuilds, replaces hormones, and repairs any injuries that may have been incurred. This is basically how researchers now understand the stress response.

STRESS IN MODERN TIMES

Modern people generally experience the stress response much less frequently than our prehistoric ancestors. In contrast, we experience a

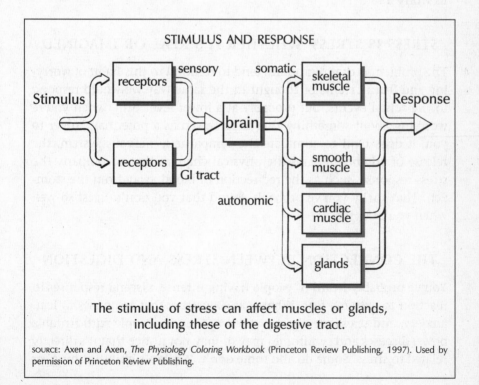

STIMULUS AND RESPONSE

The stimulus of stress can affect muscles or glands,
including these of the digestive tract.

SOURCE: Axen and Axen, *The Physiology Coloring Workbook* (Princeton Review Publishing, 1997). Used by permission of Princeton Review Publishing.

more subtle form of stress. In fact, researchers have identified these different kinds of stress as Type 1 and Type 2. Type 1 stress occurs when there's an easily definable source of stress, there may be a specific action that can be taken, and there's an accompanying physical reaction. Either you run away from the tiger, you kill the tiger, or the tiger eats you for lunch. But one way or another, in half an hour, it's all over, and then the body goes into a relaxation and repair phase. Most modern people don't experience much Type 1 stress, except for people in wartime combat situations.

What we suffer from in modern cultures is a kind of ongoing, multifaceted, vague sense of stress and worry. It's our response to the evening news and "How am I going to pay the bills?" and "Will there be social security when I get old?" and "What am I going to do with my aging parents?" and "What am I going to do if my kids get into drugs?" and on and on. You have these worries just as I do—we worry about high school shootings on the news, children dying from hunger overseas, and tragedies in our cities we feel powerless to prevent. There's a constant bombardment of bad news that sets in motion worrying and expectations of the worst. We all worry some, and some of us worry a lot.

STRESS IS STRESS, WHETHER IT'S REAL OR IMAGINED

The problem is that our bodies tend to respond to this habit of worrying and fearful trains of thought in the same way we would respond to the actual events, but probably at a lower level. Still, when you're worrying about something that is perceived as a potential danger to you, it does tend to stimulate the sympathetic nervous system, the release of adrenaline, and the physical changes that accompany the stress response, such as the redirection of blood away from the stomach. That's why you've probably found that you don't digest so well when you're upset.

THE CONNECTION BETWEEN STRESS AND DIGESTION

You've probably heard of people having intense, visceral responses in reaction to extreme fear. What that suggests is that responses to fear, anxiety, and stress are directly wired to the gut. People with irritable bowel diseases and syndromes may or may not notice that it's directly related to stress. Some do and some don't. While a significant number of people find that it's not the sole cause of their condition, it's probably one of the common triggers that tends to make most GI conditions worse. Stress seems to sensitize the GI tract to be more twitchy or crampy or to interfere with digestion in one way or another. So there's a real connection wired into our physiology and our nervous system, linking stress and digestive function. In fact, research has identified nerve fibers in the gut so extensive and complex, they sometimes call it the "gut brain."

This confirms our impression that stress responses and even emotions involve not only mental processes but a series of actual physical changes the body goes through. And many of these changes affect the functioning of the digestive tract, if only temporarily. So it's definitely worthwhile monitoring your own reactions to stress and tracking their effect on your health.

For some people, the digestive tract becomes the sensitized part of the body that functions as a kind of barometer, reflecting stress, worry, or anxiety. Whether we're anxious about a test, a job interview, or a date, we may find ourselves running to the bathroom. Not everybody has that response but it's pretty common—butterflies in the stomach, nervous diarrhea. For some people, the GI tract becomes their target organ and that's the way their body expresses excessive stress.

USING STRESS TO YOUR ADVANTAGE

You can learn to use those responses and read them, much as you would notice the oil light coming on in your car and take action to prevent problems. You can use your responses to identify the issues that cause you the most intense anxiety or worry—gut reactions. When emotional reactions affect your digestive system, you can use the same connections with your nervous and immune systems to call up the relaxation response. So if there are nerves that can make your gut feel irritable, crampy and spastic and upset, you can use these same mind-body connections to send messages to your digestive system that are soothing, relaxing, calming, and stress relieving. And that's something that you can consciously learn to do. Just as we all learn to worry, we can learn to relax.

THE RELAXATION RESPONSE

Learning some form of relaxation technique often has a beneficial effect on chronic digestive symptoms. Although these methods are deceptively simple, they can make a difference. Some people with digestive illness report that these are some of the most important things they do for their health.

 ◆ Simple breathing techniques
 ◆ Meditation
 ◆ The relaxation response (Herbert Benson)
 ◆ The body scan, which relaxes different parts of the body (Jon Kabat-Zinn)
 ◆ Imagery

Learning how to put your mind and body into a relaxed state allows the body to automatically go into that healing and repair mode. So the regular use of relaxation makes sense. Relaxation is a very direct thing that people can learn to do with a little practice.

When patients come in with conditions that seem to be made worse by stress, I encourage them to learn an effective relaxation technique and practice it diligently for a minimum of three weeks. I give them tapes that can help them learn to relax and provide information on relaxation classes. If they're having active symptoms and a really difficult problem, I suggest they set aside twenty to thirty minutes twice a day for relaxation, for a three-week trial period. Most of the people I see find that relaxation helps to relieve their symptoms. Some people find it's the most important thing they do. Others notice that it helps them feel better and relieves some of their symptoms, while they and their doctor investigate the other things that affect digestion (like hidden food allergies or undiagnosed infection).

How long does it typically take to integrate these practices? Often people get relief very quickly. But it's something that you *learn* to do. Accept that it will take a little time, just like anything that's worth doing. I usually ask people to practice a couple of times a day for three weeks. This introductory period provides a very good sense of whether or not this approach is helpful and just how helpful it can be. Knowing that it's a time-limited practice in the beginning gives people a chance to get involved and then decide for themselves, based on their own experience. These techniques are definitely worth exploring and have been used with measurable success in combating conditions as serious as cancer and leukemia.

THE INDIRECT EFFECTS OF STRESS

There's another aspect of the effects of stress on the gut—the indirect effects of stress. When people feel stressed beyond their capacity, they often find coping mechanisms that help to temporarily relieve the stress. Some of these temporary solutions may not be good for their digestion: for example, drinking too much alcohol; drinking too much coffee; overeating; eating junk food; smoking.

In our attempts to reduce stress and anxiety levels, we often indulge in habits that are more directly damaging to the digestive system. For example, someone who has digestive upsets from a yeast overgrowth will probably find he does better when he eats less sugar. When he's stressed, the cravings for sugar may be intense and the sugar seems to relieve the stress temporarily. In many cases, the wave

---

Using the Power of Imagery to Reduce Stress and Promote Healing

Alexandra was 30 years old, active and successful, but worried. She had developed signs of cancer. Several eminent physicians had diagnosed her condition as benign, but she worried that it was precancerous and wanted to know if she could do anything to make it go away.

Alexandra was intensely involved in every aspect of her life. She worked long hours, traveled frequently in her work, and kept a busy social schedule as well. She often felt tense and tired and wanted less stress in her life, though she saw that as a problem separate from her condition.

As part of our consultation, I asked her to relax and let an image of the cancer come to mind. She imagined it as rocks in a stream and was upset to see it was partially obstructing the flow. As she looked more closely, however, her perception of the rocks changed dramatically. She noticed that they were very smooth, shiny, and lustrous, and looked more like pearls than rocks. Alexandra immediately understood that, like pearls in an oyster, these nodules had formed in response to irritation and represented an attempt to protect her from further harm.

When I asked her what would need to happen for the pearls to be able to dissolve, she sensed a need to "remove the source of irritation." She made changes in her scheduling, her traveling, and her diet, and the nodules disappeared within a few months.

By paying attention to her problem in this way, Alexandra not only learned a valuable lesson in stress management but personally experienced the wisdom of her body and mind working together to maintain a healthy equilibrium. Her symptoms got her attention, and her use of imagery allowed her to understand both the meaning of her symptoms and what she needed to do to allow healing to proceed. In her case, the imagery didn't resolve her condition directly, but showed her what she could do to allow that to happen.

of uncomfortable symptoms that surface within a day make it clear that this is not the best solution.

Learning a more direct way to reduce the stress response can prevent self-damaging or self-sabotaging coping mechanisms that don't really work.

MARTIN ROSSMAN, **M.D.**, is founder and director of the Collaborative Medicine Center, as well as founder and co-director of the Academy for Guided Imagery. With David Bresler, Ph.D., he has defined and developed the therapeutic approach of Interactive Guided Imagery. He received his medical degree from the University of Michigan and is a diplomate of acupuncture. He serves as a faculty associate at the University of California at San Francisco, the California School of Professional Psychology, and John F. Kennedy University. Dr. Rossman is author of *Healing Yourself,* now in its second printing. He is an active contributor as board member or fellow of the Stanford Corporate Health Project and the Rosenthal Center for Complementary Medicine in New York. Dr. Rossman can be reached for telephone consultations through his office in Mill Valley, California, at 415-383-3197.

The Academy for Guided Imagery can be contacted at PO Box 2070, Mill Valley, CA 94942; phone 800-726-2070 or 415-389-9324; fax 415-389-9342.

11

Toxic Overload*

JEFFREY BLAND, Ph.D.

❖

The liver is a virtual chemical factory, a busy internal power plant with a central role in our metabolism. The hepatic system processes foods and liquids coming in from the digestive tract, transforms them into usable form, and breaks down the by-products. Vitamins, fats, proteins, and other nutrients are extracted and synthesized. Some nutrients are converted to stored energy. The liver is a major manufacturer and exporter, producing biochemicals such as bile and cholesterol for use by the body. It also handles toxic waste disposal and recycling by filtering out toxins from the blood. They're converted into harmless materials for disposal in stool and urine. The liver is the largest, most active organ in the body.

When we're in good health, the liver's processes work so efficiently we often don't even notice exposure to toxins—like a glass of wine or a little insecticide. When the liver is intact, we tend to be less troubled by allergies and we seem to tolerate most medications. This means our hepatic system is providing a marvelous protective screen between us and the outside world. But our liver can become overworked. It can eventually become overwhelmed by chemicals, metals, or other toxins from the environment.

THE GUT-LIVER CONNECTION

Toxins are also produced within the human GI tract. Some by-products occur from even the healthiest metabolism. These internally

*Portions of this chapter were adapted from *The 20 Day Rejuvenation Diet* by Jeffrey Bland, Ph.D. (New Canaan, CT: Keats, 1997). Used with the permission of NTC/Contemporary Publishing Group, Inc.

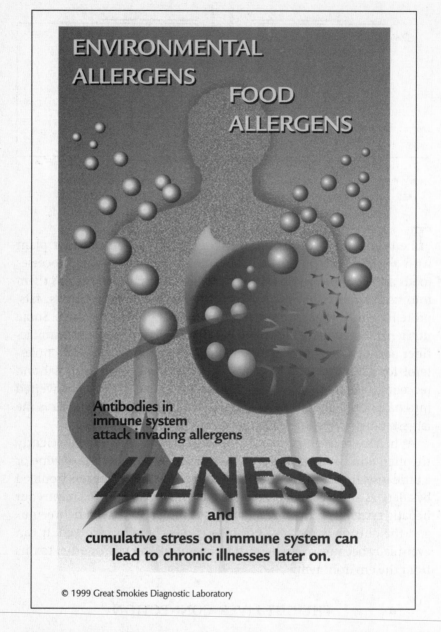

ENVIRONMENTAL
ALLERGENS
                  FOOD
                  ALLERGENS

**Antibodies in
immune system
attack invading allergens**

ILLNESS

and

**cumulative stress on immune system can
lead to chronic illnesses later on.**

produced toxins must all be processed by the liver. If food is poorly digested, it can produce ammonia, alcohol, and other chemicals in the body as a result of increased putrefaction.

The overgrowth of bacteria or yeast in the GI tract may create toxic overload that can stress detoxification. When overgrowth occurs, the

---

When the Liver Becomes Overwhelmed

❖

Jeff, a drummer in the rock group Toto, died mysteriously one August afternoon in 1992 after using an insecticide spray on the roses in the backyard of his home in Los Angeles. He was believed to have died of a heart attack brought on by an allergic response to the pesticide. The media later reported that this reaction had been aggravated by Jeff's regular use of drugs and alcohol. This type of response to toxins can occur if liver function is impaired. His death is an example of the tragedy that can occur when the liver's ability to detoxify is compromised.

---

liver may be less able to detoxify other incoming substances that would normally go unnoticed. The buildup of these toxins in the body can result in general toxicity or in specific illness. For example, research has found that an overgrowth of *E. coli* bacteria is frequently present in the stool of patients with food sensitivities or Crohn's disease.

The toxic by-products of bacteria and yeast are passed on to the liver for processing.

Metabolic toxins may account for some cases of food sensitivity. Research tends to bear this out. In addition, depressed levels of any particular liver enzyme would mean a less efficient job in breaking down certain foods.

Food sensitivity can be a cause of gastrointestinal illness. In large studies, food sensitivity has been linked to both irritable bowel syndrome (IBS) and Crohn's disease, which were effectively managed by the elimination diet. (See Chapter 20 on treating allergies.)

YOUR LIVER AS TOXIC WASTE RECYCLER

The liver breaks down toxins and renders them harmless through a series of complex chemical processes.

Phase 1

In the first step, called Phase 1 Detoxification, the liver activates a series of enzymes we will call CP-450.* When we are exposed to toxic

---

*CP-450 is short for cytochrome P450 mixed-function oxidases.

substances, the activities of these enzymes increase as part of the body's defense mechanism. Activities of other hepatic enzymes also increase. These enzymes are so vital to the body's processes, they're coded by at least 71 different genes.

The enzymes prepare toxic substances to be transformed into nontoxic form. Fat-soluble toxins are converted into more water-soluble substances that can be excreted in the urine or bile and discharged from the body. Typically the liver breaks down and re-forms chemicals that occur in the bloodstream, such as hormones, drugs, food additives, and metabolic by-products.

The result of Phase 1 is the production of a new class of compounds, intermediate chemicals. This intermediate state is just that— these compounds are meant to be converted again, in a second step, into a form the body can excrete. Intermediate compounds are often more toxic than the original substances, but they are intended for a second phase of processing.

Phase 2

In Phase 2 Detoxification, the intermediates undergo a second conversion, combining them with mineral compounds, amino acids, or other biochemicals that are water-soluble and can be excreted in urine and bile. This process of synthesis is described as conjugation. There are at least eleven different processes in Phase 2, and each requires the presence of specific nutrients and enzymes.

If the liver is unable to use the Phase 2 pathways, there will be a delay in the breakdown and processing of these toxic intermediates.

Intermediates can accumulate and begin to build up in the body as toxins. Again, they can be more harmful than the original toxins. This may occur when:

- ◆ We are ill and our liver happens to malfunction.
- ◆ The level of toxins is greater than the hepatic system can handle.
- ◆ We lack the nutrients necessary for the detoxification process.
- ◆ There is a chronic GI condition adding internally generated toxins to the liver's burden; this might result from conditions such as chronic constipation or leaky gut syndrome.

YOUR UNIQUE LIVER

Since the CP-450 enzymes are coded on at least 71 different genes, it's like having 71 possible sets of instructions. Given the many variations

---

An Enormous Variation in Liver Capacity, from Person to Person

❖

Medical studies indicate that there is a wide range in the liver's ability to break down toxins, even among apparently healthy people. I discovered the truth of this statement firsthand when I conducted a research study on liver capacity, by evaluating the liver detoxification function of members of my own company's staff. Since the people who work with me are well-informed about nutrition and keep healthy diets and lifestyle, I believed we would find little individual variation in their liver function.

I was astonished by the results. When the test challenge was administered (a small dose of caffeine), some people were able to clear the caffeine as quickly as thirty minutes—for others, it took as long as thirty *hours*. Although no one on staff had overt liver disease, there was more than a sixty-fold difference in Phase 1 ability among these normal individuals.

This tremendous variation in function probably explains why some people are so much more sensitive to their environment than others. In fact, we found that poor liver response in the testing paralleled the presence of health problems. The people on staff who had the slowest CP-450 detoxification were those with histories of allergy, asthma, and environmental sensitivity. On the other end of the continuum, those who had very active CP-450 function seemed to be the staff members who never got sick when they traveled internationally, could eat most anything, and had few health problems.

---

from person to person in the genetic markers for these liver enzymes, the potential for variation is great. When genetic instructions are expressed in any individual, enzyme activity can vary enormously. This is probably a major factor in the tremendous difference in the ability to detoxify and the speed and efficiency of liver function. This variation in the capacity to detoxify explains aspects of individual sensitivity to chemical substances, toxic exposure, alcohol, and medications.

Individual Capacity as the Basis for Individual Response

I am now convinced that people who have a poor detoxification system, for whatever reason, are much more vulnerable to their environment and to drugs, food, chemicals, intestinal infections, and the myriad of potentially toxic substances produced within the body. For example, because drugs are metabolized by the detoxification systems of the liver, differences in the capacity and speed of processing, probably explain the differing levels of sensitivity that show up as reactions to medication, or side effects.

ARE YOU A PATHOLOGICAL DETOXIFIER?

We found that liver function can be generalized into three categories:

◆ *Normal detoxifiers.* The first profile is seen in people who have relatively normal CP-450 activity and whose liver can break down and process chemicals and toxins without difficulty. These people are defined as normal detoxifiers and our studies show that about half the populations we've studied function normally.

◆ *Slow detoxifiers.* In the second most common category are people who have depressed CP-450 activity and excrete toxic by-products at a slow-to-normal rate. These are individuals we term slow detoxifiers, and they represent about one-third of the populations studied.

◆ *Pathological detoxifiers.* The last category is made up of people we describe as fast-slow detoxifiers, or pathological detoxifiers. They typically have rapid detoxification in the first stage due to increased enzyme activity. However, in the second phase, their ability to resynthesize toxins for disposal is delayed or depressed. This means that toxic by-products cannot be fully excreted or cleared as quickly as they should be. When this occurs, the toxic intermediates remain in the liver. We found that people with this profile have major adverse symptoms during the detoxification process, apparent from the toxicity of these by-products, which remain in their system too long.

We have also found that when liver enzyme activity is called on, cellular damage may result if the body is lacking essential nutrients. Important nutrients in detoxification include:

◆ *Phase 1:* the protective antioxidants such as vitamins A, C, and E, which cushion the cell against toxic by-products that can form when chemicals are broken down.

◆ *Phase 2:* nutrients such as amino acids and minerals the liver uses to reconstruct toxins and prepare them for secretion.

TESTING LIVER FUNCTION

Since functional capacity is highly individual, lab testing has been developed to evaluate the unique health status of each patient. The test results can provide the basis for personalizing a therapeutic program. This testing is one of the most valuable tools of functional medicine.

Traditionally, testing has been used to detect the presence of disease. Lab tests measure levels of biochemicals in body fluids as markers of disease. For example, a high blood sugar level indicates diabetes, and a high uric acid level is a sign of gout.

In contrast, functional testing looks at function. The goal is to detect malfunction before disease develops or damage occurs. This testing allows us to intervene earlier in the disease process, at a stage when problems are easier to reverse.

A specific functional test has been developed to assess liver capacity. The test is extremely valuable because it can identify problems with the liver earlier than traditional evaluations. In the standard liver test, enzymes are detected only when the liver has begun to break down and cell death is beginning to occur. In contrast, the functional liver evaluation measures the efficiency of liver function.

Many patients whose livers appear normal in a standard liver screen are found to have poor liver detoxification in a functional assessment. So the absence of disease does not necessarily mean the presence of healthy liver function. The loss of reserve capacity means the liver is functionally aging more rapidly than it should, losing resilience; this increases the risk of chronic health problems.

A functional liver test provides the information needed to develop a therapeutic nutritional program. This assessment can be particularly valuable, because liver function can be enhanced by providing the specific nutrients that may be lacking. Damaged tissue can also regenerate with the right nutritional support.

TREATING THE PATHOLOGICAL LIVER

To treat the fast-slow detoxifier profile without side effects, we first place people on a nutrition program to rebuild the liver system. The goal is to restore the liver's ability to perform Phase 2 detoxification. Key nutrients in restoring these functions include antioxidants; the amino acids glutathione, N-acetyl-cysteine, and L-cysteine; and trace minerals such as zinc, copper, and manganese. The burden on the liver is also reduced by decreasing fat in the diet and providing a better balance of protein, carbohydrate, and fat.

Functional testing can provide the physician with information to

Signs of Liver Overload

❖

Elizabeth's biopsy showed evidence of a fatty liver. She seems to have inherited this tendency and she's always liked the wrong foods. She's been plagued most of her life by an overweight condition that just hasn't responded to dieting. She also has diabetes and is troubled by constant fatigue. She was seen recently by a respected hepatologist who implied that until she is a liver-transplant candidate, there is little they can do. The specialist recommended trying water-soluble vitamin E, and although the vitamin has help a little, it hasn't really been enough.

Her condition is complicated by a severe candida infection throughout her GI tract and elsewhere in her body; this periodically causes her mental confusion and loss of concentration. Her detoxification process is so compromised it's impossible to give her medication for the candida. She had been treated with Glucophage to help her liver produce more insulin and stabilize her blood sugar, but her liver is now so toxic, she's been unable to tolerate the drug.

We immediately scheduled her for a liver detoxification profile so we could confirm where the breakdown was occurring in her liver's processing. We also began her on a nonallergenic rice powder supplement for one meal a day, which will provide her good nutritional support and enable her to start losing weight gradually.

With the information from the functional liver evaluation, we'll be able to tailor a program of specific nutrients and foods to help her liver begin to heal. Then she can start a weight loss reduction program with medication. She'll also be able to begin a medication that will reduce some of the excess fat in her liver (using a surprisingly effective drug called Urso developed from a Chinese remedy made from bear bile). At the same time, we'll continue to gradually detoxify her liver, decreasing the fat and restoring the capacity to detoxify. Without the ability to clear toxins, Elizabeth will find it hard to become truly well.

—Trent Nichols, M.D.

tailor an individualized nutritional program. Supplying the specific nutrients that are critical to the liver's processes can minimize damage to the body. An individualized nutrient program can improve both phases of liver function.

In many cases, we have found that this type of nutritional program can improve liver function in as little as one to three weeks. Periodic follow-up tests and exams give us the ability to tell if we're on track and how much progress is being made. Repeating the testing also provides feedback that helps us adjust the program as we go along.

NUTRIENTS THAT SUPPORT LIVER FUNCTION

Type of Nutrient	Specific Nutrient	Function
Antioxidants	Vitamins A, C, and E	Protection against damage as the toxins break down/Phase 1
Additional antioxidants	CoQ10, B_6, B_{12}, folic acid	Protective effects
Trace minerals	Copper, manganese, zinc, and molybdenum, selenium	Activity of glutathione pathway
Amino acids	Glycine (often from glutamine), arginine, ornithine, taurine	Phase 2 processing called conjugation
Supportive amino acids	NAC, cysteine, methionine	Phase 2 processing
Specific liver support	MSM (supplement containing sulfur) Glutathione	*For pathway using sulfur *Pathway using glutathione
Thioles	Found in garlic, onions, and cruciferous vegetables	Antioxidant protection
Herbs	Silymarin, ginkgo, green tea	Healing effects, antioxidants

*See your doctor to take the liver detoxification profile and learn the nutrients your body specifically needs.

MAJOR FACTORS IN LIVER FUNCTION

Liver capacity is one of the most individual functions in the body. There are so many pieces to the puzzle. Here's a review of some of the most important:

- ◆ *Heredity.* The vital liver enzymes are coded on 71 different genes.
- ◆ *Actual liver function.* In normal people, we found it can vary by sixty times.
- ◆ *Toxins from the digestive tract.* These are biochemicals from undigested food or toxic microbes.

◆ *Toxins from external sources.* These result from small exposures or intense incidents.

If you suspect that your liver is challenged by any of these factors, consider working with a physician trained in nutritional medicine. Basic lab testing is available to profile the efficiency of your body's detoxification, and identify where problems might be occurring. With that information, specific nutrients can be recommended by your doctor that will support the function and healing of the liver. If your condition is serious, you should not self-treat. The wrong choice of nutrient or herb could place a further burden on your system. Remember that your liver is one of the essential organs in the body, as necessary as your heart.

JEFFREY BLAND, PH.D., has been actively involved in nutrition-related research for twenty years and has served as director of the Bellevue-Redmond Medical Laboratory, professor of chemistry at the University of Puget Sound, and senior research scientist at the Linus Pauling Institute of Science and Medicine. Dr. Bland is the founder and CEO of HealthComm International, Inc., a leading research and development company in the field of functional medicine. He is the author of many widely read works on nutrition, including *Nutraerobics, Your Health Under Siege, Medical Applications of Clinical Nutrition,* and *The 20-Day Rejuvenation Diet Program* (Keats Publishing, Inc., 1997) and Genetic Nutritioneering (NTC Publishing Group, 1999).

HealthComm International provides information and training to health care professionals through publications and other media designed for busy practitioners, as well as regional workshops and yearly conferences on functional medicine. They can be reached at PO Box 1729, Gig Harbor, WA 98335; 800-843-9660 or www.healthcomm.com

---

12

Damage from Free Radicals*

JEFFREY BLAND, PH.D.

❖

The cascade of events that begins in the digestive tract and culminates in the liver can generate a particular kind of risk—reactive and destructive molecules called free radicals. If these dangerous reactions are not detoxified, they can ricochet through the cellular materials of the body. Oxygen-free radicals have the potential to affect the immune system and initiate heart disease, cancer, and genetic damage.

By identifying the presence of free radicals, we can work to prevent the diseases they might initiate. Preventive measures against free radical damage involve a commonsense lifestyle, with good nutrition in the bargain. These protections include eating a diet rich in fresh fruits and vegetables and good quality protein (vegetable or animal), then supplementing it with antioxidant nutrients and sufficient sleep.

OXYGEN AND OXIDATIVE STRESS

Free radicals are also described as oxygen-free radicals and originate as a series of oxygen compounds in the body. Oxygen is a paradox. It is absolutely essential to our life from minute to minute. Our bodies require oxygen for metabolism, for energy production, in aerobic processes that take place in every cell in the body. This happens in the tiny furnace of the cell called the mitochondria, which spin off energy. This energy-making activity provides the fuel for all the other activities of the body—digestion, cellular repair, immune function, the operation of the nervous system, reproduction, even the contraction of

*Portions of this chapter were adapted from *The 20 Day Rejuvenation Diet* by Jeffrey Bland, Ph.D. (New Canaan, CT: Keats, 1997). Used with the permission of NTC/Contemporary Publishing Group, Inc.

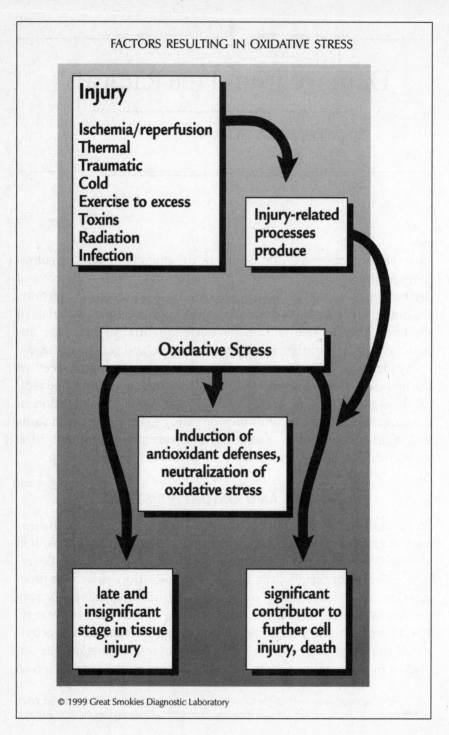

FACTORS RESULTING IN OXIDATIVE STRESS

Injury

Ischemia/reperfusion
Thermal
Traumatic
Cold
Exercise to excess
Toxins
Radiation
Infection

Injury-related processes produce

Oxidative Stress

Induction of antioxidant defenses, neutralization of oxidative stress

late and insignificant stage in tissue injury

significant contributor to further cell injury, death

A Story with a Happy Ending

❖

At 36, Michael is successful and prosperous, a self-made entrepreneur. What isn't visible is his struggle with constant low-grade pain since adolescence, from fibromyalgia. He also suffers from chronic fatigue so serious it leaves him little energy for much of a personal life. He has just enough energy to manage the thriving business he's developed, but nothing more. Michael is limited from a rich life by his ever-present health problems. What's worse is that his condition continues to become gradually worse.

Michael's case was so complex that we scheduled a series of functional tests to evaluate the issues. His pancreatic enzymes were low, which meant that he wasn't fully digesting his food. His pH reading indicated that his body was too acidic. A test indicator of inflammation in the colon was high (elevated alpha-antichymotrypsin), suggesting a possible irritation or infection.

Initial stool testing reflected the presence of the yeast *Candida albicans*, which raised our suspicion of other pathogens in the digestive tract. We scheduled another test that evaluated chemical markers to identify pathogenic microbes. This test for organic acids found signs of the bacteria *Clostridium difficile* and the parasite *Giardia lamblia*, and confirmed the candida. The first part of the treatment protocol we designed for Michael was aimed at settling down his GI tract, and within ten days this began producing the first significant improvement he has experienced in more than fifteen years.

Given the presence of so much possible inflammation, we also scheduled tests for oxidative stress, such as a measure of LDL, probably one of the best indicators of cardiovascular risk. This test reflects levels of oxidative stress, and his levels were very high. We know that large amounts of antioxidants, especially vitamin E, will be required to bring these levels down into a safe range. Consider that this is a very active person in his mid thirties, with an extremely good diet, and yet he still is showing a significantly high marker for oxidative stress. A logical question to ask would be "What is occurring to cause oxidative stress in someone this young, particularly since he has a good diet?"

We believe the answer may be found in his intestinal infections, leaky gut syndrome, and liver stress. In response to the toxic overload, his liver appears to be producing high levels of free radicals. We also found cellular DNA adducts, which measure the amount of potential DNA damage that may be resulting, an issue related to oxidative stress. His levels were unusually high. However, when we measured his T cell activity we found the levels to be low.

This combination of immune suppression (low T cell count) but high levels of oxidative stress place him at risk for more serious illness. Fortunately, he may be able to prevent potential problems, before there are signs of any form of degenerative disease. The goal is to lower his oxidative stress by clearing problems in the GI tract and to increase protective factors by working with his nutrition, diet, and lifestyle.

—*Jerry Stine, Nutritional Consultant*

our muscles. Oxygen is essential to the energy production that runs all these processes and numerous others.

The Dangerous Side of Oxygen

However, oxygen has a dark side. It can be a reactive chemical substance, and in certain forms can cause harm to the body. We know that combining oxygen with iron produces rust and eventually causes the breakdown of objects made of iron. In much the same way, certain forms of oxygen can combine with the biological materials of the body, causing them to deteriorate.

Although our bodies don't rust, they are subject to damage from a subtle form of stress from the effects of oxygen, called oxidative stress. Oxygen can cause harm by breaking down cells and tissues such as fats, structural proteins, enzymes, and genetic material (DNA). Fats can become rancid, cell walls can become brittle, and enzymes no longer work. Genetic blueprints are damaged or lost. Since the DNA is the master plan for repairing and rebuilding the body, this is like losing part of the instruction manual for the system. The breaking down of all these processes accelerates any potential for heart disease, cancer, hardening of the arteries, and Alzheimer's disease.

Oxidative Stress as the By-product of Fighting Infection

Activated forms of oxygen are released by white blood cells as one of our immune defenses against microbes to poison or "bleach" pathogens and destroy them. The "bleach" secreted by white blood cells is just like the bleach you use to brighten your clothes. Called hypochlorite, it is chemically converted in our bodies into activated forms of oxygen (superoxide, hydroxyl radical, and hydrogen peroxide), all potentially harmful. The forms of oxygen most likely to damage tissues and cells are called oxygen radicals or free radicals. Internal processes that stimulate free radical production include infection by viruses, bacteria, and other pathogens, or overstimulation of the immune response. This is a case in which the solution to one problem leads to another, the creation of oxidants. There are numerous other stressors that generate free radical production as well.

The Explosive Chain Reaction of Free Radicals

To understand the intense and random action of free radicals in the tissue, imagine a Ping-Pong table covered with mousetraps. All the traps are set, baited with carefully placed Ping-Pong balls. Then imagine tossing another ball onto the table. As that ball springs a trap, it bounces and begins a reaction that triggers a nearby trap, and then the next and the next. Eventually, all the mousetraps on the table have been impacted, with balls bouncing in all directions. This is similar to the chemical reactions initiated by free radicals.

Oxygen-free radicals are equally erratic. Since their chemical structure is unstable, the free radical molecules can destabilize other molecules on contact. Because free radicals have an unpaired electron, as they make contact with other cellular molecules, they rob the electron from the second molecule. When that occurs, it turns the second, stable molecule into an unstable free radical, which now has the unpaired electron. At this point, the original free radical has stabilized. This destabilizing process continues to move through the body from cell to cell, until it is slowed or stopped by making contact with the body's own antioxidant defense system.

Why Free Radicals Matter

If these dangerous reactions are not detoxified, they can damage cell walls, the cells' ability to produce energy, and genetic material, the DNA. They oxidize the cell wall by making the fat in the membrane rancid, changing it so that it becomes brittle like rubber or plastic overexposed to sunlight. If many cells are damaged, this creates the potential for disease. In the engine of the cell (the mitochondria), free radicals can deplete protective enzymes, decreasing their ability to produce energy. The overall effect on the body could be symptoms of chronic fatigue. When our genetic material (DNA) is damaged, it may become unable to replicate. This means the inability to make new cells, which blocks repair efforts in that particular tissue. All these effects can result in a progressive loss of functioning and increased biological aging, by affecting the health of the individual cells.

Free Radical By-products in the Liver

There is tremendous potential for free radical damage in the liver. In the first phase of detoxification, some of the toxic load is converted into substances that have free radical activity and are potentially cancer-promoting as well. As long as the second phase of detoxification can quickly metabolize this load of free radicals and carcinogens, there is no problem. Then the transformed, inert by-products are simply secreted into the bile, pass into the stool, and are excreted from the body.

However, when the reserve capacity of this second phase is exhausted, the liver can no longer buffer the body against free radicals and carcinogens. Then they may overflow and cause damage locally or leak into the general circulation, where they can create profound biochemical damage in distant parts of the body.

Oxidative Stress Can Occur Anywhere in the Body

Wherever and whenever oxygen is being used by the tissue in metabolism, there is the potential for oxidative stress. This means that without adequate antioxidant protection, damage can occur to muscles, blood vessels, lungs, kidneys, brain, joints, and any other tissue. In bone, this effect can take place as part of the process of osteoporosis.

THE MOLECULAR BOMB SQUAD

Smog	Radiation
Tobacco/Smoke	Alcohol
Medications	Pesticides
White Cell Activity	Aging

FREE RADICAL GENERATION

THE CAUSES OF FREE RADICALS

Major stressors can stimulate the development of free radicals in the body:

- ◆ Environmental exposure from air pollution, radiation, extreme cold
- ◆ Toxins and chemicals
- ◆ Physical trauma, exercise to excess, infection
- ◆ Sustained or chronic psychological stress
- ◆ Responses to stress: consuming alcohol, sleep-inducing medications, muscle-relaxing drugs, anti-anxiety medication, higher intake of fat and protein, smoking
- ◆ Biological aging

The function of your metabolism can be altered by these types of stressors. During these periods of altered metabolism, a person may suffer from oxidative stress and the body may produce more damaging forms of oxygen. The increased oxidative stress can cause chronic health problems, unless high enough levels of antioxidants are available. In times of high oxidative stress, pay particular attention to your nutrition. Make sure you don't do without food or eat a low-nutrient diet. That means avoiding fasting, dieting, or eating junk food at times when you're under high stress. Be careful if you have any of the other stressors that can trigger the explosive action of the free radicals in your body.

Essentially, when the body is producing excessively high levels of oxygen-free radicals, it is in the process of breaking itself down. The more toxic the burden and the greater the psychological and physical stress, the more potential there is for damage from free radicals. Free radicals can cause the breakdown of cell walls, protein, and even genetic material.

HOW TOXINS CAN CAUSE OXIDATIVE STRESS

Alcohol, pesticides, drugs and medications, and other chemical compounds must all be detoxified, causing increased oxidative stress on the liver and putting more demand on the antioxidant system. Even strenuous exercise can cause these effects.

Free Radicals from Chemical Exposure

Oxygen radicals are manufactured in the body following most kinds of exposure to chemicals and toxins, as well as by-products of our metabolism. Chemicals capable of generating free radicals include medications, drugs, alcohol, cigarettes, pollutants, pesticides, industrial chemicals, and heavy metals.

The Effects of Alcohol

We know that oxidative stress can come from exposure to various chemicals. Alcohol is an example. When our bodies metabolize alcohol, it results in the production of two major free radicals, super oxide and hydroxyl radicals. These biochemicals can damage the liver directly, and they can also deplete the liver of antioxidants (such as glutathione). This is what occurs in the development of cirrhosis. The damage done to the liver by long-term excess alcohol intake is not direct, but the result of oxygen-free radicals that have not been fully buffered by antioxidants.

Alcohol is metabolized in the liver by a specific family of enzymes (CP-450) that act as chemical catalysts. High alcohol intake can have a number of effects: it can deplete the enzymes and the nutrients essential to break down toxic chemicals. Without the enzymes and the protective antioxidants, oxidative damage can occur to the liver and the nervous system and eventually throughout the body.

The Effects of Pesticides

Toxic chemicals such as pesticides can also increase our level of oxidative stress. Research indicates that exposure to an organo-chlorine pesticide such as lindane increases the activity of the detoxifying enzyme system in the liver and accelerates the production of oxygen-free radicals. This can cause increased demand on the antioxidant enzyme systems of the liver. Like alcohol, lindane exposure can deplete glutathione, a principal detoxifying nutrient involved in the trapping of oxygen-free radicals in the liver.

The Effects of Exercise

If antioxidant nutrients are low in the body, even beneficial activities such as exercise can cause oxidative damage, especially exercise for extended periods or under extreme conditions. When we exercise, more free radicals are created. If we're not protected by antioxidants, these reactive forms of oxygen can cause damage. This explains some of the damage people suffer after intense exercise, such as a marathon runner who is poorly nourished or hasn't trained properly. During the race, oxidative damage to muscles can cause a buildup of toxins that can result in tissue injury which may take days or weeks to repair.

THE PROTECTIVE EFFECTS OF ANTIOXIDANTS

Promoting Stamina

A remarkable study of elite mountain climbers in the Himalayas provides new insight into the protective effects of antioxidants. During a climb of Annapurna, one of the highest mountains in the world, professional climbers were evaluated for levels of vitamins C and E and the effects on their performance.

The athletes were climbing at altitudes above 20,000 feet without oxygen, under extreme conditions. Some climbers received vitamin E supplements of 200 milligrams twice a day for four weeks, while others received a placebo of no nutritive value. The study confirmed that antioxidants have an important protective effect. Climbers who received supplemental vitamin E were able to engage in strenuous physical activity for longer periods of time without damage, apparently because they had much better resistance to oxidative stress during the climb.

Minimizing the Effects of Aging

In another study of antioxidants and the effects of exercise, vitamin E was shown to minimize age differences. Male volunteers ranging from 22 to 74 years old were tested for muscle trauma by running downhill on an inclined treadmill. The performance of volunteers who received daily supplements of vitamin E, two 400 IU capsules, were compared with those who received a placebo. The researchers concluded that supplementing with vitamin E tends to eliminate age differences. This suggests that poor response to exercise among older people may in part be affected by their nutritional status.

Knowing that modest antioxidant supplements can protect athletes under extreme conditions, plan your own program of protective nutrients and lifestyle habits. To defend against oxidative stress after exposure, the liver requires enhanced levels of fresh vegetables and fruits, antioxidant vitamins A, C, and E, amino acids from high quality protein (both vegetable and animal sources), and sufficient sleep with all its healing benefits.

REDUCE THE FREE RADICAL STRESS IN YOUR LIFESTYLE

♦ *Don't tolerate low-grade GI problems that are generating internal free radicals*. See a doctor. Get it fixed.

♦ *Get enough rest and sleep*.

♦ *Don't smoke*. When you want to quit, seek medical assistance and use a method with a proven track record such as some of the patches. It takes a while to actually clear the addictive cravings from the body, but it's worth doing. Research shows that after several years of not smoking, your risk will be about as low as someone who never smoked.

♦ *Avoid toxic exposure,* including secondhand smoke. There are 100 trillion free radicals in each puff of cigarette smoke.

♦ *Minimize indoor air pollution.*

♦ *If you work with toxic chemicals, protect yourself.* Avoid putting yourself at risk—it's not worth it in the end.

♦ *Get exercise,* and make sure you have sufficient antioxidant protection. Train intelligently.

♦ *Avoid eating refined and processed foods.*

♦ *Avoid rancid oils.* Use only fresh and highest quality vegetable oils. Discard them every six weeks regardless.

♦ *Minimize alcohol consumption.* Alcohol is now known to be a genetic and biochemical problem. If you drink heavily, get medical help from a nutritionally oriented program. (See Joan Mathew Larson's book *Seven Weeks to Sobriety,* Fawcett Columbine, 1997.)

ANTIOXIDANTS ARE YOUR BEST PROTECTION

♦ Eat fresh fruits and vegetables because they're good natural sources of antioxidants. Use organic produce whenever possible.

♦ Vitamin A, C, E, and Coenzyme Q10, and the bioflavinoids such as quercetin can provide basic antioxidant protection.

♦ Also include B complex vitamins, especially B_2.

♦ Include the subtle benefits of trace minerals such as manganese, copper, zinc, and selenium, and especially the sulfur-based supplement MSM (methyl-sulfonyl-methane).

♦ Consider the benefits of specific herbs such as ginkgo biloba, the pycnogenols such as pine bark extract or grape seed extract, silymarin, green tea, and alpha lipoic acid.

♦ Work with a nutritionally oriented physician to be tested for your levels of these vital nutrients. Your doctor can have you retested periodically to be sure you are maintaining protective levels of antioxidants.

13

How Problems with Digestion Can Cause Illness Anywhere in the Body

JEFFRY ANDERSON, M.D.

If you have digestive illness, whether it's severe or mild, it's important to know that there are new treatments available. Decades of research have resulted in new understandings of how the body works. In the New Medicine, this expanded understanding is applied to treatment through the strategic use of nutrition, nutrients, and herbal medicine, often in combination with drug therapy.

New information on the dynamics of the body make it clear that conditions in the digestive tract affect the entire system. Folk wisdom reflects this interconnectedness: "Constipation is the mother of all ills" is the saying in India. In other cultures, it is said: "Death begins in the colon."

Recent research suggests that degradation of the gastrointestinal environment is one of the primary points at which health is lost. What we now know is that the same toxins associated with GI dysfunction are frequently absorbed and distributed to other parts of the body. First they place a burden on the liver and the immune system. If liver overload occurs, there will be spillover, and some of the toxins will be passed on to other organs or tissues.

Often it's the weak link in the system that will be hit by the damage—an organ anywhere in the body that is the most vulnerable. The vulnerability may be inherited, caused by physical injury, toxic exposure, or poor diet. If the sensitive system is the lungs, toxins that originate in the gut and circulate in the bloodstream may manifest as asthma or allergies. Sooner or later, this toxic overload comes to the attention of the immune system.

♦ Circulating toxins can turn on a hyperactive immune response, leading to allergies or inflammation with their associated pain and swelling.

◆ Toxins can short-circuit the immune response, resulting in infection.

At this point, corrosive toxic free radicals are released. Hopefully there are enough antioxidant nutrients to protect the cells and key cellular structures, such as the cell wall and the energy-producing "battery" of the cell, the mitochondria.

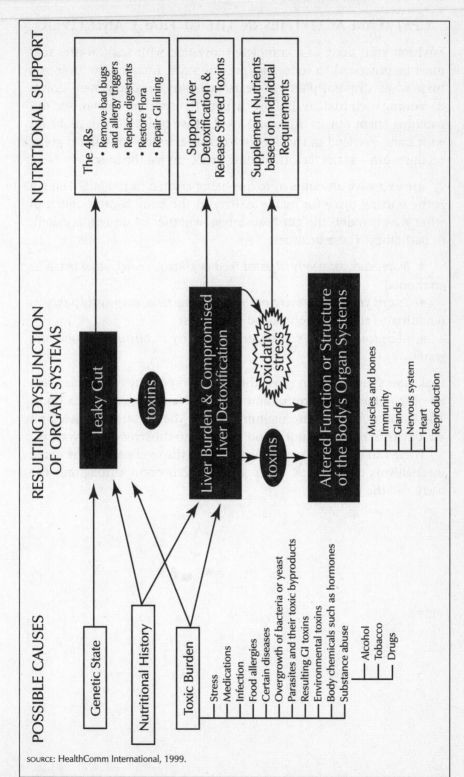

POSSIBLE CAUSES

RESULTING DYSFUNCTION
OF ORGAN SYSTEMS

NUTRITIONAL SUPPORT

Genetic State

Nutritional History

Toxic Burden
- Stress
- Medications
- Infection
- Food allergies
- Certain diseases
- Overgrowth of bacteria or yeast
- Parasites and their toxic byproducts
- Resulting GI toxins
- Environmental toxins
- Body chemicals such as hormones
- Substance abuse
  - Alcohol
  - Tobacco
  - Drugs

Leaky Gut

toxins

Liver Burden & Compromised
Liver Detoxification

toxins

oxidative stress

Altered Function or Structure
of the Body's Organ Systems
- Muscles and bones
- Immunity
- Glands
- Nervous system
- Heart
- Reproduction

The 4Rs
- Remove bad bugs
  and allergy triggers
- Replace digestants
- Restore Flora
- Repair GI lining

Support Liver
Detoxification &
Release Stored Toxins

Supplement Nutrients
based on Individual
Requirements

SOURCE: HealthComm International, 1999.

UPSTREAM ACTIVITIES IN THE GI TRACT AND LIVER

Envision your body as a complete ecosystem with toxic wastes that must be processed to restore its pristine state. Imagine the liver as a toxic waste disposal plant. It clears toxins by breaking them down, decreasing their toxicity, linking them to transport molecules, and dispatching them out in urine and stool. If we begin having problems with toxic overload in the liver, it's essential to look at what is going on upstream—at the factors creating problems for the liver.

Are excessive amounts of toxins being created in the gut? The gut is the starting place for major toxicity in the body because much of what goes through the gut is absorbed, whether by design, accident, or pathology. These include:

♦ *By-products of poorly digested food or chronic constipation* (such as ammonia)
♦ *Toxins produced by overgrowth of yeast, bacteria, or invasive parasites* (endotoxins such as alcohols and aldehydes)
♦ *Chemical pollutants, pesticides, and heavy metals* in our food and water

Leaky gut syndrome can cause the absorption of any of this material, all of it potentially harmful and intended for disposal by the body. The by-products of these malfunctions in the gut are all passed on directly through the major blood vessels into the liver portal system.

There can be health consequences from the overload on the detox mechanisms of the liver. Toxic spillover can occur throughout the body and the system.

DOWNSTREAM EFFECTS FROM TOXIC OVERLOAD

A bottleneck effect can occur if the liver is overburdened because of chronic or persistent toxicity beyond the capacity of the detoxification pathways to handle. The liver detox machinery may become stressed and compromised. It's trying to do its job, but the process may be creating even more free radicals and even more toxic intermediate chemicals.

Here are the events in the liver that can result from overload:

- Increased oxidative stress from the liver's detoxification process
- Impaired carbohydrate metabolism
- Increased immune activity and the production of biochemicals that promote inflammation
- Failure of Phase 1 Detoxification or accelerated Phase 1, which can cause increased production of free radicals
- The bottleneck effect if Phase 2 Detoxification is slow

Effects on the cells and tissues:

- The body needs to put these toxic chemicals somewhere.
- If the system can't excrete them, it will store them.
- Chemicals and pesticides will typically be stored in fat.
- Heavy metals will be stored in protein tissue—in muscles, bones, and cartilage.

Eventually some of these toxins are re-released and then stored again. When they are released, they eventually go to the liver, and the liver has to cope with them again. The liver either detoxifies them or recirculates them. If this occurs, it may cause more damage as they move through the system and then get redeposited.

The increasing accumulation of toxins can cause cellular damage. It is critical that you begin detoxifying by starting with first things first, which is the gut.

POSSIBLE CAUSES

Genetic Heritage
Nutritional History
Lifestyle Factors
Toxic Burden

- *By-products of poor digestion*
- *Impaired nutritional status*
- *Poor absorption*
- *Overgrowth of yeast or bacteria*
- *Parasitic infection*
- *Food allergies*
- *Stress*
- *Inflammatory conditions*
- *Degenerative diseases*
- *Medications*
- *General infections*
- *Contaminants in food and water*
- *Environmental toxins*

SYMPTOMS THAT CAN RESULT

◆ Widespread chronic fatigue or weakness from compromised energy production, even in the energy-producing unit of the cells (the mitochondria)

◆ Compromise of the immune system, less resistance to infection, autoimmune disorders, allergies, sensitivities, colds and flu, bronchitis, sinus infections, chemical sensitivity

◆ Problems in the muscles and joints from aches and swelling to pain or arthritis

◆ Skin disorders, including acne, dermatitis, eczema, psoriasis, and urticaria

◆ Consequences to the central nervous system and brain function: mild problems including difficulty with concentration and memory, coordination, headaches or migraines, attention deficit disorder, and in severe cases, symptoms that resemble autism

◆ Circulation of chemical toxins, causing more serious neurological symptoms ranging from seizure disorders to damage of the nervous system

◆ Decrease in hormone production caused by toxins in the body

◆ Liver damage, with compromised detox functions, possible hypoglycemia, and mood swings

◆ Specific conditions such as arthritis, asthma, or allergies that can result from the constant circulation of toxins. This can be due to toxins that compromise the immune system, causing inflammation or aggravating existing conditions. The toxins stimulate the release of an immune response with biochemicals that can set in motion a full-blown reaction.

The presence of conditions caused by the leaky gut syndrome indicate that toxins have been released from the GI tract and are out in general circulation. Then degenerative diseases such as cancer or autoimmune conditions can eventually develop.

STRATEGIES TO CLEAR THE BODY

When we talk about strategies, we mean cleansing and supporting the GI tract, the liver, and the entire system.

◆ First you detox the GI tract.

◆ Then get the liver detox systems working.

◆ And finally clean up the downstream consequences, which are toxins in the tissues and cells.

So cleaning up the gut is the starting point.

◆ Make sure that you are not constipated.

◆ That you're digesting everything thoroughly so you don't have putrefaction.

◆ Clean house. Get rid of bad bugs. Be sure you don't have toxins from an overgrowth of yeast or bacteria or some invasive parasite.

◆ Put in the good flora.

Then you can start addressing the liver detox issues.

The point is that you can't deal with the downstream conditions until you've treated the upstream problem in the gut and liver. For people with a highly toxic system, it is necessary to address the liver as well as the gut simultaneously. If you start mobilizing heavy metals and chemicals out of the tissue, unless you have dealt with the liver first, then you're just putting more demand on it.

In order for you to be more fully healthy, these concerns need to be addressed in the digestive tract, throughout your entire system, and as symptoms elsewhere in the body.

Doctors observe that some of these conditions resolve naturally as a result of clearing the GI tract and liver. When you clean up the upstream issues and the liver, then the downstream consequences tend to just go away. At that point, stored toxins can also be detoxed from the tissues and cells.

If you have any of these concerns, we recommend that you seek a qualified, compassionate health care professional who is familiar with detoxification concepts and work with him or her on resolving your digestive issues.

Part II
NEW TOOLS TO EVALUATE YOUR HEALTH

14

Testing to Rule Out Disease

TRENT NICHOLS, M.D.

❖

Testing to rule out disease is a sensible way to evaluate a health problem. If a condition is chronic or long-standing, even if the symptoms are mild, it's important to make sure there is no major underlying condition or pathology. This means ruling out a tumor or a structural problem that could be causing illness.

Of course, the more exact the diagnosis, the more focused the treatment. Developing an accurate diagnosis involves a kind of systematic "detective work" on the part of the doctor and the patient. In many cases, more than one test is necessary, to define the problem as exactly as possible.

Diagnosis is essential. When a major condition exists, treatment can't really proceed without a diagnosis. Once the problem is located and defined, treatment can be selected and begun.

BARIUM SWALLOW X-RAY FOR THE UPPER GI

While this is not the most comfortable test in the world, it is a relatively low cost basic test for any kind of gross abnormality in the digestive tract, including disorders of the esophagus, hiatal hernias, and tumors.

In this test, the patient drinks a solution that produces an image when X-rayed. A series of X-rays are taken that allow a view of the digestive tract from the mouth to the small intestine. The X-ray is read during the test by a technician and reviewed later by a radiologist and the physician. This test is useful for identifying anatomical and motility problems. It can also detect gastric or peptic ulcers. In some versions of this test, a fizzy tablet is also taken, which helps produce a clearer x-ray by providing air contrast in the image. Glucagon, an anti-motility hormone, may also be taken in conjunction with the test. Although this test can be quite uncomfortable, it typically lasts less than half an hour.

BARIUM ENEMA FOR THE LOWER GI

This is an X-ray that involves an enema procedure. This rather uncom-fortable test involves the slow injection of a highly pressurized enema into a cleaned-out colon to examine the area from rectum to the lower end of the small intestine. It is used to rule out ulcerative colitis, tu-mors (both benign and cancerous), diverticulosis, strictures, and mis-shapen, prolapsed colons (often the result of many years of poor diet and constipation). Before and after these tests, cleansing the digestive tract is important. Initially, a purge solution is taken (GoLYTELY or CoLYTE); following the test, patients are encouraged to drink a lot of water and take an antioxidant supplement to counter some of the ef-fects of the radiation exposure.

ENDOSCOPY

Endoscopy is the gold standard of GI testing because it allows a direct look at the digestive tract, providing a view of the condition of tissues and structures. Upper endoscopes, colonoscopes, and sigmoidoscopes are performed to view various areas of the gastrointestinal system.

Upper endoscopy is performed using a flexible fiber-optic tube, which may include a videoscope (a video chip on the tip). The tube is inserted through the mouth to view the esophagus, stomach, and py-loric area, as well as the first portion of the small intestine (the duode-num). The colonoscope is inserted through the anus and travels around the colon into the small intestine. The sigmoidoscope is a flexible instrument used to assess the rectum, the sigmoid (segment of the colon), and the descending colon.

All the major GI conditions discussed in this book can be evaluated to some degree through the use of endoscopy or barium swallows. The scopes are used to search out inflammation, polyps, tumors, diverticu-litis or diverticulosis, strictures, a dilated colon, or ulcers. One obvious advantage of the scopes for testing is the total avoidance of any expo-sure to X-ray radiation. Biopsies or even complete polyp removal can be performed using these instruments, often avoiding more invasive surgery. The procedures are typically performed under conscious sedation from which patients generally recover within about an hour.

ENDOSCOPIC ULTRASOUND

This instrument is an endoscope with an ultrasound transmitter on the tip that provides information through the use of sound waves, producing data that is read by specialized technicians. This type of endoscope can be used on the esophagus, stomach, colon, or rectum. The information gained from this test gives us an idea of the thickness of the muscle in the wall of an organ and whether there are any defects present. The ultrasound device can define the extent of a polyp invasion or show tumors in the muscle wall and indicate their size. If treatment is necessary, this information can help the physician plan a surgical resection or radiation therapy. The rectal ultrasound can be used to define problems in the pelvic floor for conditions such as fecal incontinence, constipation, and pelvic pain. This is particularly important in patients who have had unsuccessful surgery for urinary or fecal incontinence or multiple obstetric or gynecological surgeries.

CT SCANNING AND MRIs

These sophisticated imaging techniques, frequently used by doctors today, have now become highly perfected and refined. The MRI is based on a signal from a large magnet that interprets the density of tissue to create X-ray-like images. The CT scan utilizes multiple X-ray beams at different levels, interpreted by a computer to give cross-sectional images. The information gained from these procedures now often replaces exploratory surgery.

Both techniques rely on obtaining cross-sectional images of the anatomy that create a series of sequential images of the patient being X-rayed. The image produced provides detailed information that enables physicians to find problems that could not be detected by normal two-dimensional X-rays such as barium enemas or barium swallows.

To be evaluated, the patient lies in a tunnel-like chamber while the test is being performed. The open MRI, a newer design, doesn't require lying in a closed chamber. Basically, the MRI measures the spin of your atoms in a very sophisticated procedure that requires no radiation.

The information is generated through a signal from a large magnet that changes proton spin.

In an evaluation of the digestive tract, the MRI is sometimes limited because it's much more sensitive to movement. For images of the abdomen, CT scanning is often still better because the peristalsis of the bowel creates constant motion that can blur the image. While it takes longer to do an MRI than a CT scan, the MRI is useful in areas of the body where there is little movement, such as the liver. Consequently, the MRI is probably the test of choice for the liver because it's able to give a little more definition. One of the problems with the CT scan is that metallic objects can distort the image. For instance, surgical staples give off artifacts, an image caused by reflection on the metal, that can blur a portion of the X-ray.

LAPAROSCOPY

This procedure uses a surgical instrument that functions like a telescope, about the thickness of a Magic Marker, inserted in a small port incision in the abdomen. When diagnostic laparoscopy is performed, the abdominal cavity is first filled with air or carbon dioxide to create a space in which the organs can be visualized. Surgery can be performed using this same method, through the use of more than one port. With this technique, surgeons are able to perform fairly sophisticated surgeries without an incision, such as the removal of a portion of the colon (resection). Laparoscopy can also be used surgically in the treatment of ulcerative colitis and in the removal of colon tumors. The use of this instrument eliminates the necessity of large incisions in the abdominal wall, promoting more rapid healing.

Laparoscopy can allow the surgeon to gently shift organs within the abdominal cavity through the use of probes. This technique can be used to move, manipulate, or remove tissue. In abdominal surgery, binding scar tissue (adhesions) that may be causing pain and interfering with intestinal motility can be freed using this technique. In gallbladder surgery, an instrument can be inserted to move the liver and remove the gallbladder.

In fact, laparoscopy is now widely used by general surgeons for gallbladder removal. The apparent ease with which this procedure can be performed and the promise of quick recovery may be contributing to its overuse. If you are advised to have your gallbladder removed, seek a second opinion from a gastroenterologist. In some cases, what has been diagnosed as delayed gallbladder emptying turns out to be irritable bowel syndrome (IBS). In these situations, removal of the gallbladder will not fundamentally correct the condition.

TESTING FOR MOTILITY

The esophageal motility test is used for patients who have trouble swallowing (dysphagia) or frequent heartburn. Patients swallow a small nasogastric tube that measures the pressure at various points in the length of the esophagus.

Another test for motility is called colonic transit time. We use this test most often for patients who are troubled by constipation. The test can be performed by having the patient swallow a number of radiopaque rings in a gelatin capsule. The markers contain a material comparable to barium that creates an image visible on X-rays. The patient is then X-rayed for several consecutive days, depending on the protocol being used. The test is usually performed until all the markers are passed. The pellets go right through the digestive tract; they're not absorbed. The length of time it takes for them to move through the gut can reflect problems with colonic inertia, in which the colon has difficulty moving the stool along. If the test shows that the rings remain in the system for five or seven days, this will indicate a slowing of motility, an outlet disorder, or a generalized condition, depending on where the markers are seen. This test can also be used to measure transit time.

MEASURING HYDROCHLORIC ACID AND BICARBONATE

Doctors now measure hydrochloric acid using an endoscope to draw a sample of gastric juices from the stomach and measure the degree of alkalinity or acidity. Another way to perform this test is to use gastrin to stimulate acid secretions and then measure the response.

The test for gastric acid stimulation is most frequently used to detect hyperacidity, which is problematic in cases of *H. pylori* infections. Hyperacidity can cause ulcers or suggest the presence of gastronoma, a pancreatic tumor that causes the secretion of too much gastrin (a neurohormone secreted by the stomach) as a result of hyperacidity. In this test, pentagastrin (a synthetic gastrin) is given by injection and the acid is measured through a nasogastric tube.

In the use of the Heidelberg capsule, the patient swallows a capsule that sends back data via radiotelemetry reflecting the relative acid or alkalinity of different areas in the lumen. The information on acidity is used to detect or diagnose low output of hydrochloric acid (called hypochlorhydria) or a total lack of HCl production (called achlorhydria).

The pancreatic secretion of bicarbonate is measured by testing secretin stimulation. Secretin, a synthetic hormone, is given intravenously, and the physician measures the bicarbonate produced in a duodenum over a sixty-minute period. This tells how well the pancreas is performing. The procedure is also being used therapeutically in cases of autism, to improve pancreatic production of this enzyme and stimulate brain function by balancing secretin output and neurotransmitters.

The Comprehensive Digestive Stool Analysis is another practical test for measuring acidity and other aspects of digestive function. (See Chapter 16 for a more thorough description of this test.)

FUNCTIONAL TESTING

There is enormous value in the new functional testing. Functional assessment makes it possible to evaluate how various organs are actually performing. With this information, treatment can be designed, even if no definitive diagnosis can be made. This is particularly important in minimizing conditions at an early stage or preventing mild illness from becoming more serious. The testing typically involves small, inexpensive, noninvasive samples that can be taken at home and mailed to the lab, once they're ordered by a health practitioner. This testing can provide useful information on disorders for which conventional therapy has no readily available answers.

Unraveling the Mystery of Digestive Illness:

USING ANTIBODY TESTING

ARISTO VOJDANI, Ph.D., M.T.

IMMUNOSCIENCES LAB, INC., BEVERLY HILLS, CA

Antibody testing is an important recent development in lab technology, a resource that is proving helpful to many people caught in the riddle of digestive illness.

Antibody tests are performed through simple samples using saliva or blood. The results reflect the state of immunity within the body. The testing measures the levels of antibodies—proteins produced to defend against microbes, allergenic foods, and other foreign substances. Antibodies provide a record of immune activity against specific organisms and an accurate reflection of exactly which microbe is triggering an immune response and causing illness. With this information, treatment can be targeted much more specifically than in the past, increasing the possibility of successful therapy.

Laura's Story

Laura had been sick since childhood with low-grade GI complaints. It seemed to begin soon after she got the measles when she was four. As an adult, she contracted giardia on a trip to the mountains and suffered severe digestive distress for several years. Repeated lab tests provided no clues to her situation. When antibody testing was performed, both parasites and a viral infection were identified. Armed with a specific diagnosis, her doctor prescribed the drugs, nutrients, and herbs that helped her clear the parasite and the virus almost completely within six months.

DETECTING HIDDEN MICROBES

In evaluations for digestive disease, labs have traditionally found it difficult to detect pathogens. Inflammation or infection can be caused by numerous species of bacteria, yeast, parasites, or viruses.

Microbes can be harbored anywhere in the GI tract. The area of the tissue surface within the digestive tract is immense. If all the layers of the tiny ridge-like villi were unfolded and spread flat, it would cover an area the size of a tennis court. Imagine the number of potential hiding places for microbes. Some opportunistic organisms take full advantage of this terrain. For example, cryptosporidium can lodge and remain in the crypts (the deepest crevices between the villi). Due to this type of problem, many pathogens are not detected in lab tests. Yet the need for reliable testing is very real, as anyone with digestive illness can confirm.

TESTING THE STRENGTH OF IMMUNITY

Our understanding of the immune system holds the key that will unlock the mysteries of many diseases and disorders. Although there is tremendous variation in the causes of disease, illness usually develops only when the immune system malfunctions. One of the greatest challenges facing medicine today involves unraveling the complexities of the immune system and finding better methods to diagnose and treat its disorders.

In the last decade, the science of immunology has greatly expanded the scope of lab diagnosis. Advances in protein chemistry, the study of bacteria, and cell biology have increased our understanding of the body's natural defenses. Much more accurate testing of immune function is now possible as new biological materials and methods are developed.

An example of these innovations are the tests now available that specifically identify IgM antibodies. IgM are the first antibodies produced in our initial encounter with an invader (an antigen). Elevated levels of IgM are strong evidence of immediate acute exposure. Testing for IgM has gained recognition as an important diagnostic approach.

New technological advances have also enabled the development of a wide range of antibody tests. A variety of sensitive and specific assays have been designed that offer great accuracy and precision. These evaluations reflect reactivity to drugs, proteins, polypeptides, and large molecules. Researchers can link antibodies to radioactive tracers, enzymes, or fluorescent tags. This makes it possible to find evidence of infectious agents, even at very low concentrations in different clinical speciments.

HOW ANTIBODIES ACT AS OUR PRIME DEFENSE

The foreign molecules from bacteria or other invaders (antigens) are the ultimate target of all immune responses. Immune function is provided by a complex network of specialized organs, cells, and cell products that protect the body from microbes and other infectious agents. When a threat is detected, the body marshals a diverse army of cells and molecules that work in concert. Antibodies are generated in reaction to the antigens, to neutralize them—producing our immunity against microbes or their toxins.

Specialized protective cells roam the body, consuming the antigens they find. This process also involves chemical messengers that activate T cells. The stimulation of T cells result in the production and cloning of an entire army of various T cells and additional messenger chemicals. This in turn can escalate the mounting immune defense to a higher level of intensity.

Many antibodies are "programmed" to react to one specific invader (a particular bacteria or virus). The body has a vast database in memory of earlier invaders and can produce antibodies to match a great number of antigens. When antibodies attack an antigen, great numbers of these microscopic proteins bind to the invader to form a clustered mass called an immune complex. This serves to neutralize the action of the bacteria or virus and to clear it from our system.

TESTING FOR ANTIBODY LEVELS

Tests are now available to document antibody levels that reflect the presence of invasive microbes or allergenic foods.

Antibody testing is highly relevant in the diagnosis and resolution of many disgestive disorders. It is also a useful tool in treating autoimmune diseases. While bacteria and food antigens can directly induce disease processes, they can also cause indirect effects as autoimmune disorders. About one in four Americans suffers from some form of autoimmune condition such as ileitis, colitis, asthma, chronic respiratory problems, arthritis, lupus, diabetes, multiple sclerosis, AIDS, or immune deficiency.

Physicians who use antibody testing have found that it provides profoundly useful information. It has been suggested that this approach has the capacity to change the way medicine will be practiced in the future. Antibody testing makes it possible to intervene earlier in the disease process. Armed with this type of results, doctors can target treatment very specifically, using natural compounds and powerful medications. Early treatment can reverse problems before more serious invasive conditions develop.

Microflora Immune Competence Test
* Measures antibodies for yeast, aerobic and anaerobic bacteria, protozoa, and dietary proteins including wheat, soy, corn, egg, milk and others

Parasite Antibody Panel
* Antibodies for protozoa: *Blastocystis hominis, Cryptosporidium parvum, Dientamoeba fragilis, Entamoeba histolytica, Giardia lamblia, Toxoplasma gondii,* and others
* For helminths: Ancylostoma, Ascaris, Taenia, Toxocara, Trichuris, and others

Bacteria Panel
* Aerobic bacteria (*E. coli, Lactobacillus, Enterococcus, H. pylori*)
* Anaerobic bacteria (*Clostridium perfiringens and difficile, Bacteroides fragilis, Klebsiella*)

Viral Screens
* Epstein-Barr virus, cytomegalo virus (CMV), herpes 1 and 2, HIV, human papilloma virus, Lyme disease, Mycoplasma species

Aristo Vojdani, Ph.D., M.T. Immunosciences Lab, Inc. can be contacted at 8730 Wilshire Boulevard, Suite 305, Beverly Hills, CA 90211; phone 800-950-4686 or 310-657-1077; fax 310-657-1053.

15

Detecting Microbes

OMAR AMIN, Ph.D.,
DIAGNOSTIC LABS

Many of us have heard about illnesses caused by giardia, but we tend to overlook connections between parasites and digestive disease. According to the Centers for Disease Control, microscopic parasites probably cause more than 90 percent of all parasitic infections in the United States, and many doctors believe we may be seriously underestimating parasites as contributors to disease. Worldwide, infectious diarrhea due to cholera, amoebas, giardia, and blastocystis, among others, is the second most deadly condition, fatal to 3 million people a year.

PARASITIC INFECTION IN THE UNITED STATES

We consider this type of problem an exception in America, a rarity. Most doctors and patients don't usually think of parasites as a common cause of illness. We assume we've eradicated these problems with modern sanitation and water treatment. But research shows that parasitic infection is common, and the incidence is increasing. In many cases, these infections underlie familiar digestive illness and other conditions as well.

Symptoms of intestinal infection are not isolated or unusual. Opportunities for exposure and transmission of parasitic infection increase as overseas travel and immigration expand. Parasites are also transmitted in food processed through mass methods of farming, food manufacturing, and shipping from sources all over the world. Water treatment in huge urban systems is unable to totally eliminate contamination and periodically makes it worse.

Giardia, for instance, is often waterborne, and these infections are

---

A Case of Undetected Infection

❖

When he was about 6, Tony started having problems connected with his digestion. Tests for parasites came out negative. The doctor said it was ulcerative colitis and put Tony on a variety of medications, including steroids. However, his condition did not improve; in fact, it actually worsened. More tests were performed and a stool sample was sent to a lab specializing in the detection of parasites. A infection with *Entamoeba histolytica*, a common but virulent amoeba, was detected. Based on the information from the test results, another of Tony's doctors prescribe medication targeted at clearing the parasite and his symptoms resolved.

It is impossible to determine if the *E. histolytica* infection caused the ulcerative symptoms (which it often does) or if an earlier intestinal condition compromised the integrity of the GI lining, paving the way for the *E. histolytica* to become established. It is clear that the host-parasite relationship was a causal influence, since the elimination of the parasite was instrumental in resolving the ulcerative condition. The key component here is the proper identification of the specific parasite in the test sample.

---

on the rise. In 1997, *The Wall Street Journal* reported an average of 2 million cases annually in the United States. Giardia is also a problem worldwide. In St. Petersburg, the public water system is often contaminated by giardia.

Cyclospora, a parasite in the news, is tracked as a new or emerging pathogen; sometimes it is transmitted on imported fruit. In 1996, it was found on Guatemalan strawberries and raspberries. However, it is also domestic and common in the United States; like all infectious agents, it can be transferred in stool, on human hands, and as contaminants in food and water.

Cryptosporidium, another waterborne parasite, caused illness in more than 400,000 people in Milwaukee in 1993. Over 4,000 were hospitalized and more than 100 died. Cryptosporidium is found in the public water systems and reservoirs of many American cities. In some places, such as the San Francisco Bay Area, it is known to be transmitted by the runoff from hillsides where cattle graze, upstream from unprotected reservoirs.

What happened in Milwaukee drew the attention of the media and the public because so many people were affected. But doctors are coming to believe that all over the country, this kind of infection happens every day. Most of us live crowded together in big cities, many of us

A SAMPLE OF INTESTINAL INFECTIONS IN THE U.S. (1996)

Pathogen—% of Samples Infected	Digestive Symptoms	General Symptoms
Entamoeba histolytica—15%	Diarrhea, constipation, cramps, bloating, flatulence	Fatigue, nausea, allergies, pain, weight loss, insomnia
Blastocystis hominis—8%	Flatulence, bloating, diarrhea, cramps, constipation, poor digestion/poor absorption	Fatigue, nervous disorders, pain, skin conditions, nausea, allergies, muscle problems
E. coli (Entamoeba coli)—8%	Diarrhea, cramps, flatulence, bloating, constipation, irritable bowel	Fatigue, allergies, headache, nausea, depression/irritability, joint/back pain, skin problems
Entamoeba hartmanni—8%	Diarrhea, bloating, cramps, flatuence, irritable bowel	Nervous system, respiratory, and skin disorders, allergies, pain, nausea
Cyclospora—2%	Symptoms that come and go, bloating, flatuence, diarrhea, cramps	Fatigue, itching, nausea, anemia, headache, muscle aches, depression

SOURCE: Omar Amin, Ph.D. *Review of 644 Samples.* Phoenix, AZ: Diagnostic Labs, Inc. (1996).

travel overseas, we frequently have contact with people from all over the world, and we have many opportunities for exposure.

In a survey of samples received at Diagnostic Labs in the summer of 1996, of 644 samples, parasites were detected in more than half (378).

Among this group, we noticed a number of typical characteristics.

◆ More than half the people with infections had traveled overseas in the past five years.

◆ People traveling to Mexico and Europe had the highest risk of infection.

◆ People living in households where someone was infected had twice the risk of infection.

The Greatest Risk Factors for Parasites

❖

- Foreign travel
- Contact within the household with someone who has a parasitic infection
- Previous parasitic infection (implying relapse or reinfection)

Other causes

- Drinking tap water
- Poor hygiene
- Dining out frequently
- Frequenting salad bars
- Having a partner with a parasite problem
- Having pets
- Going camping (especially if you drink the water from streams or even fountains!)
- Working at an infant care center
- Living in an institutional setting or group home

- Of people who were infected, some had no symptoms.
- This implies that some people unknowingly act as carriers. Since they have no symptoms, they might be unaware of the problem, go untreated, and unknowingly pass it on to others.
- People infected by more than one parasite had symptoms similar to those with single infections.
- Women were twice as likely to be infected as men and to be more heavily infected.
- The most prevalent pathogens were *E. histolytica*, *Giardia lamblia*, and *Blastocystis hominis*.

DIFFICULTIES IN DIAGNOSIS

Parasitic infections have long been considered diseases of the tropics, so physicians often don't consider them when diagnosing common illnesses. Parasitology is seldom discussed in the mainstream medical journals and traditionally, there has been little reporting of parasite incidence. For example, giardia has been widely tracked by the Centers for Disease Control (CDC) only since 1987. When physicians receive their training, very little information is provided on parasitology in medical school and in professional journals. Given the lack of information and minimal clinical exposure, doctors don't usually consider parasites as a possible cause of illness, especially when the symptoms aren't confined to the digestive tract.

DIFFICULTIES IN DETECTION

Parasites have complex life cycles and are often not shed at regular intervals. In fact, three of the major parasites in the United States and worldwide (amoebas, giardia, and cyclospora) tend to be shed at irregular intervals. This means that the parasite may be present in the stool for two, three, or four days a week, but not the rest of the week. *Entamoeba histolytica* is active for one or two days, and then is not typically active or detectable the next day or two. If the stool sample is collected from a patient with one of these cyclical parasites on a day when the pathogen is not active, it won't be in the stool and obviously won't be detected by testing. However, this doesn't mean that there's no infection present. At the current time, this is a limitation for which no modern technology can compensate. Consequently, repeated samples are very important. Generally, to make testing practicable, we recommend at least two or three samples be taken on different days.

EMERGING PATHOGENS

Another problem we encounter in detection is the fact that there are so many emerging pathogens. These are new parasites, which remain insufficiently studied. For example, cyclospora was formally classified as a human parasite for the first time just a few years ago. Before that, the labs were probably seeing it, but didn't know what it was because it hadn't been described as such. Other pathogens are reclassified as they become better understood or as their virulence is observed to change. Only in the 1990s has *Dientamoeba fragilis* come to be considered capable of causing disease (pathogenic). In addition, there are some life forms in nature that make detection extremely difficult. Bacteria have been identified that can exist without a cell wall and therefore can take on many shapes. These elusive pathogens make diagnosis extremely difficult.

DAMAGE TO HUMAN HEALTH

Parasitic infection can be damaging to humans by direct injury to the tissue of the digestive tract or the liver, among other organ systems. In addition, the most destructive effects may not be caused by the parasite itself, but by its toxic by-products, which are produced unintentionally as a part of its living process. Parasites can disrupt digestive activity, interfering with the action of digestive enzymes and nutrients. In addition, parasites can compromise the human immune system in order to promote and assure their own survival.

OPTIMAL DETECTION

The most effective method of detecting parasites continues to be stool sampling. The optimal approach involves taking samples every other day, a minimum of 48 hours apart, collecting at least two or three samples.

Although some microbes such as *E. histolytica* reside in the large intestine, many are harbored in the small intestine. Pathogens such as giardia reside primarily in the small intestine, where they strongly adhere to the intestinal lining and therefore cannot usually be detected in samples from stool further down the digestive tract. For this reason, the test must include fecal matter from the small intestine in order to test as accurately as possible. The best specimen is a sample of soft stool taken from the occurrence of a diarrheal episode, because it usually contains material from the small intestine. In the patient who has constipation, the purge test is most optimal.

OTHER METHODS OF TESTING

◆ Elevated white blood count (eosinophil level) may be used as a screening tool to indicate the need for further testing.

◆ Antibody testing is also available. Antibody levels for immuno-globulin G (IgG) can indicate infection, but not whether the infection is current or previous. Repeated testing for IgM levels will show if the infection is currently active.

◆ Samples of blood serum can be evaluated to detect parasites found in the blood. However, this method is useful only for parasites of the circulatory system, not those most typically found in the GI tract.

♦ Tissue samples from biopsies of the colon or duodenum can be tested for parasitic infection, as well as tumors or pathology.

TESTING FOR YEAST

A correlation exists between the presence of parasites and the presence of candida (and other forms of fungus as well). In addition, when there is excessive candida present, the levels of beneficial bacteria tend to be lower. If there are factors present such as parasites that promote the growth of candida, it consumes the resources and the space that would have originally been allotted to the beneficial microflora (the lactobacillus and bifidus). Yeast overgrowth is also documented as a significant factor in some cases of attention deficit disorder and autism (based on the work of Dr. William Shaw and others).

A Note from the Lab

It has been our experience that some people with symptoms of digestive disease may also have an underlying parasitic infection.

Detecting and treating parasitic infections can be a complex process. For example, some organisms are classified as commensals, microorganisms that are present but don't actually cause disease (nonpathogenic). In the past, parasites thought to be harmless have included *H. pylori, Blastocystis hominis, Dientamoeba fragilis,* and even *Giardia lamblia.* In the last ten years, they have been reclassified, because we now recognize that these organisms and numerous others can cause serious infections. In fact, some can contribute to illness that can linger for years if untreated. Once the infection is found and treated, patients often improve quite rapidly.

We've also noticed that parasitic GI infections don't cause symptoms just in the digestive tract alone. The effects of many pathogens are experienced throughout the body, in any of the major organ systems. Associated illnesses can include fatigue, difficulty with mental concentration, depression, and neurological symptoms, as well as allergies, asthma, arthritis, skin disorders, and other chronic health problems.

OMAR AMIN, PH.D., is founder of Diagnostic Labs, Inc. in Phoenix, Arizona. He is a professor of parasitology and a Ph.D. graduate of Arizona State University, where he relocated after teaching at the University of Wisconsin for twenty years. He is an internationally recognized authority, with more than a hundred major publications, extensive worldwide field research, and international teaching experience. He has been a Fulbright scholar and has received numerous research grants for his work. Dr. Amin is available for professional consultations with health care practitioners and will also answer patients' questions directly.

Diagnostic Labs, Inc. offers laboratory testing for the detection of human parasitic infections; practitioners and patients can contact the lab at 3530 E. Indian School Road, Suite 3, Phoenix, AZ 85018; phone 602-955-4211.

16

Testing in Preventive Medicine*

THE INSTITUTE FOR FUNCTIONAL MEDICINE

❖

Functional medicine focuses on evaluating and treating the dynamic processes of the body. How do each of the systems function? How can we assess them? How do we intervene to correct them when they're out of balance? This approach provides a rational, thoughtful way of practicing medicine.

The goal is not just to heal symptoms, but to normalize function—to restore the capacity of organs, tissues, and cells. In this context, health is seen as more than the absence of disease. It's the state of positive vitality unique to each person, health on every level from the cell to the whole person.

Functional testing evaluates and measures this physical and biochemical functioning. Since problems can be detected earlier, when they're less serious, they can be addressed through less invasive means. Treatment often involves changes in nutrition and lifestyle to restore health.

BIOCHEMICAL INDIVIDUALITY

We are each unique. It's obvious that we have unique personalities, fingerprints, and genetics. And while it's apparent that your shape, size, and capabilities are your own, so the functioning of your chemistry and organ systems have characteristic patterns individual to you. For example, your liver may be large or small, with an extensive or a more limited functional capacity. It may be highly active or sluggish,

*Adapted from *The Fundamentals of Functional Medicine* (1997). Written and published by the Institute for Functional Medicine, Gig Harbor, WA. Used by permission.

healthy or struggling. A familiar example is the highly individual capacity to handle alcohol.

In addition, these patterns of functioning aren't static and don't always remain the same. Shifts in function occur long before disease is apparent. So this testing looks at your unique patterns, but also provides a snapshot of how you're functioning at any given time. For example, a person who is never troubled by liver problems might find himself or herself challenged after heavy exposure to chemicals.

Our liver is frequently called on to detoxify a wide range of substances, including digestive by-products, toxins from bacteria, alcohol, hormones, medications, caustic chemicals, and heavy metals. Functional liver testing can show how well the detoxification process is working. When problems are detected before major damage has occurred, specific nutrients and herbs can be recommended to heal tissue and restore function.

DIAGNOSING PROBLEMS BEFORE DISEASE OCCURS

Functional testing can provide doctors with the information they need to intervene before disease develops. Traditionally, diagnosis has been defined as "the art of distinguishing one disease from another." Clinical diagnosis has been described as "diagnosis based on the symptoms . . . *irrespective of the changes producing them.*" In contrast, the new functional testing explores the changes that precede illness, and that is where therapy intervenes.

For example, a test has been developed to assess the barrier function of the intestinal lining, to diagnose the leaky gut syndrome that occurs when the gut becomes too permeable. This particular test answers the question "Is the GI barrier intact and able to keep out harmful microbes and allergens?" The goal is to reduce hyperpermeability and slow the leakage of bacteria or oversized food molecules that could trigger allergies. This can minimize reactions and calm inflammation. Intervening in this process can also prevent the symptoms and conditions that can result from leaky gut such as allergies, arthritis, or asthma.

You can see from this example that a functional approach focuses not only on the end result but also on the dynamic processes that precede and underlie illness. Functional testing provides diagnostic tools that can locate many subtle problems in functioning. Like a good mechanic running a diagnostic on your car, once the practitioner understands what's malfunctioning and why, they can begin to correct it.

TESTING AND TREATMENT IN FUNCTIONAL MEDICINE

Tests have also been developed to assess digestion, find signs of serious allergies or inflammation, and measure levels of free radicals and the status of metabolism. In addition, functional testing can track many aspects of your body chemistry: levels of hormones, nutrients, or body chemicals that serve as signals of malfunction or disease, considered biochemical markers. You can imagine how useful it is to have this kind of specific information available through simple, low-cost testing.

The emphasis here is not only on treating disease but also on raising the capacity of the organ systems, with special emphasis on the systems where illness is first initiated—the GI tract, the liver, and the glands. Strategies often include rebuilding GI flora and barrier function, reducing the toxic burden on the liver, and restoring the rhythm of the glands that produce essential hormones.

This testing empowers your doctor to address small problems before they cause major problems. Getting this information early makes it possible to intervene earlier in the disease process. Harmful dynamics in metabolism and organ function can be shifted using food and nutrients, lifestyle, environmental factors, and mind-body medicine prescribed to fit your unique needs. Restoring function can rebuild inner health.

Food Allergy Testing

SIDNEY MacDONALD BAKER, M.D.

When using nutritional medicine to treat digestive illness, two simple questions are key in understanding health problems: Could there be a deficiency or an unmet need for an essential nutrient? Could there be a toxin or allergen that should be avoided or eliminated?

Avoid is the key word in the second question. If our bodies are burdened by the metabolic costs of detoxification, it makes sense to lighten the burden on our system. Wash your hands before dinner. Stay away from poisons. Eliminate allergens from your diet.

ELIMINATION DIETS

Using an elimination diet means avoiding the offending substance (or substances) before it has a chance to become a burden to your body. Not only may we be challenged by food intolerance, but most of us also suffer some consequence from eating apparently healthy foods against which our immune system has taken a "negative attitude."

One way to discover whether or not the elimination of certain foods may be the key to feeling better is to just avoid them for at least seven days. Foods we eat frequently that can be allergens, include cereal grains and milk products, breads and fermented foods, oranges and other citrus fruits, spices, eggs, coconut, fish and shellfish, tea, coffee, and so on.

But what if you go to all that trouble to eliminate foods and miss something that just happens to be your problem, such as potato or tomato or peppers? Sometimes a test can be quite useful in sorting out the problem and giving you a short list of likely possibilities. It's also important to know that there is no perfect test. None will identify foods that could trigger your symptoms throughout your lifespan.

That said, there is testing available that can take away some of the guesswork.

The test I find the most useful measures IgG antibodies to foods. Antibodies are proteins produced by the body to combat bacteria or harmful microbes, offending foods, or other threatening substances. IgG antibodies are associated with responses to foods that we sometimes call food sensitivities or delayed food allergies. The reason for testing for IgG is that abnormally high levels of the antibody are an indication that the immune system is responding abnormally and too aggressively to a particular food. This type of evaluation is known as an IgG ELISA Test.

We have found that this test is quite valid when done at a laboratory with reliable methods. In certain medical situations, it is an essential tool in the treatment of patients with complex chronic illness. However, this test is technically tricky and lab directors have told me that they have tried to set it up and could not get consistent results. John Rebello of Immuno Laboratories in Fort Lauderdale, Florida, has perfected a technique that produces results that are reliable by the strictest definition of laboratory dependability. Moreover, his tests are the only ones subjected to scientific clinical studies in which patient success is based on the lab results (*Townsend Newsletter,* January 1998).

RESEARCH ON ALLERGY TESTING

Proper scientific studies are based on the assumption that all participants are the same. From this standpoint, it can be difficult to design research that looks at the very different reactions of individuals in response to allergens such as food, pollens, or molds.

To study food intolerances, we posed the question "Do tests for IgG antibodies accurately reflect the reactions caused by particular foods?" In order to answer the question, we conducted a series of double-blind, placebo-controlled studies. Reactivity was evaluated for each individual through blood tests that measured their particular levels of IgG antibodies. Then we divided patients into two groups and randomly assigned avoidance diets based on real scores or diets in which participants avoided nonproblematic foods. In summary:

- Group A avoided foods found to be *reactive* through allergy testing
- Group B avoided foods found to be *nonreactive* through the testing

The study was arranged so that neither the patients nor the doctors knew which participants were really on a real allergy avoidance diet. To learn which group did better, we asked the study participants to report their symptoms. The symptoms included problems typically associated with food sensitivity, as well as any and all general health concerns, such as:

- Digestive concerns
- Headaches
- Skin disorders, including eczema or inflammation
- Respiratory problems like wheezing or congestion
- General symptoms—anything from fatigue or sleep problems to hyperactivity or other issues

As patients began feeling better, the scores that reflected their symptoms began to drop. The group who avoided the foods identified as reactive by testing improved by one-third. For those who avoided nonreactive foods, symptoms dropped by only one-fifth. Here's how the symptom scores looked after the first four weeks of the study.

	Initial average symptom scores	Scores after 4 weeks on the diet
Avoided reactive foods	5	3
Avoided nonreactive foods	5	4

All the participants in the study did a little better! The intention to heal is powerful and accompanies any change we make. Since diet is one of the biggest lifestyle changes most people ever commit to, big results can occur. However, the patients who did better were those who were avoiding actual food intolerances that had been confirmed by the antibody testing. They fared far better than those who were avoiding nonreactive foods. The experiments were an elaborate way of showing that allergy testing really works.

It is understandable that an elimination diet has some powerful nonspecific effects in relieving symptoms. If you want to feel better, go on a diet—any diet! If you want to approach the problem of food sensitivities seriously, testing to see which are your reactive foods and which are your safe foods before changing your diet can save you some confusion.

The test also identifies foods that are nonreactive, which may be especially important in chronic illness with excessive and inappropriate immune activation. This type of condition has been associated with conditions such as autoimmune disease, chronic fatigue syndrome, and hyperactivity. In these cases, it seems important to know which foods tend to trigger the *least* immune reactivity. For some health conditions, IgG testing can provide so much information on the origin of the problem that I believe it would be negligent to ignore this diagnostic option.

SIDNEY MACDONALD BAKER, M.D. 40 Hillside Road North, Weston, CT 06883-1514; phone 203-227-8444, fax 203-227-8443, e-mail: sbaker@snet.net, http://www.sbakermd.com

17

How to Find Out What's Working and What Isn't

JOHN FURLONG, N.D.

To practice truly preventive medicine, we have to know when to intervene. We need to be able to identify that crucial period when health is beginning to slip away, before the damage has been done.

We now have many of the pieces of the puzzle in our hands—the basis for truly preventive medicine. Basic yet sophisticated new lab tests are able to reflect the uniqueness of individual biology. We know much about how the body works; we know much about what *should* be happening and which nutrients assist with various dynamics within the body. Now functional medicine combines the research of the past two decades on body chemistry and processes and applies it to the scientifically known aspects of disease. The success of our therapies and the safety of this approach are clear to both patients and doctors.

These tests help us find inflammation, overly aggressive immune responses, poor digestion, and hormone problems; they all fit in the model of functional, preventive medicine. We also have the tools to intervene in these processes effectively with nutrients and herbs, minimizing the use of synthetic medications. It's clear that medicine has made enormous progress in the development of pharmacology and technology, essential in heroic intervention against acute injury and disease. In contrast, when we're working preventively, we find the time-honored relationships between what we eat, how we think, how much we exercise, and whether we reduce stress continue to be the most powerful modifiers of the disease process. We can adjust these aspects of our lives, knowing that the results will be naturally in accord with our physiology.

You are the person most likely to benefit from this new preventive

When the Complaint Is Fatigue

When John visited his doctor, he expressed concern about the frequent fatigue he felt throughout the day. He was also troubled by chronic and severe bronchitis. His history showed that he had worked in a plasticizing plant for a number of years.

Because of the possibility of chemical exposure at work, his doctor order a liver detoxification test. When the results came back, the main abnormality the test showed was in one of the Phase 2 Detoxification pathways (for glutathione), which was *below* the low end of the normal range. His level was the lowest of all the detoxification profiles I've ever seen. Glutathione has the job of detoxifying a wide variety of chemicals, including plasticizers. We realized John was probably depleting his body's stores of glutathione through his workplace exposure, and that's why his level was so exceptionally low. He was also tested for antibodies to certain plasticizing chemicals and the tests indicated levels 50 percent higher than the normal range for one, and twice normal for the other. It's unusual to get two tests that reflect a problem so clearly. Not only had he been depleting glutathione in the liver, he'd also been overstimulating his immune system, often associated with chronic fatigue, due to the frequent chemical exposure.

The kind of information we learned on John's test was directly applied in designing his treatment. His doctor chose to provide nutritional support for glutathione processing by suggesting John take the amino acids from which glutathione is made, which are glycine, cysteine, and glutamic acid, or N-acetyl-cysteine (which has been well documented for its detoxification support). In some cases, reduced glutathione itself is used. A complete spectrum of antioxidants (vitamin C, E, selenium, and carotenoids) was also recommended, since glutathione depends on some of these for its conversion back to an active form.

When problems with this aspect of liver function occur, it's important to take them seriously because glutathione has the job of detoxifying many common chemicals, including medications such as Tylenol, tetracycline, and penicillin; nitrosamines (by-products of nitrates in foods such as luncheon meats); toxic elements; and certain pesticides, such as organophosphates. Fortunately, John's theraputic program shows every promise of bringing about a good result.

In John's case, we had two kinds of testing evidence that pointed to his chemical exposure as the source of a fatigue problem. Chronic fatigue can occur with exposure to chemicals because they put a burden on the immune system and the liver. The hope is that over time, John's condition can be reversed through the avoidance of the chemicals and nutritional support of his liver detoxification function.

medicine, being able to avert severe disease when the first signs of illness are present. Functional tests can help your doctors understand you better, enabling them to recommend therapies specific to your situation and get to the root cause of many kinds of illnesses. See your preventive or functional practitioner before things get out of hand and you'll reap many benefits. You may even find you feel better than ever before!

THE CDSA (COMPREHENSIVE DIGESTIVE STOOL ANALYSIS)

This simple test, obtained from one to three stool samples, gives some twenty different measures. It assesses how food is utilized by the digestive system and the absorption of fats. The test also indicates the levels of bacteria and yeast, and the by-products of bacteria (both good and bad) in the colon. These assessments together provide a window into our digestion, an area we often overlook, but one essential for good health.

For instance, the test can show low levels of an enzyme from the pancreas called chymotrypsin. If this enzyme isn't being secreted at the right level, our ability to absorb proteins may be impaired. In some cases, this is the cause of symptoms such as a failure to gain weight, gas, and bloating, and may relate to arthritis. The CDSA also reports on fats found in the stool. Although unabsorbed fats are normally quite low, when they are elevated, they can point to gallbladder problems, and difficulty in absorbing vitamins such as A, D, and E.

You can see from just these two examples that looking at twenty markers can provide a wealth of useful information your doctor can use to help you feel better. Some of the test results are used to determine which supplements may best enhance digestion, avoiding unnecessary and ineffective guesswork. The choice of the right nutrition for your unique body chemistry can make a real difference. This means the right selection of vitamins and minerals, flora, and food tailored to your unique situation. Rebalancing good bacteria can frequently alleviate symptoms such as irritable bowel syndrome and improve most problems in the GI tract, from constipation to colon polyps to Crohn's disease.

Another important marker assessed in the CDSA is beta-glucuronidase. This is an enzyme produced by certain bacteria that essentially sabotages some of the detoxification work performed by the liver.

When it's present in the GI tract in excessive amounts, it can release toxins bound by the liver back into the body. High levels of this enzyme have been found in some cases of colon cancer; although the test is not telling us that cancer is present, it *does* seem to indicate an environment in the gut where cancer may be more likely to develop.

The test also measures levels of N-butyrate, a substance that provides the gut lining cells with the energy to maintain themselves. This is no small job, since our body regenerates these cells about every four days. If N-butyrate is low, it indicates that the cells are in a constant state of semi-starvation. Then our body can have difficulty nourishing and repairing the colonic lining. This marker, if low, may also serve as a warning sign of risk for colon cancer.

INTESTINAL PERMEABILITY

The intestines have two very different jobs to do. One the one hand, they must allow us to absorb nutrients, vitamins, and minerals from our food. On the other hand, the intestinal cells must act as a barrier to bacteria, large protein molecules, and potential toxins that would cause problems if allowed to pass into the bloodstream. This dual function is central to our good health. And fortunately, it can be measured easily.

This test measures the degree of intestinal permeability in the small intestine. It answers the question "Has the intestinal wall become too permeable, allowing toxins, allergens, and bacteria to enter the bloodstream?" The procedure involves drinking a solution containing two harmless compounds, lactulose and mannitol. Lactulose is a larger molecule. Mannitol is very small. Because these molecules tend to pass through our system undigested, a urine collection can reflect how much of each substance is passing through the gut barrier into the bloodstream.

Many factors can affect this gut barrier. In some people, just eating a food that triggers their sensitivities can affect the barrier function, causing hyperpermeability, and the ratio of lactulose to mannitol found in the urine will increase. Similarly, when people have Crohn's, parasitic infections, or other conditions, the ratio of lactulose to mannitol can be affected.

This is a test to identify the integrity of the small intestine and how well it's likely to function and repair itself. So the information gained can help a physician determine how much wear and tear are affecting the small intestine. Periodically during treatment, this test can easily be retaken to gauge how well a person is responding to the therapy. If the test results show improvement with treatment, the doctor is on the right track!

If intestinal permeability is abnormal, there are several strategies to assist with repair. Nutritional approaches have proven quite effective and may involve specific nutrients (such as L-glutamine, vitamins A and fish oil capsules, vitamin C, folic acid) and the avoidance of reactive foods. Once offending factors such as parasites, yeast, or abnormal bacteria are addressed and the gut receives the nutrients it requires, the healing can be quite rapid. As the intestines regain their usual resilience and their proper barrier and absorptive functions are restored, many symptoms can resolve. Doctors see good responses to this approach in conditions such as allergies, general abdominal discomfort, irritable bowel syndrome, autism, and behavior problems in children. Even more severe problems such as Crohn's disease have a greater likelihood of healing when intestinal permeability is normalized. A simple test, yes, but one that provides exceedingly important information!

CANDIDA CULTURES AND ANTIBODY TESTING

Many of you have heard of the problems associated with the overgrowth of intestinal yeast, most commonly the candida species. In the case of yeast, there are two important issues to consider. First, an overgrowth of candida is *not* the same thing as a systemic yeast or fungal infection. A systemic overgrowth is usually seen only in people whose immune systems are significantly impaired due to conditions such as AIDS or the use of certain medications. Second, a low level of yeast is *normal* and for most people presents no great problem.

There are, however, many people who have overgrowth of the candida organisms in the gut, the mouth, and occasionally throughout the digestive tract and in women, in the vagina. Usually this is the result of major or repeated antibiotic therapy and a poor diet, high in sugars and low in fiber. Yeast don't typically invade the body in the way a strong bacterial infection would, but they can overtax the body's immune system and can result in reactions in important organ systems such as the liver and ovaries.

How are these problems identified? Questionnaires can provide clues to the presence of yeast overgrowth, but more definitive testing is done by culturing the yeast from stool or sampling the blood to look for antibodies against the yeast.

Stool Testing for Candida

Since the yeasts tend to grow easily and abundantly in the intestines under the right circumstances, sampling the stool to attempt to grow the yeast (culture it) represents a practical means to determine the amount of yeast present. The stool culture measures the relative abundance of living yeast in the lower gut that are capable of growing and reproducing. In addition, the culture can be used to test antifungal products that can kill that particular strain of yeast and determine the most likely medication or herbal product that can help eradicate the yeast. This capacity for sensitivity testing is very important since some yeast, like bacteria, are becoming resistant to certain treatment agents. So culturing for yeast tells us which organisms are present at what levels, and which drugs and herbs are most likely to eradicate them.

Blood Tests for Candida

The body's immune system may react too strongly to yeast and cause more problems. One means to determine if this is happening involves examining the blood for short and long-term responses to candida yeast. One blood test can look at all these factors. IgG is the most prevalent antibody, and if it's elevated in the blood, that indicates that there has been an ongoing exposure to the yeast which has activated the immune system. The presence of the IgM antibody reflects a more short-term immediate response to yeast. A third antibody, IgA, is tested because elevated levels serve as a marker for superficial yeast infections. This kind of infection is typically countered by surface anti-

---

Treating Yeast Infections

❖

I have personally seen patients who sought my help after a year of treatment for yeast with a commonly used prescription drug with only minimal response. We found through stool testing that they had highly active yeast infections (testing at the highest level reported of 4 +) and that the particular organism was resistant to the prescribed medication.

bodies made by immune cells in the gut lining. In addition, if there is a large burden of yeast and the body is unable to clear it well, there will be candida antigens (proteins) found in the blood. This is different from finding live yeast in the blood, but still reflects a lot of extra stress on the body.

Finally, the liver has a part to play in all this. If the yeast is present and causing problems, the immune system should recognize it. Antibodies typically stick to the yeast cells and/or proteins and the liver should be clearing these from the circulation. If there are yeast antigen-antibody complexes (clusters), it can indicate a situation in which the liver is overburdened or the immune cells are being suppressed, allowing these reactive combinations to circulate in the bloodstream, stimulating immune activity where it may not be needed. This is also important to know, since an overstimulated immune response can sometimes cause additional problems in the body, such as arthritis.

Yeast overgrowth is important to identify, because it may play a part in a large variety of illnesses—fatigue, allergies, changes in the menstrual cycle, difficult with thinking and learning, and of course, irritation of the intestines. Since the questionnaires and popular literature list so many symptoms of yeast infection, many doctors are doubtful that the syndrome really exists, especially since they are used to thinking of yeast overgrowth as a process that occurs only in extremely ill patients. The results of the test show the level of immune activity necessary to control this normally innocuous microbe. The findings can illustrate the depth to which the yeast has been able to get a foothold in the body. This provides the practitioner with the means to treat yeast overgrowths most effectively and the information they need to help a wide variety of patients.

LIVER DETOXIFICATION

The liver is a miraculous organ. It's the only key organ that is capable of regenerating itself. Its important work includes immune surveillance, digestive secretions, and detoxification.

One of the liver's unique functions is the detoxification of substances absorbed into the bloodstream from the gut. The liver receives virtually all the blood flow coming from the intestines. Since our gut and liver never quite know what interesting things we're going to challenge them with, they have developed the ability to detoxify or deactivate a huge variety of substances and chemicals. This comes into practical utility when we drink a glass or two of wine. The alcohol is broken down to acetaldehyde, which is eventually processed and excreted as water and carbon dioxide. This process requires a number of enzymes and a lot of energy from the liver cells. They perform this type of activity for virtually all medications, many food components, and any of the lovely waste products coming from the bacteria and yeast in the intestines. No wonder the liver is a crucial organ!

Since good liver function can mean the difference between health and disease, there's real value in knowing how well it's able to perform. The liver detox profile looks at five key enzyme systems the liver uses to detoxify chemicals, drugs, and digestive by-products. This assessment is called a challenge test, because small doses of common substances are taken to test the liver's ability to respond (in this case caffeine, aspirin, and Tylenol). This gives the practitioner a gauge of how much stress the liver is under and how its activities can be further supported in specific terms. By testing the liver's response to low-grade metabolic stress, the practitioner is able to determine if certain supplements, or even foods, should be avoided or should be added for nutritional support.

This type of testing is extremely useful for people who have frequent fatigue or who have had unusual reactions to medications or supplements. I also strongly recommend it for people whose work exposes them to strong chemicals (such as solvents, varnish, petrochemicals, or polyurethane) and for autistic children. Some people find that their system protects them and keeps them free of symptoms with such exposures, but at a certain cost to the liver. The test also provides the basis for customized nutritional support, identifies whether nutrients are being depleted, and may identify people with imbalanced enzyme systems. By addressing the quirks and requirements of the liver and minimizing the *sources* of exposure (like gut bacteria, chemicals, or medications), you can minimize the wear and tear on the crucial enzyme systems in the liver.

An additional benefit to the liver challenge test is an assessment of oxidative stress. The process of oxidative stress is potentially harmful to the body. It's a stressor to which *all* our cells must respond or be damaged. Excessive exercise, smoking, alcohol, and medications all contribute to the formation of highly potent molecules known as free radicals. These unstable molecules can damage many different systems in the cell and can ultimately cause cell death. When the body is lacking antioxidants, free radicals can increase and damage cells. The cumulative damage can cause disease or even cancer under certain conditions. The adequacy of individual antioxidant nutrition can be assessed by evaluating how much free radical activity there is in response to the aspirin challenge. Inflammatory conditions such as lupus, arthritis, and even heart disease have significant components of oxidative stress. These conditions can often be improved by supporting the antioxidant capacity using the information gained from this insightful test. Protective nutrients include carotenes, vitamin C and flavonoids, vitamin E, and minerals like selenium and zinc.

TESTING FOR OXIDATIVE STRESS

The test for oxidative stress is actually part of the complete detoxification profile, or it can be ordered separately. Oxidative stress is another aspect of the detoxification issue. With this test, we're challenging the body just a little by giving a small dose of aspirin. The test is be used to measure free radicals that are produced as the body metabolizes the aspirin. Free radicals are highly active molecules that can be compared with a superball bouncing around in a room very rapidly, hitting walls, lights, whatever happens to be there. The energy of the free radical is not necessarily a problem if there's enough "cushioning" in the tissues surrounding its activity. Free radicals are generated from day-to-day activity such as exercise or metabolizing foods and generally don't create any problem as long as there are adequate levels of antioxidants from the diet or a supplement.

Problems can occur if too many free radicals are being generated, which is known to occur often in conditions of inflammation, such as rheumatoid arthritis. In these situations, the amount of free radicals being produced is excessive and the body typically doesn't have the reserves to cope. To use the superball image, instead of having one ball bouncing around causing occasional damage, there may be the equivalent of having fifty, so all kinds of things are subject to damage. In this situation, excessive free radical damage can occur.

The other situation that causes problems is when there's not enough antioxidant protection, even in the presence of normal free radical production. In this case, the normal wear and tear of free radicals on the body is experienced as excessive because the protection is lacking. This can happen when antioxidants are depleted. It may happen when one antioxidant is taken in excess or taken without the others, unbalancing the way the body handles free radicals. This may be the effect seen in the Scandinavian study on smokers who were given beta-carotene alone—some of the participants actually had a greater incidence of lung cancer.

The value of tests like the oxidative stress test is to detect excess production of free radicals and make changes before problems occur. Two of the chemicals that result from the aspirin challenge serve as markers of how much free radical damage this small dose of aspirin has generated. These chemicals can be measured in urine, and if those levels are high, we know the person is very susceptible to free radical activity. If the levels are normal, then we know he or she is not particularly susceptible to free radical damage and has adequate stores of antioxidants. The test also includes an examination for other important markers, including lipid peroxides in urine. In addition, we measure blood levels of three antioxidant protectors, which are extremely important. This provides a well-rounded picture of the level of protection available against free radical damage.

JOHN FURLONG, N.D., is a naturopathic physician, trained at Bastyr University in Seattle. His experience in medicine ranges from hospital care to holistic health care. He was a founding member of a collaborative health center in Connecticut, where he provided services in nutritional, homeopathic, and botanical medicine, and detoxification. He also founded the People's Health Alliance, a nonprofit organization promoting public education in natural approaches to healing. He is currently assistant director of education at the Great Smokies Diagnostic Laboratories.

Great Smokies Diagnostic Laboratory offers a variety of diagnostic testing, including tests described above; educational materials are available to both patients and practitioners on health, preventive medicine, and functional testing through their Client Services Department, 63 Zillicoa Street, Asheville, NC 28801-1074, or by calling 800-522-4762 or visiting their web site at www.gsdl.com.

18

Assessing Inflammation and Immunity

WILLIAM TIMMINS, N.D.

❖

Functional medicine and testing are based on the view that our body's chemistry can reflect important information on how our system is functioning. The concept of biochemical individuality suggests that each person has somewhat unique metabolic patterns that can be interpreted to determine his or her nutrition and health needs. Functional treatment involves carefully evaluating personal history, testing to assess the body's capacity to function, supporting the body with optimal nutrition, minimizing harmful environmental factors, and restoring metabolic balance.

TRADITIONAL DIAGNOSIS AND TREATMENT

Traditionally, physicians have used lab tests to confirm the source and degree of illness. However, many symptoms can't be associated with a specific disease, particularly in the early stages of an illness. So there are situations in which disease can't be diagnosed using the traditional model of evaluation.

The word *dis-ease* means "without ease." People with undiagnosed and untreated conditions are truly without ease. A patient's chief complaint may be only that he or she has no energy and is unable to carry out day-to-day activities. Until recently, doctors have lacked the tools to identify the underlying causes of these types of health problems. As a result, it's been difficult to develop treatment for conditions that weren't linked to specific diseases, but were associated with processes in the body that were malfunctioning. Even patients whose illnesses have been accurately diagnosed may not fully heal if only the symptoms of their illnesses are being treated. The ultimate underlying cause may remain unidentified.

FUNCTIONAL DIAGNOSIS AND TREATMENT

The goal of the functional medicine practitioner is to measure the body's processes and treat the dysfunctions that are causing the disorder. If normal functioning is restored throughout the system, symptoms can resolve as the body naturally heals and returns to a state of wellness. The degree of healing may also depend on whether functional diagnosis and treatment is provided before serious damage has occurred.

Only a few years ago, the scientific tools needed to accurately assess various aspects of body function did not exist. Functional medicine was correct in theory, but lacking in diagnostic science. Today we have the practical ability to measure a wide range of processes vital to every system in the body.

After taking a careful health history and reviewing symptoms, testing is done to determine whether a particular process is within normal physiological range. If this function is not within normal range, it's viewed as the cause or a contributing factor of illness. When indicated, additional testing can be done to measure other related factors.

MONITORING THERAPY

Functional diagnostic testing strongly influences the way treatment is carried out. This approach provides the information needed by the practitioner to develop a viable course of treatment. Further testing helps the practitioner monitor the progress of the patient's response and guides the adjustment of treatment.

MEASURING OUR IMMUNE DEFENSE

Testing for Secretory IgA

WHY THIS TEST IS IMPORTANT: Have you ever wondered why food contaminated with bacteria such as toxic *E. coli* can cause severe illness in some people and not others? In part, the answer is found in the ability of our digestive system to defend against infection.

Many people are amazed to learn that the digestive tract, throat,

Using Functional Testing and Treatment

❖

Jeanette came to us soon after cancer surgery, seeking help to rebuild her immunity. Functional testing showed poor absorption and also inflammation in reaction to gluten (a component of wheat). In addition, her adrenal glands were struggling and her vital hormones were clearly out of balance, due to stress, blood sugar imbalance, and the GI condition. When we tested her adrenal function, the results indicated that her cortisol was far too high and her DHEA was depleted. This type of pattern is known to compromise antibody production (especially SIgA), as well as cellular immunity (typically NK killer cells), and this was confirmed in Jeanette's test results. Her hormone levels reflected an elevated cortisol at night, which indicated that her body wasn't shutting down, unable to shift fully into a rest-and-repair cycle. Her melatonin production was also out of cycle, further disturbing her sleep patterns, which wasn't helping her immunity either.

Based on this information, we first elected treatment to heal the inflammation in the GI tract from the gluten intolerance. Our other initial goal was to restore normal adrenal function. Jeanette showed marked improvement in the following months. Because of the seriousness of her history, we have continued to monitor her progress for the past two years. A summary of the changes in her cortisol levels and DHEA during this time are summarized below. You'll notice the skewed hormone levels when we first saw Jeanette. We've been especially encouraged by the improvement in her DHEA function.

Test	Normal Range	1996	1997	1998
Total Cortisol	23 to 42	44	28	30
DHEA	2 to 10	2	7	8

In Jeanette's case, normalizing adrenal function has allowed the return of normal immune response. Supplements and changes in diet and lifestyle have recovered the healthy function of her GI tract. Normal adrenal/melatonin function has restored her to a positive sleep cycle.

and mouth hold our defense against potential pathogens, including bacteria, viruses, parasites, fungus, and invasive forms of yeast. The saliva in our mouth and the mucus throughout our entire digestive system contain protective antibodies—secretory IgA (SIgA). These antibodies play a key role in blocking the invasion of unhealthy organisms; they function as our first line of immune defense.

HOW SIgA CAN BE MEASURED: In recent years, functional tests have been developed to assess the strength of our secretory IgA. A simple saliva test can be used to measure SIgA levels in the mouth/throat and a stool test can be used to measure them in the gut. Although SIgA in each area can be evaluated independently, lab testing has shown that there's a strong correlation between antibody levels registered from the mouth/throat area and from the intestinal tract. Since saliva testing can be performed with relative ease, this is a good first step in assessment.

HOW THE RESULTS CAN BE USED: If the SIgA level measured in oral saliva is depressed, there is a high probability that it will also be low in other mucus-producing areas of the body. Low levels of SIgA suggest the value of additional testing to rule out infection or inflammation, which can cause nutritional deficiencies and toxicity.

TESTING FOR THE PRESENCE OF INFLAMMATION

A Marker for Inflammation in the Small Intestine

WHY THIS TEST IS IMPORTANT: Testing for alpha-antichymotrypsin reports a marker that indicates if inflammation is present, primarily in the small intestinal. High levels of this marker reflect the need for further testing to determine the cause of the inflammation.

MEASURING THIS METABOLIC MARKER: A stool sample is used to detect and measure this metabolic marker.

HOW THE RESULTS CAN BE USED: Whenever inflammation is present, it is important to find the cause and prevent further problems. Inflammation in the small intestine can be triggered by reactions to gluten, lactose, or sucrose; delayed food allergies; or upper GI parasites such as giardia, cryptosporidium, or amoebas (for example *Dientamoeba fragilis*).

A Marker for Inflammation in the Large Intestine

WHY THIS TEST IS IMPORTANT: This marker (lysozyme A) typically indicates whether inflammation is present in the large intestine. It can reflect a number of conditions, including irritable bowel syndrome (IBS), inflammatory bowel disease (IBD), and colon cancer.

MEASURING: Lysozyme can be measured through a stool test.

HOW THE RESULTS CAN BE USED: The information from this test can be used to direct follow-up testing or treatment. The test can be repeated to evaluate the success of treatment.

Testing for the Presence of Infection

WHY THIS TEST IS IMPORTANT: High levels of nitrate (nitric oxide) reflect the presence of infection in the body. Nitric oxide is released to enable our white blood cells to attack invading organisms. Although this biochemical has a beneficial function, excessive nitric oxide can promote generalized inflammation and can cause damage to muscles and joints.

WHAT IT MEASURES: The test measures levels of nitric oxide as a metabolic marker in urine.

HOW THE RESULTS CAN BE USED: Elevated levels of nitric oxide indicate the need for further testing to determine the source of the infection or inflammation. They also suggest the importance of supplementing with antioxidants to reduce inflammation. Decreasing nitric oxide levels will reduce the potential for damage to muscle tissue and joints.

EVALUATING OUR STRESS RESPONSE

Testing for DHEA

WHY DHEA IS IMPORTANT: DHEA is often referred to as the mother hormone of the body, and we produce more of this essential hormone than any other. In combination with cortisol, it's involved in the regulation of virtually all aspects of body function. Both are secreted by the adrenal glands, the source of our defense response to the stressors of life (both external and internal). In order for us to cope with digestive illness and support immune defenses, DHEA levels must be maintained so healing can proceed.

HOW DHEA CAN BE MEASURED: This test is performed through simple saliva specimens.

HOW THE RESULTS CAN BE USED: Abnormal DHEA levels can interfere with immunity, energy production, skin regeneration, bone health, sleep quality, and thyroid function. If we have evidence of adrenal hormone levels, that can provide the basis for developing a therapeutic program. The levels can easily be rechecked through future saliva tests, guiding strategies to promote or supplement DHEA gradually until it returns to the normal range.

Measuring Cortisol Levels

WHY CORTISOL IS IMPORTANT: Cortisol is the primary hormone that directs immune function, and it works in harmony with DHEA. These hormones also regulate the production of the cells that secrete SIgA (the immunocytes). If cortisol and DHEA values are out of balance, a depression of SIgA can ultimately occur. Therefore, when SIgA levels are low, it's important to look at adrenal function. This can reflect excessive physical, mental, or emotional stress.

Stress is handled by our sympathetic system, in response to both intense events (the fight-or-flight mechanism) and low-grade ongoing stress. Our parasympathetic system does the repairing, restoring, and rebuilding. A critical balance exists between the two systems. When we are responding to stress too much of the time, it can overload the sympathetic system and lead to adrenal exhaustion. If illness is present, it's essential to identify and correct any depression of our adrenal hormones, to maintain our body's ability to heal.

HOW CORTISOL IS MEASURED: One way to measure cortisol levels is through a simple home test that samples saliva. This provides us with a real-life assessment of the effects of stress on the adrenals.

HOW THE RESULTS CAN BE USED: Restoring the normal balance of cortisol and DHEA will help the body produce more immunocytes and therefore improve secretory IgA levels. Measuring cortisol and DHEA can also identify adrenal dysfunction, and treatment strategies can be developed to restore normal function, optimizing health and immunity.

DETERMINING DIGESTIVE STATUS

Measuring Reactions to Gluten

WHY THIS TEST IS IMPORTANT: Reactions to gluten can be devastating for anyone who has inherited gluten intolerance. This condition is especially common in people with northern European and Scandinavian heritage. The body's response can cause severe inflammation in the small intestine, a breakdown in the mucosal lining. The damage from gluten may be so extreme that it can create allergies to numerous other foods, and secondary illnesses may develop. The number one problem that results from gluten intolerance is malabsorption, which can lead to severe nutritional deficiencies and resulting illness.

MEASURING GLUTEN INTOLERANCE THROUGH GLIADIN ANTIBODIES: This test, using a saliva sample, measures the immune response to gliadin (gluten protein). Positive test results indicate gluten intolerance.

HOW THE RESULTS CAN BE USED: Gluten intolerance is known to be associated with inflammation of the small intestine and with malabsorption. People with a gluten intolerance often find that once they're on a 100 percent gluten-free diet, within as little as two months there can be a normalization of the SIgA defenses and a major reduction in inflammation. As inflammation decreases, the ability to absorb nutrients will increase, improving nutritional status.

Measuring Milk/Dairy Intolerance

WHY THIS TEST IS IMPORTANT: This test provides essential feedback regarding a person's ability to handle dairy products in general. Allergic reactions to milk and other dairy-based foods have been associated with symptoms such as diarrhea, constipation, chronic fatigue, and arthritis, and can lead to leaky gut syndrome. It can also cause irritation and inflammation of the GI tract, damage to the villi in the gut lining, and the reduction of the immunocytes that produce SIgA. People who are sensitive to milk proteins (casein and lactalbumin) are usually also lactose intolerant. Dairy allergy that's not addressed can lead to illness elsewhere in the body, including respiratory problems and sinus infections.

HOW DAIRY PROTEINS ARE MEASURED: This is a saliva test that measures the response to mixed milk proteins. If an immune reaction is detected (the presence of antibodies), this means the body is mounting an attack against milk protein in an allergic response.

HOW THE RESULTS CAN BE USED: A positive result on this test means there is an allergy or a sensitivity to dairy products. In that case, it's important to avoid all milk and dairy products. With the complete avoidance of dairy, the symptoms subside quite quickly.

The Metabolic Profile

WHY THIS TEST IS IMPORTANT: This diagnostic test assesses the status of our own unique body chemistry. At any given time, our chemistry reflects the stability or compromise of our health. If our biochemistry is brought back into balance through the use of nutrients, the foods we eat, and our lifestyle, healing can occur naturally.

WHAT THE TEST MEASURES: This test measures body chemicals that reflect:

- Energy production and oxygen metabolism
- Deficiencies in B-complex vitamins, amino acids, and minerals
- Brain function reflected in neurotransmitter metabolism
- Liver function, particularly how well a person is able to neutralize and expel toxins
- Specific needs for antioxidants and other nutrients
- Digestion and absorption problems
- How efficiently the body is metabolizing and using the nutrients from food
- How effectively the body is metabolizing carbohydrates
- Markers for dysbiosis where there is an overgrowth of yeast, microscopic parasites, or bacteria
- Signs of damage to cells

HOW THE RESULTS CAN BE USED: This test can be used as a key diagnostic tool for chronic health problems. It is helpful in customizing individual treatment programs. This view of the body's processes at the level of the cell allows us to look at problems that might interfere with our ability to take the fuel from the food we eat and convert it into energy.

The test's chemical markers may reflect nutritional deficiencies. This information can be used to address specific needs for vitamins, minerals, antioxidants, amino acids, and dietary changes. Diet therapy and supplements can play a vital role in restarting or rebalancing the metabolism.

The metabolic profile provides clues about where to intervene in complex problems, by giving an overview of how the metabolism is functioning. It can show whether cells are being destroyed, malfunctioning, or functioning normally. With this information, more serious health problems can often be prevented or reversed.

WILLIAM G. TIMMINS, N.D., is founder and director of San Diego's Bio-Health Diagnostics. He received his degree in naturopathy from the International University of Naturopathic Sciences and cofounded two of the nation's first integrative healthcare centers. A lecturer, former host of two weekly radio programs, and national physicians' consultant for clinical and research laboratories, Dr. Timmins maintains a busy patient practice in nutritional consulting while conducting independent research and providing professional training on functional diagnostic testing. More than a decade of helping his patients has enriched and confirmed his theories in the real-life measurement of his work's success.

Dr. Timmins and BioHealth Diagnostics provide nutritional consulting, and individualized wellness and longevity programs; for professionals, a wide array of audio- and videotapes are available, as well as seminars, and patient and doctor educational programs in the clinical applications of functional diagnostic testing. BioHealth Diagnostics in San Diego can be reached at 800-570-2000.

Part III

NEW STRATEGIES FOR INNER HEALTH

19

Remove, Replace, Restore, and Repair*

JEFFREY BLAND, PH.D.

❖

STEP 1. REMOVE

- Common food allergies or sensitivities (see Chapter 20).
- Bad bugs—candida or bacterial overgrowth or parasites (see Chapter 21).
- Problems from viruses (see Chapter 22).
- Minimize environmental toxins and also digestive toxins (see Chapter 23).

STEP 2. REPLACE

See Chapter 24.

- Betaine hydrochloride (hydrochloric acid)
- Enzymes (animal-based or plant-based)
- Bicarbonate (which enables the enzymes to work)

STEP 3. RESTORE BENEFICIAL FLORA

See Chapter 24.

- Probiotics—*L. acidolphilus* and other probiotics.
- Provide prebiotics if starches and sugars are tolerated. Nourishment for the beneficial microflora such as FOS (fructo-aligo-saccharides) and inulin (in Jerusalem artichokes, dandelion greens).

*Adapted from *The Fundamentals of Functional Medicine* (1997). Written and published by the Institute for Functional Medicine, Gig Harbor, WA. Used by permission.

- Increase fiber and monitor the response. Soluble fiber such as oat bran increases butyrate and other essential fatty acids. Nonsoluble fiber such as cellulose is best tolerated by some.
- Increase resistant starch in the diet to reduce acidity, and raise fatty acids. See *Breaking the Vicious Cycle* by Elaine Gottschall.
- Monitor level of starches and sugars (see Chapter 31).

STEP 4. REPAIR

See Chapter 25.

- Provide nutrients to heal the GI mucosa: vitamins A and C, B_5 (pantothenic acid), B_6 (pyrodixine), the amino acid L-glutamine, and the mineral zinc.
- Support the immune functions of the GI tract: vitamin A to nourish antibody production.
- Continue to avoid allergens and irritants: certain drugs (such as NSAIDs), alcohol, and foods that trigger allergies.

20

Minimize Food Allergies

MICHAEL ROSENBAUM, M.D.

❖

Why are we concerned about allergies? Allergies and sensitivities are often linked to digestive problems. When the offending food is discovered and removed, people improve. So a small investment of time and effort can produce big results.

The process of treating people for food allergies basically involves discovering and then eliminating the food that triggers allergies. Among the basic treatments for food allergies, elimination is probably the most important. The primary therapies include:

- ◆ The elimination diet
- ◆ The rotation diet
- ◆ Desensitization
- ◆ The use of digestive enzymes with meals

Once people see how great they feel without the symptoms, it becomes almost effortless to give up the foods that cause symptoms, because they know how they'll feel if they go back to eating it.

BASIC THINGS YOU CAN DO TO DISCOVER YOUR ALLERGIES

The Food Challenge

One of the best means of testing for food allergy is the home food challenge test. In this test, people usually go through a brief period of withdrawal from any allergenic foods they have eliminated. We usually wait until the seventh day before introducing suspected foods so that they have had four days of withdrawal and then perhaps three positive days after that. From the seventh day on, people can test one food at a time by reintroducing it into their diet.

Typically, this test is done at lunchtime, when a large amount of a particular food is consumed as the only food in a "mono-meal." If there are no obvious symptoms within thirty minutes to an hour, the person can repeat half of the amount of the meal again and then wait three to six hours. The food should be tested at a time when you are not at work and your attention is not being diverted, when you can focus on yourself. If there's no clear reaction after three to six hours, often the reaction will manifest on awakening the next morning. People may feel even worse upon awakening and feel very much hung over. And if the response is really powerful and uncharacteristic, that could also be a sign of delayed food response.

In these situations, wait until the reaction has completely subsided before testing another food. If you want to expedite your recovery, then you can take something like milk of magnesia to force the food out of your system completely. Otherwise, you may have to wait two or three days until you are totally over the first reaction and ready to test something else. Allow your system to clear thoroughly. The home food challenge test is often considered the gold mark standard for food allergy. It's best done when you have enough time and attention.

The Pulse Test

The pulse test (or Coca Test) is named after Dr. Coca, a famous allergist at Columbia University in the 1920s. He found that when people with food allergies ate an allergenic food during the sensitive period, they could experience an increase in their pulse rate of at least 12 beats a minute. Determine your baseline pulse over a period of a week. If you find that your pulse has gone up to least 12 to 16 beats per minute when you consume the offending food, that serves as a positive test. Most people will not get all the symptoms of allergies at once, but often they will get some of them within an hour of ingesting an allergic food and usually within three hours.

Dealing with Reactions

Bicarbonate can often be used by itself to treat an accidental food allergy reaction. When feeling unwell after a restaurant meal, consider taking Alka-Seltzer Gold, which can sometimes dispel the symptoms completely within five minutes. The theory is that some food allergies may be caused by a food that is not totally digested. There is proof now that a lot of food is not fully broken down when it is absorbed, especially if a person has a leaky gut. Food particles that are not totally digested may be absorbed. If they are proteins, the theory is that they can cause an allergic reaction that may trigger the entire spectrum of food allergy responses. When you add extra digestive enzymes and some bicarbonate, the food can be broken down more thoroughly. This approach is most helpful for someone whose body doesn't produce enough enzymes or enough bicarb.

HOW TO USE THE ROTATION DIET

Some people with serious food allergies choose to rotate foods every four days. The rotation diet offers major benefits: it allows you to minimize your exposure to any one food and it makes it just a little easier to observe the foods you may be reacting to.

When people are reactive to a wide range of foods, it's not enough to simply eliminate one or two foods. The best solution is to rotate many different foods to make sure that no one food is repeated too often and to assure a variety of foods in the diet. In a rotation diet, any food that is eaten one day is usually not repeated for another four days. So you devise a diet with foods that are eaten together for day 1, day 2, day 3, and day 4. Then day 1 is repeated on the fifth day and day 2 is repeated on the sixth day and so forth. In that sort of diet, you want to put foods together that you like to eat together. So you have a list of starches and flesh protein foods and vegetables and fruits and beans. And you make sure that whatever is consumed together stays together on that day.

Another important aspect of these diets is the rotation of food families. The principle here is that foods fall into biological families. For instance, lemons, grapefruits, oranges, and limes are all in the citrus family. There is a percentage of the population whose allergies are more severe and who must do a more careful food rotation. In these cases, foods can be grouped by food family. Lemons and oranges might be eaten on Monday and Friday, but limes and grapefruits would be taken on Wednesday and Sunday. In that way, you can actually eat food in the same family four times in one week.

A Rotation Diet for Severe Allergies

People with severe food allergies may need a seven-day rotation. These are people who are still reactive to food on a four-day rotation diet. In one sense, the seven-day rotation is much easier because the days of the week never change. What you eat on Monday is always what you eat on Monday. If you require this diet, it can be used to your advantage. For example, you can devise a menu so that what you eat on Saturday and Sunday is always the same and that way you can design very nice meals for the weekend. Every day remains the same.

People with a lot of allergies may find that some of their allergies are permanent. In this case, they need to completely eliminate these foods from their diet so that they are not even in the rotation. Then they would eat everything else on a rotation basis. Most foods would be taken every four days. However, a few foods might be eaten on an every-seven-or-eight-day basis, depending on the level of sensitivity.

It's helpful to remember that cooked food is less allergenic than raw food. Cooked tomato sauce tends to be less allergenic than a raw tomato. The same is true for applesauce in comparison with an apple. That may explain why some people are allergic to apples but can eat applesauce. And another basic principle is that people tend to be more allergic to foods in cold weather than in warm weather. So there may be more reactivity in the winter than in the summer months.

USING DIGESTIVE ENZYMES

Pancreatic digestive enzymes or pancreatin—depending on the strength of the product, from one to three tablets can be taken either toward the end of the meal or even fifteen or twenty minutes after the meal. This is based on the theory that pancreatic insufficiency is one of the causes of food allergies.

Bicarbonate can be taken after the enzymes. The bicarbonate helps the pancreatic enzymes to work by creating the necessary alkaline environment. One of the bicarbonates that has been used a lot is Alka-Seltzer Gold because it has no aspirin in it. It's a combination of sodium and potassium bicarbonate.

Apparently people with food allergies may not be producing enough pancreatic digestive enzymes or perhaps not enough bicarbonate. If you replenish vital digestants and nutrients, digestion can improve, the food particles are broken down more finely, and fewer reactions result. Another perspective on of food allergy proposes that the problem may involve not only the size of the food particle but also the lining of the gut and the leaky gut syndrome (see Chapter 7).

TESTING BY AN ALLERGIST

There are a number of ways to medically test for food allergies. Some people lack the time or inclination to do accurate home challenge testing.

Skin Testing

Another way to test for food allergy is skin testing. There are different kinds of skin tests.

♦ *The prick or scratch test* used by most allergists is notoriously inadequate for the testing of food allergy and tends to produce inaccurate results (false negatives and false positives). The test findings often don't correlate very well with what we see in the food challenge tests.

♦ *Intradermal testing* involves injecting the allergen underneath the skin (raising a small bubble), rather than just scratching the skin. This method tends to be more accurate.

♦ *Skin testing to find the degree of individual sensitivity.* There's another form of skin testing that was devised by the very famous allergist Dr. Rinkel during the 1940s and further developed by Dr. Joseph Miller in Alabama. The idea here is to determine not just whether a person is positive or not positive, but to find the exact level of sensitivity that an individual has to that food so a specific treatment dose or antidote can be created for that person. In this evaluation, intradermal skin tests are performed, but varying dilutions are used for each allergenic food. As part of the test, two or three or more injections of each specific food are given, each injection in a different concentration (dilutions of one to five). At the end of the testing, the antidotes for all foods causing allergies can be put together in one formula. Injections of the antidote can be given on an individual schedule, depending on the severity of the allergy. Some people take them every day or even several times a day. Others get injections twice a week.

Treating Allergies with Simple Antidotes

Another technique is to give these doses under the tongue (sublingually). In that case, the doses are usually taken two to three times a day. The length of treatment depends on the case and the person. The therapy may be given for one or two years, or it may be required indefinitely. People are usually retested about once a year to see if their doses have shifted. This particular technique of testing is used more by ear, nose, and throat physicians rather than traditional allergists. Traditional allergists do not typically give an antidote treatment for foods (such as desensitization), whereas Dr. Rinkel and Dr. Miller certainly did, and they found the method to be very helpful.

THE ELIMINATION DIET

Unmasking the Allergy

Often you can predict the foods someone will be allergic to if he or she says, "You can take anything out of my diet, Doctor, but please don't ask me to give up chocolate." It is possible to crave bread or corn or peanuts—any food. Taking a medical history for food allergies involves asking people about the foods they love and crave the most and what they would miss the most if they had to give it up. Often the food that is craved the most is the food that is triggering allergies.

When a food is eliminated, a process of unmasking occurs in which a person may feel worse rather than better. They may actually go through a period of withdrawal very similar to the withdrawal experienced by people with alcohol or drug addiction. This period of time usually lasts about four days. Often on one or two of those days, patients will crave the very foods that have been removed from their diets and may have uncomfortable symptoms such as diarrhea, aches, pains, a runny nose, or fatigue. That is the unmasking or the withdrawal effect.

Overcoming the Allergy—What to Do and What Not to Do

During the withdrawal period, the person becomes resensitized to that food. In other words, the numbness that built up during tolerance goes away, and the person becomes much more sensitive to that food. After the four days of the withdrawal period, the person enters a supersensitive state. For the next three weeks or so—usually until the end of the month—there are another twenty-six days of being super-sensitive. During that period, if a person eats the food he or she is sensitive to, there will be an exaggerated reaction to the allergenic food that is much greater than when the person was eating the food every day.

When we are eating an allergenic food every day, our body masks our reaction. We may feel numb and be unaware of any reactivity. When the allergy is unmasked and we become sensitive once again, then a strong response can be elicited. We may become as sensitive as we would have been as a baby.

It's important to be very strict for the first four weeks. I have had people who were very careful for two weeks, then said, "Well, I've been invited out to a dinner party and I've been so good for two weeks. I'll treat myself—after all, it's only one meal." And then they may get extremely sick. A markedly exaggerated reaction can occur, which could include almost any kind of response, but it is usually unmistakable. Mental symptoms—your mind may suddenly go totally blank. Extreme fatigue may come on abruptly. Intense muscle aches and pains or headache could occur suddenly. The symptoms could be anything abdominal from nausea and vomiting to diarrhea or extreme gas. It could be a skin rash or even hives. It could be a rapid pulse. This period of heightened sensitivity typically lasts at least four weeks. Once it is over, it is usually possible to rotate these foods back into the diet without creating a reaction.

HEALING THE LEAKY GUT SYNDROME

Allergically sensitized foods can be the result of *or* the cause of leaky gut.

In one form, oversized particles are absorbed directly into the lining cells of the GI tract, so things penetrate the cell far too quickly. There are not enough guards or sentries available for protection. Bigger particles that shouldn't get through go right into the cell in transcellular absorption.

The other kind of leaky gut is one in which particles penetrate between the cells (paracellular). There are pores between the cells. If the lining is incomplete or damaged, there may not be enough cells to go around and particles sneak in between the cells and get into the bloodstream and the system. I would imagine that either of these malfunctions could contribute to food allergies.

There are various ways to correct a leaky gut. One of the theories is that it's caused by dysbiosis, by parasites, by yeast, or even by a major overgrowth of normal bowel flora. There are a number of nutrients you can take for leaky gut syndrome that might result from food allergies.

Zinc is one of the primary nutrients I use because it's critically important for growth and wound healing. Zinc is essential to the cells that have rapid turnover, particularly the lining cells of the GI tract. These cells are replaced about every four days, so zinc can be rapidly depleted in the body. In addition, zinc levels tend to be going down in the American diet. In older people especially, it is not unusual to find evidence of zinc deficiency. Among its many functions, zinc also increases the release of vitamin A from the liver. If you are zinc deficient, you may actually have a nice storehouse of vitamin A in the liver and be unable make use of it.

Vitamin A is the other vitamin essential to digestive health. It is responsible for the integrity of lining cells of all the mucosal surfaces of the body, including the entire digestive tract. It is also necessary for the production of the secretory IgA, the antibodies that protect the GI tract.

Glutamine is one of the hallmark nutrients now used to treat leaky gut. It raises the levels of growth hormone vital for wound healing and new protein synthesis. For that reason alone it may play an essential role in restoring the lining of the gut. And glutamine itself is often used as a fuel by many of the cells in the body in place of glucose.

MSM, a form of the mineral sulfur, is an exciting nutrient that produces encouraging results. It tends to be very soothing and healing to the entire digestive tract. It helps to prevent oxidative stress throughout the GI tract and it's also supposed to prevent pathogens from adhering to the gut wall—potentially harmful bacteria, yeast and parasites.

DGL (deglycyrrhizinated licorice), is a type of licorice that has had the glycerin removed. It's also very soothing to the upper GI tract and may help to promote healing and get rid of leaky gut.

Growth factors are another kind of substance that is gaining wider recognition. They have been used to treat all kinds of GI disorders, including colitis, Crohn's disease, and irritable bowel syndrome. Growth factors are found in DGL, glandular products, and peptides (the building blocks of protein). Sea Cure is a peptide product extracted from predigested white fish. The effect on conditions like irritable bowel syndrome can sometimes be very profound.

As a doctor, the other important way I help people heal leaky gut is through stress reduction. Stress raises cortisol output and excess cortisol can cause ulcers and impair the lining of the gut. So stress reduction is also a very important treatment for leaky gut and may be a factor in some allergies as well.

21

Clearing Bad Bugs

THE TEAM

❖

If you've been sick for a while and don't have a diagnosis, review this chapter carefully to see if any of the symptoms or patterns here match your experience.

Doctors of nutritional medicine are now finding that microbes are often the underlying and undiagnosed cause of many health problems. The microbes may be undiagnosed parasites, an overgrowth of yeast or bacteria, or even viruses. They can cause illnesses that don't seem to relate to the digestive tract, including allergies, asthma, arthritis, or even neurological problems. These problems are frequently overlooked by most doctors and gastroenterologists. Research by the Centers for Disease Control (the CDC) shows that far more than 90 percent of the parasites found are microscopic—invisible to the naked eye and difficult to detect in the lab without special expertise. We offer strategies from a number of knowledgeable practitioners:

- ◆ Find out if bad bugs are the problem
- ◆ How to get rid of them
- ◆ Strengthen your immunity to guard against future infections

How Often Are Parasites a Problem?

TIMOTHY KUSS, Ph.D.

The United States is now also seeing an increasing prevalence of parasite-related problems. Worldwide, more than one billion people are infected with parasites. But the problem is also a lot closer to home. In Milwaukee, in 1993, over 40,000 people were sickened by the mi-

All They Did Was Drink the Water

◈

Helen and Dave went camping for a long weekend and brought the children. They noticed the warnings in the park not to drink the water in the fountains (giardia, it said). But they never dreamed the water served in the roadside diner would cause problems. After all, they were in America, not the tropics. When they got home, everybody got sick. A flu, some kind of bug. After a few days they all got better. Except Helen.

Helen had Montezuma's revenge—diarrhea that just wouldn't stop. She counted the days. Surely it would stop in a few days. She went to the doctor. No apparent cause.

Days stretched into weeks, and weeks into months. She went to another doctor and another. Then she went to a psychiatrist who had a lot to say about her childhood. But none of that had any effect on the diarrhea.

She couldn't digest anything but oatmeal, so her weight dropped pretty low. She could no longer work; in fact, she couldn't really leave the house for very long. Her energy was gone. She still cooked for the family—as it turns out, a major mistake. Her world had telescoped down into a narrow little life—no job, no travel, no dinner parties. No food, no alcohol, no sex.

The months turned into years. Surely she'd get better! But the diarrhea continued. She looked like a death-camp victim—skin and bone, 82 pounds. The doctor had run a stool sample. Dave asked him to do another, just in case. It had been over two years. The report came back with "Giardia. Known to cause persistent diarrhea."

Helen took the drug and within ten days things started to turn around. The diarrhea slowed, then stopped all together. And she could eat again. She didn't have those constant stomachaches and that awful feeling of being toxic that she couldn't really explain to anybody. Dave did some research at the medical library and found there was another drug that was useful as well. Three months after the first medication, Helen took the second. Within another three months, she was almost well! She could eat anything. She called the state college and enrolled. By fall, she was immersed in a full-time graduate program. It was all just a memory.

A happy ending. For Helen, yes. But not for Dave. What neither of them knew at the time is that parasites like giardia are transmitted on human hands and in water and food. Whenever she cooked for Dave and handled the food, the bug could be passed along to him. Dave didn't get diarrhea, but he did get the infection. And in the end, he came out worse than Helen. As the doctor says, "When it comes to parasites, don't pussyfoot around. Get tested and get treated."

croscopic parasite cryptosporidium. Of these, over 4,000 were hospitalized and at least 100 died.

In a national survey, about one in seven people were found to have parasites. The review was conducted in 1976 by the Centers for Disease Control. Almost half a million samples were reviewed (450,000). If the survey had been conducted today, the figures would probably be quite a bit higher—maybe twice as high, about one person in three—due to more advanced lab techniques and increased incidence.

Parasitic disease is on the rise due to many factors, including

♦ Increased international travel
♦ Immigration
♦ The manufacturing and shipping of food internationally
♦ Worldwide urban crowding
♦ Restaurant food handlers as a major source of parasite dissemination

These trends are occurring on a massive scale that makes monitoring difficult. World travel, migration, transport, and trade occurs on a level unheard of at any earlier point in history. People, animals, food, even ships are all potential mediums for the transport of microbes. As the CDC points out, disease is only a plane flight away from anywhere in the world. Ships that discharge balast can transmit an entire microbial population, which then infects the shellfish and sea life in that area, spreading contamination such as cholera.

People may be unknowing carriers. In tropical regions, people inherit immunity developed over generations of adaptation to the microbes of that particular area. They themselves may be free of symptoms, but then may transmit the disease through personal contact or food handling to others who have not developed these immune protections.

THE MOST COMMON SYMPTOMS OF INFECTION BY PATHOGENS

Typical GI symptoms include recurrent diarrhea, alternating diarrhea and constipation, constipation alone, bloating and gas, abdominal pain or cramps, nausea, loss of appetite, or food cravings. These are often accompanied by poor digestion and poor absorption. General weakness or fatigue, which no amount of rest relieves, may be a sign.

Many physicians do not recognize how dangerous these organisms can be. They may be life-threatening or the cause of chronic illness.

Parasites Can Cause Illness Anywhere in the Body

OMAR AMIN, Ph.D.

In a survey of people found to have parasites in their stool, the Institute for Parasitic Diseases found they also had a variety of associated conditions.

◆ *Entamoeba histolytica*—fatigue, nausea, allergies, pain, weight loss, insomnia

◆ *Blastocystis hominis*—fatigue, nervous disorders, pain, skin conditions, nausea, allergies, muscle problems

◆ *E. coli (Entamoeba coli,* the parasite rather than the bacteria)—fatigue, allergies, headache, nausea, depression/lack of concentration/irritability, joint/back pain, skin problems

◆ *Entamoeba hartmanii*—nervous system, respiratory, and skin disorders, allergies, pain, nausea

◆ *Cyclospora*—fatigue, itching, nausea, anemia, headache, muscle aches, depression

FREQUENTLY SEEN MICROBES

◆ *Yeast, such as candida, normally found in the GI tract,* can overgrow and consume too many of our resources

◆ *Bacteria that normally reside in the body (aerobic, oxygen-loving types)* may overgrow due to imbalances caused by antibiotic overuse or misuse, or acute viral or bacterial infections that kill off some of the more vulnerable beneficial species, leaving others that are more hardy.

◆ *Other internal bacteria (anaerobes, the kind that thrive without oxygen)* may overgrow; these are less well known and harder to diagnose because they don't survive in the presence of oxygen.

◆ *Bacteria that come in with food and water, causing food poisoning and dysentery,* such as salmonella, shigella, or *E. coli.*

◆ *Parasites,* like giardia, in food or water can invade the body and take up residence.

◆ *Viruses* can also invade the body and survive in the cells for years (see Chapter 22).

Candida

OMAR AMIN, Ph.D.

The overgrowth of *Candida albicans* is well known to practitioners of nutritional medicine. What is less well known is the fact that candida infections often accompany parasitic infections. The energy drain on the system by the parasite tends to provide an opportunity for the candida.

An overgrowth of candida can cause physical symptoms. It can also decrease the beneficial bacteria. Researchers have found a definite relationship between the higher levels of fungal spores and lower levels of the desirable bacteria. This means the microorganisms are competing for the same limited space and finite supply of nourishment, in the closed ecosystem of the digestive tract. If there are factors that promote the growth of candida, it consumes the resources and the space that would have originally been allotted to the beneficial bacteria (lactobacillus and bifidus). These flora then decrease, limiting their positive role in the digestive process. Lab testing frequently demonstrates this change in balance.

Which came first? The decrease in the friendly flora or the overgrowth of candida? Stable flora are observed in very young children and it is true that candida is normally present in the gut of most people as a harmless coexisting organism (a commensal). However, if yeast becomes the dominant gut flora, it can become a destructive pathogen and take over in the digestive ecosystem. If the population of candida becomes too large and its strength and virulence increases, candida can cause considerable damage, especially in immune-compromised patients. The yeast can migrate to other tissues and become systemic candidiasis. Once candida becomes blood born and systemic, then every organ system is at risk. Systemic candidiasis can cause serious damage, particularly to the reproductive system in females once it develops as a chronic urogenital infection.

With candida results at low levels, if there are no symptoms, the patient is not treated. However, when a parasite is present (for example, an amoeba such as *E. histolytica*), even a low level yeast overgrowth is to be taken much more seriously, since it could become a moderate overgrowth or worse within a day.

Candida is sometimes a factor in ADD and autism. Overgrowth of candida and other species of yeast, particularly in children, due to overuse of antibiotics and sugar in their diet, can lead to the formation in the gut of abnormal organic acids, which are neurotoxic and have been associated with both attention deficit disorders and autism.

Specific Microbes

TRENT NICHOLS, M.D.

♦ Amoebic dysentery—*E. histolytica*—is an acute and chronic disease caused by the organism *Entamoeba histolytica,* which can affect the colon, the liver, and other organs. It can cause diarrhea or constipation, cramps, gas, and bloating. An estimated 5 percent of the U.S. population is infected by amoebas. It tends to be even more prevalent in South America and Mexico and is more frequently diagnosed in people who are traveling from tropical regions.

Occasionally, this pathogen can cause amoebic abscess of the liver. The sufferer will be extremely ill and typically have a history of travel to a tropical country, symptoms of bloody diarrhea, extreme discomfort, distention, and pain over the upper right abdominal area. Liver involvement or the presence of a cyst in the liver would be diagnosed by a CT scan.

♦ *Giardia lamblia* can cause diarrhea, cramps, and bloating, and is seen in patients with a history of drinking untreated water from camp sites, lakes, or rivers. Giardia is difficult to diagnose because of its variable life cycle; evaluation is usually done through stool testing or biopsy, but it may require several tests before a positive diagnosis is made. Giardia may also be diagnosed through antibody testing in blood, but the organism doesn't always match the antibody profile and may even be missed in this subtle testing.

Doctor's note: Giardia is the parasite treated most frequently in my practice here in Pennsylvania. It is pandemic worldwide because water supplies frequently contain giardia, particular those in wilderness areas.

♦ *Cryptosporidia* is becoming much more prevalent in the United States. It has only been recognized since 1976 as a cause of diarrheal disease in humans; before that, it was thought to only infect animals—such as pigs, calves, and mice. Cryptosporidium is transmitted through water and animal hosts including reptiles and birds. Both cryptosporidium and microsporidia are frequently contracted by AIDS patients.

♦ *Blastocystis hominis* is an intestinal protozoa. Patients who test positive for blastocystus do not always have symptoms. Symptoms may include diarrhea or severe constipation, weight loss, cramping, flatulence, or bloating. In the recent past, this microbe was considered to be nonpathogenic (an organism not causing symptoms). However, microbiologists have found that there are two different strains of blastocystus. One is believed to be tropical and quite virulent; some reports indicate that about a fourth of the people with blastocystus have this condition as a long-term chronic disease.

♦ *Microsporidia* is another pathogen observed in AIDS and immunodeficient patients, with symptoms of malabsorption, weight loss, and severe watery nonbloody diarrhea.

A number of other parasites have been recognized or reclassified as "emerging pathogens" in the recent past. This indicates either a change in the virulence of the microbe (their strength and ability to cause harm) or a change in our assessment of them as a potential medical problem. Other pathogenic parasites include *Dientamoeba fragilis*, cyclospora, and *E. hartmanii*.

HOW TO FIND MORE INFORMATION ON YOUR OWN

One of the resources doctors use to track the status of emerging pathogens is Medline, the online database of the National Library of Medicine at the National Institutes of Health. Medline is now accessible to the public as well, through the World Wide Web at www.nlm.nih.gov. To search millions of medical journals in an instant, go to Medline Plus and follow the instructions. You can make sure you're searching the right key words by checking the library's special MeSH headings.

Anaerobic Bacteria

RICHARD KUNIN, M.D.

The friendly bacteria in your body produce fatty acids that are essential to gut health. These fatty acids include butyrate, the preferred fuel for the colon, made by the beneficial bacteria from sugars. When we see an absence of butyrate in the stool, we may have indirect evidence that the body is not fermenting sugars properly.

Although current testing measures only the aerobic flora, the anaerobes make up more than 90 percent of the flora in the colon. Since stool samples pick up only the aerobic organisms, most of what we're seeing in lab tests is like the life on the surface of the pond. It tells you a lot about the condition of the pond, but it doesn't tell you everything that is in the pond.

Clearly part of the problem that we're running into is that people's aerobic organisms are crowding out the anaerobic organisms when there are chronic GI disorders. As far as I know, these are questions that remain unanswered.

Candida and the overgrowth of harmful bacteria can produce an abundance of toxic organic acids that have been linked to depressive illnesses, bipolar depression, and schizophrenia.

More on Anaerobic Bacteria

W. A. SHRADER, JR., M.D.

In the treatment of allergies and digestive illness, when the therapy is not effective, it is often because of overgrowth or infection—dysbiosis. People who have very complex problems may have undiagnosed dysbiosis. Often their symptoms are simply chronic fatigue.

We've found that a useful approach to gastrointestinal problems is to first treat with antibiotics and other therapies for pathogenic organisms and then provide allergy treatment (see Chapter 38). Most all the gastrointestinal problems we've been seeing seem to respond to this approach. Our treatments have addressed bacteria such as klebsiella and proteus.

We found that in certain cases, patients had an overgrowth of bacteria that wasn't showing up on lab tests. With some patients, the bacteria turn out to be anaerobes—microbes that live in the digestive tract without oxygen and are not detected in the presence of oxygen, such as bacteroides and *Clostridium difficile*. To date, there are only indirect ways to identify anaerobes by testing for the metabolic by-products of the bacteria. We use these tests as the basis for drug and allergy therapy and typcially see significant improvement.

Testing Indirectly for Anaerobes

There are currently a number of ways to indirectly gain information on anaerobes:

- Antibody testing—Immunosciences Laboratory
- Organic acids testing, the marker for *Clostridium difficile*— Metametrix and Great Plains Lab
- Monitoring metabolic by-products—butyrate levels in the GI tract, because they are made by the beneficial anaerobes. Butyrate levels are reported on the Great Smokies Diagnostic Lab CDSA report and also on the vitamin and mineral panel of Vitamin Diagnostics, New Jersey. (See the Resources section for information on all these labs.)

This area of testing is still under development and will continue to be refined in the coming years. Currently we use it to obtain indirect information on anaerobic bacteria.

CHRONIC VIRAL INFECTION

There is evidence that some viruses and even certain viral vaccines are now thought to damage GI lining cells, leading to eventual inflammatory and degenerative diseases of the gut. Many viruses that enter the body through the GI tract can cause systemic disease or disease in other organs. If the GI flora, digestion, or physiology are disrupted, this can lead to impaired gut function and allow viruses easier access to the body.

Parasitic Infection:
How Do You Know You Have a Problem?

JERRY STINE

In the case of parasites, lab work can be very constructive. Testing for parasites rarely finds parasites that aren't actually present (a false positive); this is almost unheard of.

- Parasites can be extremely difficult to detect.
- It's very common to get a report with no findings (a false negative) when there actually are parasites present.
- It is usually not adequate to trust a negative diagnosis on the basis of just one stool test. Labs will typically request two or three samples.
- There must be multiple stool collections.
- When checking the levels of friendly flora on lab tests such as

the CDSA, an absence of *E. coli* suggests the presence of a parasite.

♦ If the person has been sick for a long time and nothing shows on the stool testing, it's worth doing additional testing for the chemical by-products or antibody trails created by different pathogens. Never lose sight of the fact that the symptoms and history may tell you as much as the lab work.

Lab Testing

♦ Stool testing—Institute of Parasitic Diseases (IPD), Diagnos-Techs, and university labs nationwide

♦ Candida—Great Smokies Diagnostic Lab, IPD, and Diagnos-Techs

♦ Organic acids, possible by-products of candida and harmful bacteria, testing by Metametrix and Great Plains Lab

♦ Antibody testing—Immunosciences Laboratory and Diagnos-Techs

♦ Markers for inflammation—Diagnos-Techs and Functional Medicine Center

INTEGRATIVE TREATMENT: CLEARING BAD BUGS

Removing pathogens or eradication refers to programs to clear or kill a harmful microbe, a pathogen. Clearing the GI tract can also mean minimizing the overgrowth of a microbe that is normally harmless (a commensal) but which is taking over the ecosystem of the digestive tract and crowding out beneficial bacteria.

The most destructive of the pathogens are generally the parasites, usually single-celled protozoa. The most common overgrowth is probably yeast, particularly the candida species. There are some bacteria that can also overgrow, although yeast are still the most common. *H. pylori* bacteria is the pathogen most often associated with problems in the stomach, with stomach ulcers, another example of a target for eradication.

Objective

♦ *The objective of eradication is to kill off the targeted microorganisms as completely as possible.* It's very important to have a clear idea of the most effective drugs to use in eradication because the drug therapies are very particular to specific organisms. A few of the drugs such as metronidazole are widely used and appear to be losing their effectiveness. Multiple drug therapies at high doses can improve results. It is essential to be very thorough and resolute in the treatment, because any pathogens that survive tend to become stronger.

◆ *Prepare for treatment.* For someone who is weakened by chronic illness, this may mean going through a period of strengthening before taking the drug. It may also involve a functional liver exam (the kind given by Great Smokies) to be sure the person's liver can handle the medication. In addition, it may involve treating family members or a partner to be sure that the microbe is not simply passed back and forth through food handling or intimate contact.

◆ *Organisms that survive drug treatment are stronger than those killed off in the first days* of the treatment. Therefore, it is important to finish the full course of the antibiotic. Again, the objectives are to get a clear lab diagnosis and have a committed program of drug therapy.

Treat Decisively

Once the decision is made to proceed, you must proceed with considerable strength to make sure you are killing everything that's there. *H. pylori* is in a similar category to the parasites. Very aggressive therapy is recommended to make sure it is eradicated so that the patient is not left with a stronger species than they started with.

Special Considerations

There are two major considerations.

◆ *The first is to have the clearest, most comprehensive diagnosis before treating.* Know what is being treated for.

◆ *The second is to use the strongest, safest drug therapy available.* Often the best approach is a combination of drugs and herbs— typically a course of one or more drugs followed by a carefully chosen program of treatment with herbs. One may be specifically targeted against the pathogen drug and the other may be a systemic medication, backed up by some botanical product.

Drug-Resistant Microbes

There is always some downside to using a set of powerful antibiotics. However, the risk of not completely eradicating the parasites and being left with an even stronger version of what you tried to kill is generally worse, because the remaining parasites will be resistant. An example is giardia. In the United States, it now appears that about 40 percent are resistant to Flagyl, and that's probably often the result of drug doses that are too low or never finished.

In the case of candida and some of the other organisms that tend to overgrow, we have a different situation. It's not that difficult to get rid of candida, but keeping it from coming back can be a problem. It is important to remember that improving GI immune function is the real key when it comes to the overgrowth of organisms like candida. It also involves looking at some of the other steps in the digestive repair process. (See Chapter 25 on restoring and repairing the GI tract.)

Integrative Treatment: Using Drugs and Herbs Together
TIMOTHY KUSS, Ph.D.

As important as antibiotics are in the treatment of pathogens, antibiotics can only be taken for a specific period of time. They can't be taken indefinitely; some are too harsh for the lining of the GI tract or cause nausea unless taken with food. Others may cause certain side effects. Once a course of antibiotics has been completed, it can be helpful to take herbs, which are milder, to prevent reinfection and keep any residual candida under control. Every time food is consumed, measures must be taken to address dysbiosis.

HERBAL REMEDIES

Even though the herbs are natural substances, they are antibiotic (destructive to microbial life) and must be treated with respect just as a drug would be.

The herbs are best begun gradually. Take one herb the first day, preferably in the morning and preferably on a weekend, on a day set aside, so that if a cleansing effect results, the dosage may be adjusted or the herb may be stopped before the workweek begins. The second day, also take one of the herbs. Then increase to two a day, and keep this level for two days, building up to four a day—one twenty minutes before each meal and one at bedtime.

If too strong a dose of herbs is taken, a headache may occur, a sign

---

Parasites and Candida—Sample Program
Jerry Stine

History
- The Health Profile (score of 50 or above is significant)
- GI, skin, or upper respiratory symptoms are key (need not be acute)
- Emotional or mental complaints
  —Anxiety or depression
  —Spacey, foggy-headed, poor memory
- Possible exposure
  —Travel to third world countries
  —Exposure to contaminated drinking water, lakes, rivers
  —Exposure to infected family member
  —Eating out at restaurants

Lab Work
- Testing for markers of inflammation, protective antibodies—Immunosciences Lab
- Stool culture—Institute of Parasitic Diseases
- Functional Liver Detoxification Test (impact on liver)—Great Smokies Diagnostic Lab

Stage 1. Strengthening
- Improve nutrition, decrease starchy diet (40-30-30 Fat Burning Nutrition)
- Supplements—individual
- Reduce toxins in personal environment
- Duration—until improvement is seen

Stage 2. Treatment
- Drugs as prescribed by a physician
- Recommended herbs during and after treatment

Follow-up
- Rehab program—see Chapter 25

---

of toxicity. Occasionally this is the sign of a healing crisis, but it may also be a sign that the herb is too strong or disagrees in some way. Stop the herb and retry it in a week.

DIE-OFF

The die-off reaction can be counterproductive in many cases because you're killing off microorganisms (yeast, fungus, protozoa) at a pace quicker than the eliminative organs—the liver and the GI tract—can competently handle. That can be disruptive to the entire body because the eliminative resources must be utilized to minimize the ill effects of the microbes.

Additionally, you have disrupted the microbes themselves, so they can actually migrate (transmigrate) and affect other areas of the body that they had not previously been affecting. Further, the toxins that are released must also be handled by the eliminative organs. The kidneys, liver, and intestinal tract can become overwhelmed. The toxic by-products could circulate and recirculate through the blood and lymphatics causing possible die-off symptoms such as fatigue, achiness, fever, and difficulty concentrating, sometimes resembling a mild case of the flu.

The appropriate dosing is important: Microdosing may be helpful in the early stage of treatment. Begin by increasing the dosage gradually in order to prevent uncomfortable die-off. Then proceed to the full dose for the entire duration. Conventional medicine and herbal medicine are both used too quickly, too aggressively. Low dosing has the potential to create a generation of microbes that are drug resistant, having survived the initial dose.

Dosage must be determined in part by body type and by body weight. A. S. Wheelwright, a famous herbalist, suggested that people tend to have either robust or sensitive body types. The robust types are large-boned, hearty, and rarely sick. However, because they do not experience low grade symptoms, they may develop cumulative illnesses. Sensitive body types are more delicate and tend to be more prone to chronic illness.

Another consideration in dosing is the condition of the liver. This can be determined by a functional liver panel.

DIGESTANTS

One strategy to complement other therapies is to take digestants between meals to improve digestion and perhaps even digest some of the bad bugs.

◆ *Betaine hydrochloride.* Other people with parasitic infections don't have enough hydrochloric acid in the beginning, opening the gateway to the pathogen.

◆ *Pancreatin (pancreatic digestive enzymes).* In some cases, enzyme

HERBS THAT CAN BE USED TO FOLLOW DRUG THERAPY

Plant-Based Supplements*

Artemisia	Pau d'arco
Echinacea	Tannic acid (Tanalbit)
Olive leaf extract	Ayurvedic tincture (AP-Mag)
Cat's claw	Grapefruit seed extract (NutriBiotic)

Mineral-Based Supplements*

Elemental iodine (Paracidin)	Bismuth (Pepto-Bismol)
Sulfur-based (MSM-methyl sulfonyl methane)	

Antiparasitic Formulas

VRM 3 (Wormseed)—Systemic Formulas	Biocidin—Biological Research
Parex Intensive Care—Metagenics	Verma Key—Unikey
Tricycline—Allergy Research Group	Para-Relief—Prevail
Para-Guard—Tyler	Ag-CIDAL—Allergy Research
ParaGONE—Brenda Watson	Clear—Awareness (cleansing formula)

SOURCE: Omar Amin, Ph.D., Institute of Parasitic Diseases, and the Team
*Green herbs can be alternated with mineral-based supplements or bitter herbs.

production becomes compromised as a result of the pathogen (in a self-protective mechanism).

Digestants are useful to some—they aid in digesting protein, so taking them between meals may actually help digest the pathogens in the gut. However, some people report the development of moles or spots of pigmentation following heavy use of pancreatin. So it may be a universal healer—a silver bullet—and it may be a potential toxin.

Nutrition
LEN SAPUTO, M.D.

The health of the mucosal lining of the gut is important in maintaining our resistance, and immune resistance is a powerful determinant controlling which microflora can survive. It is easy to understand that nutritional support for the cells of the gut mucosa is necessary to maintain our most effective defense mechanisms. Some important nutrients that are often used to support gut nutrition and repair include:

- A good multivitamin with minerals
- Vitamin A, 10,000–25,000 IU per day (not for premenopausal women)
- Special nutrients like L-glutamine, phosphatidyl choline, essential fatty acids, magnesium
- Antioxidant support with vitamin C, coenzyme Q10, lipoic acid, glutathione, ginkgo biloba, grapeseed extract, vitamin E, beta-carotene
- Epidermal growth factor
- Bioflavonoids like quercitin
- Immune stimulants such as deglycyrrhizinated licorice, *Saccharomyces boulardii,* beta 1,3 glucan, inositol hexaphosphate, echinacea, astragalus, and thymus extract
- Consider juicing with vegetables (one to two quarts per day of fresh veggies)

BAD BUGS AND BEYOND

If the problems are caught early enough and the treatment is resolute enough, this may be enough. The person may be restored to his or her normal way of life, and this entire experience becomes something like a bad dream.

However, some people find that they do not recover after the very first round of antibiotics. People in this situation will want to consider adding:

1. Treatment to support the whole body and the immune system.

2. A major therapy such as acupuncture, once a month or once a week, as affordable.

3. A lab analysis of general nutrient levels, since the deficiency of one or more essential nutrients has been found to block healing. This has been reported in the medical literature in many thousands of studies.

4. Other systemic treatment, such as treatment with thymus extract or intravenous vitamin therapy to boost the immune response.

5. Remove other drags on the immune system, such as food allergies (see Chapter 20) and environmental toxins (see Chapter 23).

6. Rebalancing lifestyle (see Chapter 28) and gentle exercise (see Chapter 43).

7. Increased attention to self-nurturance to reduce stress (see especially Chapters 44 and 47). Maintain a meaningful life while you and your doctor, working together, sort through the options to find the right combination that heals you.

22

The Problem of Viruses

RICHARD A. KUNIN, M.D.

❖

Whenever possible, use preventive strategies to avoid viral infection. Removing a virus is extremely difficult. We have fewer treatments for viruses, and among the microbes, viruses tend to be some of the most pathogenic and virulent. Our main strategies against viruses at this point are primarily avoidance, and maintenance of strong immunity. Since most viruses are transmitted by contact, personal hygiene is ultimately the best defense.

Viruses are mysterious infective agents. They are capable of passing through filters that retain most bacteria (such as your water filter). They are usually not visible through the light microscope, which meant for years we were missing them in the lab until the electron microscope was invented. Viruses contain only DNA or RNA, but not both, which is why they are incapable of growth or reproduction apart from living cells. So they must seek out a host in order to grow and multiply. They have a protein coat, which is what our immune antibodies identify in order to detect them.

When it comes to the digestive tract, we often think of the bacteria that cause food poisoning such as salmonella or *E. coli*. But we should also be taking viruses seriously. When we have the flu, we remember all over again how formidable viruses can be. Viruses are an ongoing problem because they mutate and new strains emerge. This should motivate us to sustain our nutrient levels, preserve our immunity, and maintain basic hygiene.

A REVIEW OF THE DIGESTIVE TRACT

Mouth

Cold sores (herpes and aphthous stomatitis) are usually caused by the herpes virus. Lowered immune resistance is a big factor. Treatment with a liquid sodium selenite gargle three times per day for five days can be soothing. Vitamin C gargle has also been helpful. The amino acid lysine has been found effective in the case of herpes mouth ulcers and along with Vitamins A, B complex, E, and the mineral zinc tends to be generally preventive of cold sores.

The lymphoid tissue in the tonsils and adenoids (also known as Waldeyer's ring) is a common site of viral and bacterial invasion and combat. Most sore throats are relieved by the local application of vitamin E. The synthetic d-alpha-tocopherol is better tasting, though recent evidence suggests gamma-tocopherol may be a stronger antioxidant. The low 100 IU dose is usually appreciated for its soothing qualities and anti-inflammatory effect. General immune enhancers include echinacea, goldenseal, vitamin C, garlic, and pau d'arco.

Stomach and Upper GI Tract

Inflammation in the upper intestine by viruses and other microbes usually sends a signal to the lower tract via the nerve networks of the bowel. This can promote bloating and disturb motility along the length of the gut.

Intestinal viruses (enteroviruses) often cause intestinal complaints, even though they are especially identified with respiratory tract symptoms. In fact, they can also cause neurological symptoms.

Paralysis is associated with several of the enteroviruses: Coxsackie A7, echovirus 4,6, enterovirus 71, and polio viruses 1–3. The Coxsackie virus group B is also known to cause inflammation of the brain, heart, lungs, and pancreas, leaving some of the children with Type I diabetes. Herpangina syndrome is a painful rash on the palate and pharynx in children, and is caused by the Coxsackie virus. Persistence of Coxsackie viral infections is known to occur and may be a cause of chronic fibromyalgia and chronic fatigue syndromes. One clue is that such infections induce interferon alpha and beta production in the infected cells which can be measured by blood tests.

Epidemic intestinal viruses, such as rotavirus, Norwalk virus, astrovirus, and adenovirus 40 and 41 that cause gastroenteritis typically travel in epidemics. This makes diagnosis a bit easier. Adenovirus usually expresses itself as pneumonia, with diarrhea as a frequent accompaniment. Poliomyelitis begins with nausea and diarrhea and can be mistaken for flu. Paralysis occurs in only a small number of cases, so misdiagnosis is common.

Measles in the GI tract is important because it can persist and cause reinfection, even years or decades later. It has been reported in the dendritic immune cells of the intestine, but this finding remains controversial. However, it is known that the measles virus binds to receptors on T cell lymphocytes (the CD46 receptors). Binding to the receptor inactivates the T cell and also appears to suppress transmembrane signaling by the lymphocytes, inhibiting the activation of nearby immune cells.

This causes localized immune deficiency and would explain some cases of chronic inflammatory bowel disease in which measles appears to cause inflammation indirectly, by creating vulnerability to secondary infection. Such infections might involve microbes that are normally noninvasive, but which cause symptoms due to the local immune suppression induced by the latent measles virus. Because the secondary infection can be caused by any of a great number of microbes (yeast, bacteria, or parasite species), the syndrome is extremely individual and the diagnosis elusive.

It is helpful to know that the invasiveness of measles (virulence) is reduced by vitamin A (retinol) in the circulation. By that token, it makes sense to measure vitamin A levels and treat bowel disease with vitamin A at restorative doses. Of course, vitamin A is essential for immune response in general, and as an integral part of cellular healing. In addition, the use of Monolaurin, which contains lauric acid, a fatty acid that binds to the fatty coat of the measles virus, is also worthy of consideration in treating dysbiosis of the intestine.

Lower Small Intestine (Ileum) and Colon

There remains a surprising amount of confusion over the role of viral infection in chronic bowel disease. From my own clinical observation and experience, I am inclined to consider the herpes virus as an additional inflammatory factor, especially since this family of viruses is notorious for reinfection under conditions of stress or tissue inflammation from other, unrelated causes. Herpes I and II both thrive when the host defenses are down and serve to amplify inflammation and aggravate the damage to the bowel lining at such times. There is undoubtedly interaction between food allergy and viral infection—both ways.

The Liver

Inflammation of the pancreas and liver are common in viral illness. Hepatitis virus A, B, and C and hepatitis due to the Epstein-Barr virus (the cause of mononucleosis) can all cause loss of appetite, nausea, vomiting, bile retention, and impaired digestive function that can go on for weeks, months, or years. The use of N-acetyl-cysteine 500 mg, milk thistle 300 mg, lipoic acid 100 mg, and ascorbic acid 1000 mg— all taken three times per day for a couple of weeks has been associated with remarkable recoveries.

These viruses can often be measured in blood by testing for antibody levels (titer) for IgG antibodies (gradual onset) and IgM antibodies (acute episode).

Anal and Perineal Area

Venereal warts are caused by viral activity in the anal area and are becoming more and more common. They can be difficult to eradicate. When the venereal warts become enlarged and covered by a fibrous coat, they are best removed by a CO_2 laser. (Preventive measures: Sexual contact is the means by which this infection is acquired and spread to others. Condoms tend to be generally preventive.)

Herpes viruses are especially common in the anal canal and associated with hemorrhoids, rectal prolapse, and perineal blisters. Treatment with Monolaurin capsules taken orally and local salve or cream are a safe adjunct in quelling herpes infections and deserves a trial for at least a week. Doses up to five capsules three times per day have been helpful in my experience. Local application of skin cream containing lemon balm (melissa), lysine, or lithium have all claimed success. Of course, if herpes antibody tests are positive, the use of antiviral agents such as acyclovir (Zovirax) is standard. I prefer Monolaurin, however, due to its safety, its lack of adverse effects, and its broad spectrum of activity against lipid-coated viruses.

RICHARD A. KUNIN, M.D., is founder and president of the Society for Ortho-molecular Health-Medicine, and he has been active in private practice in nutritional medicine and psychiatry since 1963. He took his medical degree at the University of Minnesota and was an NIH Special Fellow in neurophysiology at the Stanford University. Dr. Kunin is a diplomate in psychiatry and has served as an instructor at Cornell University School of Medicine and the College of Osteopathic Medicine of the Pacific, and was consultant to the state of California in mental health research. He is the author of the bestsellers *MegaNutrition* and *MegaNutrition for Women,* and he has given more than sixty presentations worldwide on a wide variety of topics in nutrition. Dr. Kunin has a private medical practice in orthomolecular health-medicine in San Francisco and can be reached at 415-346-2500.

The Society of Orthomolecular Health-Medicine can be contacted at 2698 Pacific Avenue, San Francisco, CA 94115, or by calling 415-922-6462.

23

Avoid Toxic Exposure

JEFFRY ANDERSON, M.D.

❖

For the average American, toxic exposure is subtle and yet ever-present. To avoid ongoing exposure, you will need to think about the source of your water, the safety of your food, chemicals in everyday products, and so on. The primary concept of environmental medicine is to diminish the load—the burden on your body—and to stop further exposure. Some people tend to be more sensitive to toxins than others. Both low level and intense exposure can cause a wide variety of symptoms in the GI tract and throughout the body.

Worth the Effort

❖

Sarah had been sick for about fourteen years. She knew she was getting better a little bit at a time, but the source of her GI inflammation remained an unknown to both Sam and her doctors. When she began reading up on pesticides, the size and extent of the problem overwhelmed her and she decided to eat more organics. Since her menu was quite restricted, it wasn't hard to switch over, so she began buying everything organic—just as an experiment. She was astonished to realize that her symptoms were better! Clearly not the whole answer, but eating food free of chemicals seemed to reduce the inflammation—perhaps 10 or 15 percent.

She was so encouraged that when she learned fluoride can also be an irritant, she switched toothpastes as well and began using baking soda and hydrogen peroxide. To her amazement, more improvement! And the improvement has lasted. Definitely worth doing.

MINIMIZING LOW-LEVEL EXPOSURES

Chemicals in Water

As many as 45 million Americans are supplied with tap water that fails to meet basic health standards. This was the finding of the Environmental Working Group (EWG) in a review of federal and state records for 1994 to 1995. Updated studies indicate that our water continues to be contaminated from multiple sources. Here's what the EWG found: Over 25 million people used water contaminated by bacteria, with over 12,000 system violations! Another 5 million had lead levels above standard, meriting more than 3,500 violations. Inadaquate treatment was a problem for 20 million consumers.

Federal and state sources also reflect contamination with chemicals and pesticides in the water of a million people. But a separate EWG study, focused just on agricultural states, found that more than 14 million people used tap water routinely contaminated with five major herbicides.

The Centers for Disease Control and the U.S. Environmental Protection Agency have advised anyone with a compromised immune system to consult a physician before drinking ordinary tap water. The American Water Works Association, a trade group for water utilities, advises all individuals with the HIV virus to boil tap water before drinking it.

SOURCES OF EXPOSURE: Water often contains fluoride (added for the prevention of cavities) and chlorine; by-products of chlorine interaction (THMs); pesticides, herbicides, and inorganic fertilizer chemicals such as nitrates; heavy metals including lead; petrochemical derivatives, PCBs, and dioxins; and radioactive compounds, such as radium, radon, and uranium, as well as organic matter and bacteria.

SOLUTIONS: Clearly, this is a complex subject. One ideal water source is bottled mountain spring water tested for purity and rich trace mineral content, stored in glass; ask the vendor to send you a copy of the results on their water testing. If you decide to buy a water filter or filtration system, you'll probably want to do some reading and talk with more than one vendor. If you have specific requirements or well water, have your water tested before you select the filter. Each system offers benefits and has drawbacks. Reverse osmosis (RO) filters remove more contaminants from the water than any other system. Ceramic and carbon block filters are both respected as decent filters. Microwater units that alkalinize water appear to be useful in reducing an acid state in the body.

INFORMATION ON YOUR MUNICIPAL WATER
◆ Call your county water system
◆ EPA's Safe Drinking Water Hotline: 800-426-4791

WEBSITES THAT REPORT ON WATER QUALITY ACROSS THE COUNTRY, BY STATE AND COUNTY
◆ Environmental Defense Fund www.scorecard.org
◆ Environmental Working Group www.ewg.org

INFORMATION ON YOUR BOTTLED WATER
◆ International Bottled Water Association (IBEW) in Virginia; 800-WATER-11. Bottlers of water need to meet certain standards to be part of the IBEW.
◆ Request testing information directly from the vendor before you purchase monthly service.

TESTING YOUR TAP OR WELL WATER
◆ Clean Water Lead Testing, Asheville, NC 704-251-6800—inexpensive lead testing
◆ Spectrum Laboratories, St. Paul, MN: 800-447-5221—lead, bacteria testing
◆ Suburban Water Testing, Temple, PA: 800-433-6595—lead, coliform bacteria, fluoride, nitrate, and other substances

INFORMATION ON WATER FILTERS
◆ *The NSF International Consumer Guide to Drinking Water Treatment Units (Filters)* 1–800-NSF-MARK. $6.00 shipping and handling
◆ The Water Store, Kentucky: 800-290-0095; California: 888-437-9668

BOOKS AND ARTICLES ABOUT WATER ISSUES AND FILTER OPTIONS
◆ *Consumer Reports,* July 1997
◆ A'o, Lono Kahuna Kupa. *Don't Drink the Water.* Kali Press, 1996.

ENVIRONMENTAL ADVOCATES
◆ Environmental Working Group—San Francisco: 415-561-6698; Washington, DC: 202-667-6982
◆ Clean Water Action: 202-895-0420

MINIMIZING TOXINS IN YOUR WATER

Source or Filter	Advantages	Disadvantages
Tap water Call your water district and check www.ewg.org	Inexpensive, available, may be good; boil for fifteen to twenty minutes to remove chlorine, bacteria, some parasites	Chlorine, fluoride, heavy metals, THMs; can contain cryptosporidium, giardia, and other parasites and their cysts
Bottled water Request testing information from vendor before ordering water service; sources of water include natural spring, distilled, or filtered municipal water; check label	Usually tested and prefiltered; spring water may be a good natural source of minerals	Soft and even hard plastic containers off-gas toxic compounds including plasticizers (phthalates), vinyl chloride, bisphenol-A (an endocrine disrupter); glass is still best
Ceramic carbon filters Two-step filtration— compacted activated carbon and porous ceramic	Removes most bacteria and parasites, cysts, sediment, chlorine, some radioactive pollutants, most solvents, pesticides, and chemicals, some heavy metals	Doesn't remove fluoride or certain heavy metals, viruses or very small microbes
Carbon block, activated carbon Check manufacturer's specifications	Removes chlorine, solvents and pesticides, some radioactive contaminants	Doesn't remove bacteria, heavy metals, some radioactive compounds, asbestos, or fluoride
Mechanical filters, some impregnated with silver compounds	Filters out debris, bacteria, large parasites and cysts down to 1 or .5 microns; bacteriostatic— also kills some bacteria	Does not remove chlorine, fluoride, asbestos, THMs, most volatile chemicals, including solvents or pesticides, or heavy metals

MINIMIZING TOXINS IN YOUR WATER (continued)

Source or Filter	Advantages	Disadvantages
Reverse osmosis filters	Removes almost everything, except radon, pesticides, and volatile organic chemicals; to compensate, many systems come with add-on carbon filtration units	Also removes good minerals and makes water "lifeless"; may supplement with unit to add minerals back in; requires periodic filter change or back-flushing with chlorine; can outgas plastic compounds into water, requiring additional filtration step
Granulated, activated charcoal, typically in small portable filters and some prefilters	Better than no filtration; removes THMs, chlorine, mercury, some chemicals, large parasites, particulates	Doesn't remove bacteria or protozoa under 4 microns; asbestos, most radioactive compounds, some heavy metals, or fluoride
Alkaline water, with granulated activated charcoal prefilter, impregnated with silver; can be linked to carbon block for additional filtration	Can restore normal acid-base balance in the body and aid detoxification; may be linked with another filtration system as a pre-filter	Same limitations as other granulated charcoal filters; best in combination with a pre-filter; misses viruses, fluoride, chemicals, and heavy metals
Shower filters	Removes some chlorine that off-gases while you shower	

Pesticides and Other Chemicals in Our Food

SOURCES OF EXPOSURE: The U.S. uses a fifth of the world's pesticides—over 4.5 billion pounds a year, all sources totaled. Specific pesticide use in the U.S. has averaged from 1.2 to 1.5 billion pounds a year, yearly for the past twenty years. In developing nations, many pesticides banned here and in Europe are in common use. Worldwide, use of specific pesticides is 6 billion pounds every year.

About half of our produce and a third of our grains are reported by the FDA to have pesticides residues. However, by their own report, 90 percent of wheat samples tested contain residues. And the Environmental Working Group found that illegal pesticide levels on imported produce tended to be about twice as high as those reported—averaging 7 percent on some, but contaminating as much as 50 percent of the crop in other cases (in 1992 to 1993 records)

Meat, dairy products, and poultry may have traces of pesticides, hormones, antibiotics, tranquilizers, steroids, or other drugs. Fish and shellfish may contain mercury, lead, arsenic, cadmium, chromium, and chemicals such as dioxins and PCBs.

LEAST EXPENSIVE STRATEGY: Residues on some vegetables can be minimized by peeling. Buy produce in season as possible, since imported produce tends to have higher levels of residues and more illegal residues (since pesticide laws are less strict than ours in some countries). Some fruits and vegetables have been found to be typically low in residues when tested. Others consistently test high, sometimes because of the way they must be grown or stored. These are to be minimized or bought organically.

MOST THOROUGH STRATEGY: If you have access to certified organic produce and products, that's definitely the best option. You will taste the difference and you may even notice a difference in your health. In part, this is because truly organic products are not only free of pesticide residues, but are also raised in soil that is more nutrient rich. Testing has shown increased nutrients in organically-raised vegetables from 50 to 200 percent! Although organics tend to be a little more expensive, you may come out ahead because of reduced health care costs.

SOURCES OF INFORMATION

- National Resources Defense Council, Washington, DC: 202-289-6868; or San Francisco: 415-777-0220
- Environmental Working Group—San Francisco: 415-561-6698; Washington, DC: 202-667-6982
- *E Magazine,* subscriptions—Marion, OH: 800-967-6572
- Mothers and Others, New York: 888-ECO-INFO; San Francisco: 415-433-0850
- National Coalition Against the Misuse of Pesticides (NCAMP), Washington, DC: 202-466-2823
- Pesticide Action Network of North America (PANNA), San Francisco: 415-541-9253

WHEN ORGANICS AREN'T AVAILABLE

Strategy	Specifics
Wash vegetables thoroughly.	Vegetable washes (usually based on coconut oil) appear to be helpful; dish detergent got mixed reviews as a vegetable wash.
Peel fruits and vegetables.	High residues on skin or outer leaves can be reduced by peeling. Fruits: apples, bananas, grapefruit, oranges, pears. Vegetables: lettuce, corn (mixed reviews).
Buy in season.	Imported vegetables have higher residues in testing and more violations, since some chemicals allowed are illegal in the U.S.
Avoid foods that test very high for residues of known or illegal toxins.	Fruits: strawberries, peaches and other stone fruits, grapes. Vegetables: celery, bell peppers, green beans, spinach, leafy greens, cucumbers. Staples: wheat (90%), rice.
Avoid produce frequently treated with systemic toxins.	Systemic toxins are absorbed and can't be washed off. Toxins in animal products are systemic by nature. In plants, they're found in produce such as broccoli, cabbage, celery, cauliflower, cucumbers, green beans, lettuce, potatoes and other root vegetables, spinach, tomatoes. Fruits: grapes, cantaloupe and watermelons, peaches and other stone fruits, strawberries.
Know the source of seafood.	Buy your seafood from a source you trust; inquire; keep up with current information to see what's safe.
Shop wisely.	Buy grains in bulk; support your local cooperatives and buying clubs.
Shop selectively.	Buy the most important foods organic—baby food, dairy products, meats, staple grains such as rice and wheat.

Low Level Exposure to Toxins in the Home and Garden

SOURCES OF EXPOSURE: Solvents such as turpentine, paint and paint thinner, paint and wax strippers, spot removers, degreasers, gasoline. Pesticides in home and garden bug sprays, pet sprays, flea collars, and pest strips have been consistently linked to higher rates of cancer.

SOLUTIONS: If your exposure is from the home or garden, it may mean changing the products you use, shifting to organic gardening and nontoxic solutions to household maintenance. A number of excellent resource books can guide you in solutions. Some of the books, for example, offer simple, nontoxic alternatives to household cleaning products. Others provide solutions to complex problems, such as building materials or furnishings. Mail-order catalogues can be useful when purchasing specialty products.

◆ Reframe your expectations. If you and your family want to be safe from toxic exposure, you may not be able to have an effortless, picture-perfect lawn with no crabgrass. On the other hand, consider the possibilities. Minimizing the use of toxins on your lawn may mean planting hardy weed-resistant species of grass, or going for a more natural look by putting in a rock garden or planting part of your yard in wildflowers or ivy.

◆ You can have a wonderful garden using the clever techniques of integrated pest management. These strategies minimize the use of toxins and also nurture the land and the environment. Plant flowers and crops that repel pests, develop healthy soil, mulch for weeds, alternate your crops (intercropping) and rotate them, water your garden deeply and frequently, and encourage natural predators (a ladybug farm!)

SOME HELPFUL READING

Moses, Marien. *Designer Poisons*. San Francisco: Pesticide Education Center, 1995—in-depth review of the research on toxins, including the dangers they pose to children

Berthold-Bond, Annie. *Clean and Green*. Ceres Press, 1994. *The Green Kitchen Handbook*. HarperCollins (1997)

Organic Gardening, Rodale Press, Emmaus, PA: 800-763-2531—magazine and books

RESOURCES

The Bio-Integral Resource Center (BIRC), 1307 Acton, Berkeley, CA 94706, 510-524-2567; www.birc.org

Unknown Low-Level Chronic Exposures, such as Fluoride in Toothpaste, and Chemicals in Cosmetic Products

SOURCES OF EXPOSURE: Many everyday personal products contain additives that can be harmful to the GI tract, including fluoride (in most toothpastes); toothpaste additives—propylene glycol (major constituent of antifreeze!), sodium lauryl sulfate, DEA (di-ethanolamine). People who are highly sensitive will find that inhaled substances from fabric softeners, colognes, and even scented laundry detergents may make their GI symptoms worse. Some familiar products are actually quite toxic: for example, lindane is still widely used as a treatment by prescription for lice in children, despite its known neurotoxicity and bioaccumulation!

Become informed about which additives are toxic and then read labels avidly. Consider shifting to simpler products—those without coloring, scents, or complex chemicals. Most health food stores carry a line of safe, nontoxic toothpastes, shampoos, deodorants, and cosmetics. Even there it is important to read labels; for example, some brands of toothpaste in the health food store now contain fluoride. When you note the caution on toothpaste labels, you'll notice that the toothpaste manufacturers label fluoride as a toxin and caution not to allow children to swallow it! Since these products are widespread, a realistic goal is not total avoidance but minimizing exposure.

USEFUL READING

Steinham, David. *The Safe Shopper's Bible: A Consumer's Guide to Nontoxic Household Products, Cosmetics, and Food.* Macmillan, 1995.

RESOURCES

American Environmental Health Foundation, Dallas, TX: 214-361-9515—catalogue of environmentally safe products

Effects of Mercury Amalgam Fillings

Mercury (along with silver and tin) are found in dental fillings (mercury-silver amalgams). These metals may promote antibiotic-resistant gut bacteria and cause harmful overgrowth (dysbiois); species include klebsiella, citrobacter, and proteus. Mercury is released from dental fillings continuously in very small amounts, but can accumulate in the body in dangerous amounts. Mercury-silver amalgams have been outlawed in Europe and Scandinavia for several decades.

SYMPTOMS: People with long-standing multiple mercury-silver fillings (dental amalgams) often suffer diverse generalized problems associated with chronic low level toxicity from mercury and tin (another component of amalgam). Typical symptoms include problems with the nervous or immune systems, metabolic disorders, as well as GI dysfunction.

SOLUTIONS: Consider having your amalgams removed and replaced if possible.

REFERRAL SOURCES

◆ Foundation for Toxic-Free Dentistry, PO Box 608010, Orlando, FL 32860

◆ Environmental Dental Association: 800-388-8124. For book orders, call EDA at 619-586-7626. To receive a list of alternative dentists, send a stamped, self-addressed envelope with 55¢ postage. Mail to EDA, PO Box 2184, Rancho Santa Fe, CA 92067. Enclose $3.

COPING WITH LONG-TERM OR HIGH INTENSITY EXPOSURE

Sick Building Syndrome

These exposures are frequent or long-term, such as one might get on the job, and are characterized by poor ventilation and a high level of synthetic materials, such as certain paints, some synthetic carpets and underpadding, adhesives, formaldehyde, sealers, waxes, disinfectants, cleaning agents, photocopier solution and toner, pesticide applications, and PCBs (from older electrical equipment, fluorescent light transformers) in tightly insulated buildings that lack adequate ventilation and outdoor air exchange. Environmental testing can be obtained for some of the potential allergens and toxins in the home. This may include testing indoor air for formaldehyde and other toxins outgassed from various materials such as Sheetrock, particle board, insulation, and synthetic carpeting.

For example, the pesticide of choice for termite control was traditionally chlordane (an organochloride) until it was banned because of its extreme toxicity. Many homes were treated with chlordane for decades, from the 1950s through the 1970s. It was often injected into the soil under the house. Like DDT, it persists, and since it has a half-life of centuries, it continues to be released. Chlordane causes low level chlordane toxicity, contaminating the breathable air inside the treated house. So if you live in a house built before 1980, check any records on termite treatment. It can also be detected by testing the soil under the house.

SOME HELPFUL READING

Dadd, Debra. *Home Safe Home*. Tarcher/Putnam, 1997—resource for a safe environment

Rogers, Sheri. *Chemical Sensitivity*. Keats Publishing, 1995—a good review of health effects

RESOURCES
American Environmental Health Foundation, Dallas, TX: 214-361-9515—
    catalogue of environmentally safe products
The Cutting Edge, Southampton, NY: 800-497-9516—product catalogue
Bio-Designs by Allergy Resources, Broomfield, CO: 303-438-0600—
    product catalogue

Occupational and Industrial Exposures

EXPOSURES: These concerns are often associated with the use of
chemicals on the job, such as pesticides (agricultural and pest control
workers and landscapers); solvents (building trades); PCBs, dioxins,
and hundreds of thousands of other chemicals (heavy industry, chemical manufacturering); and petroleum and its by-products (the petrochemical industry).

ACUTE, INTENSE EXPOSURE FROM A SINGLE INCIDENT: An intense occupational exposure, an industrial accident, or a spill can involve solvents, pesticides, agricultural activities such as crop dusting and aerial
spraying, petroleum spills, and other sources of exposure.

BOOK RESOURCES—
From Medical Libraries, Environmental Groups, or Publishers
Handbook of Pesticide Toxicology. W. Hayes and E. Laws, eds. Academic
    Press, 1991.
Human Health Effects of Pesticides. M. C. Keifer, ed. Hanley & Belfus, 1997.
Rea, William. *Chemical Sensitivity.* David Lewis Publishing, 1996.

DIAGNOSIS OF MILD OR INTENSE EXPOSURE

There are a number of tests available to detect the presence of toxins
in the body or assess their effects. These tests apply to health conditions that result from long-term exposure, whether low level, moderate, or of high intensity. Some of the tests may also apply to acute,
short-term exposures.

ASSESSING ENVIRONMENTAL FACTORS IN ILLNESS: There are objective
lab tests that can be very useful in diagnosing both digestive and systemic illness with an environmental component. A detailed history of
environmental exposure is key to determining the probable sources.
Remember, many toxins and pollutants accumulate over a lifetime
(stored in body tissues), and can have both additive and synergistic

effects (one magnifying another). Certain chemicals can accumulate in what is known as the total load; or the total body burden of toxins. Therefore, it's important to begin assessing and minimizing all your exposures. Once you begin to think in this way, you'll also want to use this approach to protect your children, by avoiding exposures from birth (or even before!).

Testing GI Consequences

There are a limited number of tests of the gastrointestinal system that provide objective markers of gut damage. Unfortunately, there are no available practical affordable tests for heavy metals specifically in the gut.

- ◆ Secretory IgA in mucus, stool, or saliva
- ◆ Intestinal permeability, which tests for leaky gut syndrome
- ◆ Digestive stool analysis (CDSA) to measure digestion and absorption
- ◆ Measures of liver function—the functional detox panel (Great Smokies Diagnostic Lab)
- ◆ Testing for parasites and candida or other microbes, which tend to occur more often when the integrity of digestion has been stressed and challenged by toxins.

These tests are all discussed in greater detail in the testing section, Chapters 14 through 18. If the GI testing identifies a problem area and you have evidence for the presence of toxicity, there is a strong possibility that the exposure to toxins has compromised your digestive function. This provides the basis for developing a strategy. When there is a high likelihood that environmental influences are contributing to your illness, seriously consider seeing a good environmental physician. Check with the American Academy of Environmental Medicine, a source for referrals at 215-862-4544, (fax) 862-4583.

HEAVY METAL EXPOSURE

The metals involved are mercury (Hg), lead (Pb), cadmium (Cd), chromium (Cr), nickel (Ni), tin (Sn), arsenic (As).

Sources/Patient History

- ◆ *Devices or materials placed in your body:* mercury/silver dental amalgams (mercury, tin); remnants of orthopedic surgical procedures (stainless steel screws, pins, plates, nails, wires—nickel).

♦ *Residential/commercial:* paints (old—lead, marine, masonry—mercury); rodenticides, fungicides, pesticides (mercury, arsenic, thallium), old plumbing, with brass fittings or soldered lead joints.

♦ *Industrial/occupational/hobbies:* soldering, welding, foundry work, jewelry making, artist's materials, especially paints (cadmium); multiple industries.

Testing: Toxicological Assays

♦ *Hair analysis (quantitative):* Inexpensive, but not always accurate or reliable.

♦ *24-hour urine:* Measures actual content of body (quantitative) by output of toxic metal(s). More expensive, but very accurate and reliable. This assessment can be enhanced by administering a pharmaceutical *chelating agent* (such as DMSA, DMPS, or penicillamine) by injection or by mouth that "pulls out" heavy metals bound in tissue, acting as a specialized molecular magnet. This is called a *chelation challenge.*

♦ *Blood testing:* Most appropriate for acute or high intensity occupational or industrial exposures. Not applicable to long-term low level or mid-level exposures.

♦ *Biological marker assay:* Measures key metabolic products in blood, urine, or stool of hemoglobin synthesis and breakdown (called porphyrins) and associated enzymes, often abnormal in type or amount due to heavy metal toxic damage, and can produce serious neurological, dermatological (skin), and metabolic symptoms.

PESTICIDE EXPOSURE—LOW-LEVEL OR INTENSE

Due to the extremely wide use of many diverse types of pesticides, these chemicals are virtually impossible to avoid (they include insecticides, fungicides, herbicides, rodenticides, agricultural fumigants, and structural fumigants/wood preservatives). Although pesticides are composed of a wide range of chemical types and molecular structures, almost all share similar toxic effects on tissues and organs. Many classes of these chemicals are designed to be toxic to the nervous systems of insects, and are toxic to the human nervous system as well. They can also cause problems to our gastrointestinal and respiratory systems; many of these chemicals are clearly toxic to the immune system, others are documented to be harmful to bone marrow, and many are cancer-promoting.

Organophosphates and Carbamates

These chemicals, most frequently used as agricultural and residential insecticides, degrade rapidly in the soil, where they're broken down by microorganisms, but can persist for weeks on "inert" surfaces such as wood, metal, stone, or concrete. They are very difficult to measure directly in the tissue or blood. These classes of pesticides include malathion, parathion, chlorpyrifos, Diazinon, aldicarb, and carbaryl.

HOW THEY HARM: They can damage the body by inhibiting an enzyme that is essential to the function of the entire nervous system (acetylcholinesterase, or AChE).

TESTING: Markers in the body chemistry for AChE are relevant to both acute and long-term exposure. They can be measured through a blood test in plasma (less expensive but less accurate) or red blood cells (more expensive and highly accurate). In acute and chronic exposures, significant depression of AChE can occur.

Organochlorines

Organochlorines include DDT and chlordane, which have been illegal for a number of years but are still found in abnormal levels in most individuals tested, due to slow breakdown. For this reason, high levels of DDT and chlordane can still be found in a large percentage of the population. Common organochlorines currently in use include lindane, dieldrin, and hexachlorobenzene, among others.

These widely used pesticides are characterized by slow breakdown and long persistence in the environment and the body (years or decades). Exposure can occur through water, food, air, or skin absorption. Although we don't yet know all the mechanisms by which they work, we do know for certain they are endocrine disrupters, even in minute exposures. These toxins have the greatest impact on fetal development, growing children, and adolescents. Organochlorides are also known to be carcinogens. They are all neurotoxins, and the organs most vulnerable to this damage are the brain, liver, kidneys, heart, and reproductive tissue. Organochlorides have been found to inhibit essential energy-dependent functions in the cell.

Other classes of chemicals characterized by relatively slow breakdown include herbicides, chlorphenoxy acids (such as 2,4-D and 2,4,5-T) and nitrophenolics (including DNOC and DNBP). Other classes of chemicals that share certain characteristics with organochlorines include industrial chemicals such as PCBs and dioxins. These chemicals also tend to persist in the environment, are highly toxic to the nervous system, and are known as endocrine disrupters.They are actively used in manufacturing and continue to be released into our environment as contaminants.

General assessment includes measurement of organ/tissue damage or dysfunction. Markers for toxics can be measured in blood or in fat, which provides direct measurement of chemical or by-products of breakdown (metabolites). A fat biopsy is especially important in accessing chronic exposure.

SOLVENTS

Solvent exposure is common in the household and in certain occupations, especially painters, artists, people working in the field of electronics, in the petroleum industry or gas stations, gardening or landscaping.

Testing involves direct measure in urine or blood, or through a biopsy of fat tissue. This is particularly important for both solvents and organochloride pesticides.

- ◆ Biological markers, which measure damage done by toxins
- ◆ Measures of the integrity of the immune system—levels of antibodies and T and B cells
- ◆ Specific tests to measure neurological function—brain scans, PET scans, EEGs, neuropsychological performance tests

You may find you have underlying damage from long-term low level exposures, as inflammation and dysfunction can continue even after the day-to-day exposure has been eliminated. Although the day-to-day exposures may be eliminated, you may still have the toxins in your body, stored in fat and tissue (chemicals and pesticides) or in bone (heavy metals). Until you completely detoxify, you will probably continue to have problems.

So eliminating the external sources of exposure is important, and you may feel better rather quickly. But to get totally well, you may need to go through a more long-term detox to get rid of what has already accumulated in your body. The goals are to eliminate the toxins you may already have accumulated, which are already doing damage, and to lighten any additional burden from your current environment. Toxins stored in the body can continue to challenge digestion and overload the liver. If you have developed chronic degenerative diseases in addition to the GI problems, it is essential that you absolutely eliminate toxic exposure. Otherwise, it becomes extremely difficult to overcome these problems.

RESOURCES

Chemical Injury Information Network: 406-547-2255; website http://bizcomm.com/CIIN. Provides a newsletter, bibliography, and a research service on chemical injury.

American Environmental Health Foundation, Dallas, TX: 214-361-9515. Extensive catalogue of environmentally safe products including extensive listings including home and garden, personal care, furnishings, building products, water filters, and books.

= 24 =

Replace Digestants and Restore Flora

THE TEAM

❖

It's essential that we digest foods thoroughly. If the food goes through the small intestine poorly digested and if leaky gut occurs, the leakage of these by-products makes our body a little more toxic and reactive to sensitivities. In the colon, we want to avoid the putrefaction that can occur if food isn't fully digested.

In this chapter, we'll look briefly at each of the major elements of digestion—enzymes, hydrochloric acid, bicarbonate, friendly flora, as well as the function of the glands. Why are they important? What can we do to replace and restore them?

ENZYMES IN THE MOUTH

WHY IT'S IMPORTANT: Starch digestion begins in the mouth, through enzymes in saliva.

WHAT TO DO: The first step is to slow down and savor your food. Chewing well enables the food to mix with saliva and be broken down small enough to be well digested.

STOMACH ACID, ENZYMES, AND BICARB

WHY THEY'RE IMPORTANT: Stomach acid (hydrochloric acid, or HCl for short) protects us from bad bugs before they become a problem. Stomach acid begins the process of protein digestion and is one of the signals to the pancreas for enzymes and bicarbonate. The pancreas secretes our basic enzymes: lipase (fats), protease (proteins), amylase (starches), and others with specialized functions. It also provides the bicarbonate that neutralizes stomach acid, and insulin, to regulate our blood sugar, which goes directly into the bloodstream.

Strategies to Provide Digestants

1. Get testing to see how your body is functioning.

2. Hydrochloric acid can be supplemented—with great care—using a product from the health food store. If used carefully, this can help in the short term, but is not always a long-term solution. Both enzymes and bicarbonate can also be supplemented.

3. The function of your pancreas can be supported with glandular supplements.

4. You can also improve pancreatic function by taking the best possible care of your pancreas.

MEASURING HYDROCHLORIC ACID, BICARBONATE, AND ENZYMES

Conventional Methods

♦ *Hydrochloric acid (HCl) production* can be measured as part of an endoscopic exam, by drawing a sample of gastric juices. This test can also be performed with a hormone stimulus, pentagastrin.

♦ *HCl production* can also be tested using a Heidelberg capsule; in this test, the patient swallows a capsule that sends signals back via radiotelemetry to detect low output of hydrochloric acid.

♦ *The pancreatic secretion of bicarbonate* is evaluated by giving secretin, a synthetic hormone, intravenously and measuring bicarbonate output over a 60-minute period.

♦ *A 72-hour fecal fat analysis* tells how well the pancreas is supplying the enzyme lipase to digest fats. This test can be performed by any major lab.

Alternative Testing

♦ *The Comprehensive Digestive Stool Analysis (CDSA)* is another practical test for measuring acidity and other aspects of digestive function.

♦ *Testing for overgrowth in the small intestine* (the CDSA, a candida evaluation from Diagnostic Labs, or other testing). An overgrowth may mean the pancreas is not totally doing its job.

◆ *Testing for a marker for inflammation in the small intestine—alpha-antichymotrypsin.* Very low or high levels of this marker may reflect low enzyme production.

SUPPLEMENTS

Hydrochloric Acid

◆ Hydrochloric acid is available as betaine hydrochloride in most health food stores. In some cases, that addition helps digestive problems. We encourage you to add betaine hydrochloride under the supervision of your doctor, because if you take too much, it will cause heartburn.

◆ When you begin any new supplement, be sure that is the only addition to your diet for at least one to two weeks so you can more easily identify unwanted effects.

◆ If you take only one capsule and that causes heartburn, it may mean you already produce too much acid. Take no more, and check with your doctor.

◆ The labels recommend dose of 1 to 2 capsules with meals. Remember that we're all different—the nutritional requirements of a 100-pound woman are quite different than those of a man who weighs 200 pounds.

Any time you get heartburn following the use of betaine hydrochloride, it usually means you are taking more than you need. Check with your doctor and be sure to cut back the dose.

Pancreas Glandulars

If your pancreas is struggling, taking betaine hydrochloride may only be a short-term solution. Some people feel better in the beginning, because they finally have enough stomach acid for digestion, but less well later on because the pancreas is still struggling. Another solution favored by complementary practitioners is to take a good quality product that supports the healing of the pancreas. These are extracts called glandulars and are available from vitamin companies in health food stores and reputable mail-order companies. Reliable suppliers of glandulars include Allergy Research Group and Standard Process.

Take Good Care of Your Pancreas

Our pancreas produces enzymes, bicarb, and insulin. Knowing how essential these functions are, please be sure to take the best possible care of your precious pancreas. The easiest way is to cut down on sweets and refined starches.

Our ancestors ate whole food. The hunters ate meat and plants and the farmers that followed them ate whole grains as well. So our pancreas didn't evolve to handle sweets and simple starches. When we eat that kind of food, it's a shock to the pancreas and requires a huge blast of insulin. If we eat too many sweets too often, we can actually cause diabetes—what the old-timers called sugar diabetes.

The solution is to eat foods that don't trigger insulin, that are low on the glycemic index. (See Joyce Daoust's *40-30-30 Fat Burning Nutrition* or *The Zone* by Barry Sears.)

How We Become Low on Digestive Enzymes

An infection by microbes is known to actually suppress enzyme production. This is a survival strategy on the part of the microbe. In addition, our modern diet tends to be very stressful to the pancreas. This is unfortunate, because the pancreas has a major role in both digestion and the regulation of blood sugar. Without enough enzymes, you can't fully digest your food.

Enzyme Supplements

Some practitioners use the results from the CDSA to tailor enzyme supplements to the needs of the patient. Enzyme products favored by practitioners include Protozyme, a German enzyme product from MarcoPharma (available by mail order from Smart Basics); Creon (an entera-coated product) or Ness (both available only through doctor's offices); or N-Zymes 10, a multiple vegetarian-based enzyme product available from the health food store.

The question of which type and brand of enzymes to purchase is a huge one. There are vegetarian enzymes and those extracted from animal sources (pancreatin). Some vegetarian enzymes are produced by a mold-growing process, so for mold-sensitive people, this is not the answer. Pancreatin, a frequently used animal-based multiple enzyme product, is generally extracted from animals in the slaughterhouse, and some individuals report the development of spots of pigmentation following heavy use of pancreatin. If you favor vegetarian enzymes, ask about the manufacturing process or consider ordering Protozyme, a product known for low reactivity. If you want to use pancreatin, spend the extra money and buy a top quality brand. The same quality issues apply to glandulars.

The Use of Bitters to Stimulate Digestion

There are a wide variety of digestants on the market. A traditional strategy is the use of gentian to stimulate our own hydrochloric acid secretion. Gentian is available in bitters, a liqueur that has been made in Europe for centuries. Angustora Bitters can be purchased in many liquor stores. Health food stores also carry European bitters. Gentian root can also be purchased in bulk, ground, and put in capsules, and taken twenty minutes before meals to promote digestion.

Bicarbonate

Another strategy to encourage digestion is taking bicarbonate after a meal (Alka-Seltzer Gold, which is bicarbonate without aspirin). This can sometimes dispel the symptoms completely within five minutes. When you add extra digestive enzymes and some bicarbonate, the theory is that the food will be broken down more thoroughly. This approach is most helpful in someone whose body doesn't produce enough enzymes or enough bicarb.

THE IMPORTANCE OF BENEFICIAL FLORA

Beneficial flora turns out to be so significant, it is even proving useful in the management of HIV. Research on AIDS has found a link between those who remain in remission and those who supplement their friendly flora. It may be that keeping down pathogenic bacteria in the gut frees up the immune system to deal with other issues.

However, out of more than 1,400 articles over the course of fifteen years on the nature of probiotics and their safe and beneficial uses, there are at least two dozen reports of lactobacillus causing serious infection, including a few by acidophilus. The majority of these cases have been identified in transplant patients (more than twenty patients, mainly liver), recent surgery (fourteen), cancer (six patients), diabetes mellitus (four), and ostomy (one). Researchers indicate that this is a very uncommon condition. Balance this against the knowledge that there are literally tens of thousands of people who have been monitored in research studies and found to have specific benefits with no problems.

As with any supplement, food, or other substance you take into your body, make the addition of a probiotic product or yogurt the only major change for that week. If you are scheduled for surgery, you may wish to cut back on your supplement or at the very least discuss your use of probiotics with your doctor.

TESTING

There are several ways to test for flora.

◆ *Measure flora levels directly* with a test such as the Comprehensive Diagnostic Stool Analysis (Great Smokies Diagnostic Lab).

◆ *Check for an overgrowth of yeast (candida), bacteria, or parasites.* Whenever there is an overgrowth or parasitic infection, you know that the levels of flora are depressed.

The status of the flora can be an indicator of how severe the overgrowth is when the problem is due to anerobic bacteria, which are not usually measured directly, or caused by a parasite that isn't showing up on the tests. The lactobacillus are the most vulnerable and are generally destroyed first, then the bifidus, and then *E. coli* (the benign forms). If the *E. coli* are gone, you have real problems and can assume there is a serious disruption in digestive function. The loss of beneficial flora can be caused by the use of medications or by the presence of a parasite. A parasitic infection that significant must be treated. If the bifidus is gone but the *E. coli* have survived, the problems tend to be more moderate.

Disruptions in gut flora patterns are very individual and can vary greatly. Some people are deficient in certain species of lactobacilli, others in bifidobacteria or beneficial *E. coli*. The only way to know for sure is to have the flora levels checked through stool cultures, ordered by your health care practitioner. Once flora levels are established, it is easier to know what kind of probiotic cultures to take to rebuild your flora.

SUPPLEMENTING FLORA

Although there are currently more than 1,400 studies on *Lactobacillus acidophilus* alone, we still don't have all the information on the best way to supplement flora. Still, we do know that replenishing the good bacteria helps most people become better able to resist illness. There is very extensive research on the benefical effects of supplementing with lactobacillus, particularly *Lactobacillus acidophilus* and *Lactobacillus plantarum*, as well as the yeast *Sacchromyces boulardii*.

Yogurt

It appears that yogurt can provide a dietary supplement of flora. Although current research suggests that it's only a temporary replacement, we know that people from cultures in which yogurt is a staple often have a history of being long-lived. We do know flora tend to diminish in yogurt due to storage and refrigeration. The best products are fresh yogurt made locally or homemade, as well as supplements.

The first consideration with yogurt is to be sure you don't have a dairy allergy (IgE) or a delayed allergy or sensitivity. In some intermittent allergies, yogurt can be tolerated every fourth or every seventh day. People who cannot tolerate cow's milk yogurt may want to try goat's milk yogurt. Tolerances are always totally individual.

Certain brands agree better with specific individuals. Some people, for example, find excellent results with yogurts that are also high in bifidobacteria, such as Brown Cow yogurt, available nationwide. Be sure to read labels and track your responses.

If you are dairy intolerant, excellent yogurt can be made at home with your favorite soy milk.

Yogurt can be useful following antibiotic therapy, illness, digestive upsets, in response to stress, before and during long distance travel. *Lactobacillus acidophilus* is the culture found in most yogurts. Others also contain bifidobacteria, another major resident of the GI tract. *The other bacteria that are found in yogurt can be indirectly beneficial but are not primary residents of the GI tract. Streptococcus thermophilus* and *Lactobacillus bulgaricus* exist only briefly in the human digestive tract after being consumed. However, they do produce lactic acid, which encourages the growth of other friendly bacteria.

Supplements

RESEARCH ON SUPPLEMENTING WITH PROBIATICS

◆ Ulcerative colitis was treated with eight different strains of acidophilus and bifidobacteria, causing long-term remission of symptoms in twelve of fifteen patients in a small study at the University of Bologna.

- A four-year review of the safety of lactobacilli among people in southern Finland of more than 3,300 blood culture isolates found no case in which lactobacilli appeared to be the cause of infection.

Lactobacillus DDS is one of the most well-studied acidophilus strains and is available nationwide in health food stores. It has been documented to survive storage in dry form in the capsule on the shelf, to produce viable cultures in the gastrointestinal tract, and to boost GI immunity.

Bifidobacteria is one of three major beneficial bacteria in the digestive tract. Some people find them quite health promoting. Clearly the last word is not yet in on the optimal ratio of any of the flora. Bifidus is contained in some fresh yogurt cultures, such as Brown Cow.

Sacchromyces boulardii, a natural-occurring yeast that is a close relative of the yeast used in baking, is another frequently recommended supplement. It stimulates the production of secretory IgA by the gut lining. There is a tremendous amount of research indicating that this yeast in supplement form can improve the course of GI illness:

- Traveler's diarrhea was effectively treated with *S. boulardii* in a group of 95 German patients. Of these, 67 percent had failed to respond to previous antidiarrheal or antibiotic drugs.

- Colitis associated with *Clostridium difficile* responded well to the use of *S. boulardii,* which was used in conjunction with the antibiotics vancomycin and metronidazole in a study at the University of West Virginia.

- *S. boulardii* was found to prevent diarrhea in critically ill tube-fed patients in a French study.

Soil-based bacteria are gaining attention as viable GI flora. They are also known as homeostatic soil organisms (HSO). See, for example, *Beyond Probiotics* by Ann Louise Gittleman, Keats (1998). HSO are an addition to the usual probiotic agents such as lactobacillus and bifidobacteria. Some people find they make a moderate difference. In other cases, they may be quite important and anecdotal success has even been reported in a patient with Crohn's disease after the patient had tried virtually every treatment program and many supplements.

HSO produce superoxide dismutase, a free radical quencher, and stimulate the production of alpha-interferon, a key immune system regulator. They also stimulate the production of human lactoferrin, which helps absorb iron and interferes with pathogenic bacteria. The theory is that in times past, vegetables and plants from the soil were

less sanitized and people regularly took in soil-based organisms cling-
ing to their food. An interesting study in England found that when
people began buying their vegetables in supermarkets, health declined
somewhat. The researchers suggested that the removal of all traces of
soil-based organisms could be a factor. You will continue to hear more
about this in the future. Note that some products contain an extract
of wheat grass, so if you have any suspicion of celiac disease or wheat
intolerance, these particular products are to be avoided.

Lactobacillus plantarum is another beneficial strain that has produced good outcomes in research studies. Children with recurrent abdominal pain took *Lactobacillus plantarum* 299V; of these, 60 percent
experienced a decrease in pain over the four-week period, in a study
at the University of Nebraska. Irritable bowel syndrome treated with
L. plantarum found rates of improvement of 67 percent to 90 percent,
in a study conducted in a Polish hospital. Those who used drug therapy instead improved by 30 percent and those who took the placebo
showed no improvement.

COMPLEMENTARY NUTRIENTS

Colostrum (freeze-dried from goat's or cow's milk) is a rich source of
secretory IgA and other immunoglobulins to replace deficient gut immunity. It is also available with added lactoferrin.

A strategy that clinicians are finding helpful is to take colostrum in
combination with a probiotic. Since colostrum can cause symptoms
in dairy-intolerant people, if you are sensitive, try half a capsule only
with your probiotic. Watch for new colostrum products coming out in
the future.

Lactoferrin is one of the primary components of colostrum and the
second most abundant protein in colostrum. It stimulates the immune
system, is antiviral and antibacterial, and has been found to selectively
block the absorption of iron by tumor tissue while releasing iron to
the body.

NAC (n-acetyl cysteine) is also important in reestablishing normal
flora because it helps decrease the toxicity of abnormal bacteria while
rebuilding normal flora.

Researchers recommend adding a complex carbohydrate called
FOS (fructo-oligo-saccharides), which tends to support the growth of
certain beneficial flora, although people who are carbohydrate intolerant may experience gas and bloating.

PRODUCTS THAT HELP TO RESTORE BENEFICIAL FLORA

Purpose	Product	Company
Probiotics	Megadophilus (DDS strain) Bifidus	Natren (health food stores)
	Replete	Interplexus—Smart Basics
	Soil-based organisms	Health food stores and others
	Probiotic Complex, Vital 10 and other formulas	Klaire Laboratories—Wellness Health Pharmaceuticals
	Lactobacillus plantarum	Allergy Research Group (public can order direct)
	Ultra Dophilus, Ultra Bifidus, Ultraflora Plus—with colostrum	Metagenics (doctor's offices only)
Colostrum (immunoglobulins that promote healing)	New Life Colostrum	Health food stores
	Wheyplex	Interplexus-Smart Basics
	Probioplex	Metagenics (doctors' offices)

WHAT THE RESEARCH HAS FOUND

In general, research does show that acidophilus can boost gastrointestinal immunity. Recent studies found major benefit in the use of flora supplements to treat GI conditions. Although there are studies that have reported no benefit, there appear to be many more studies that have found probiotics to be a safe and effective therapy or supplement to treatment. Be sure to ask your health care provider about how to best explore this underappreciated supplement. Always remember that your need for specific probiotics and your response are totally individual.

25

Repair the GI Tract

THE TEAM

❖

How can we restore beneficial microflora and repair the gut lining? How do we support healing in the GI tract after an event or an illness in which the gastrointestinal environment has been disrupted? This disruption can include routine antibiotic therapy. How can we strengthen the entire system when there has been a chronic GI problem? And how do we heal the leaky gut, to increase the integrity of the GI tract and decrease allergies?

The Strategy: GI Repair

JERRY STINE

A rehab program is used after antimicrobial programs, particularly after very aggressive attempts to clear out parasites. It could apply after being hospitalized for surgery. Most often, it's used when there has been a heavy program of antibiotics or other medication that may have disrupted the GI environment and the flora.

There are several objectives under rehabilitation. One goal is to restore the beneficial microorganisms, the normal microflora of the GI tract. Another goal is to facilitate and support the healing of the gastric mucosa, to support the growth of new lining cells. A third goal is to normalize the function of the gastrointestinal immune system.

The duration and intensity of the GI problems will define the extent of repair efforts. A mild example is seen in a relatively healthy person with no history of chronic unwellness who has had an episode of antibiotic treatment. A relatively mild and simple rehab program that may take only three or four weeks would be very adequate here. At the other end of the spectrum is the person who has had many years of chronic illness in which problems with digestive malfunction or dysbiosis have been major factors. In someone with problems of this intensity, the rehab program may take several months, perhaps six to nine months in really advanced cases. It depends on the original stresses on the GI tract and how long-term the condition has been.

The areas addressed in any of these rehab cases are:

♦ *Test for allergies* to make sure there is rotation or complete elimination of trigger foods from the diet.

♦ *Effective replacement of microflora* is more effective when accompanied by immunoglobulin supplements. Adding immunoglobulins to the flora usually substantially improves results.

♦ *Include nutrients that encourage the healing of the cells of the GI tract,* or that protect those cells, or both, such as N-acetyl-glucosamine, L-glutamine, slippery elm.

♦ *Slow or shut off inflammation,* particularly inflammation of the gut but also hypersensitivity generally speaking.

♦ *Deal with long-term malabsorption and any actual malnutrition* that has occurred as a result.

We are looking at supplements that promote repair—vitamins, minerals, amino acids, and fatty acids. All of these features are components of the rehab protocol. Keep in mind that these protocols often follow an eradication protocol. Eradication is treatment to minimize an overgrowth of yeast or bacteria, or to remove invasive parasites. Although this type of treatment is necessary in many cases because of some kind of parasite or overgrowth, it can actually add metabolic damage. This is because antimicrobial drugs tend to be indiscriminant, knocking out both the harmful pathogens and the beneficial flora. In addition, medications may aggravate sensitivity in the gut lining.

The repair phase must be worked out carefully on a case-by-case basis. And the rehab phase is the most lengthy, the most complicated, and the most important stage in returning the person to normal health, or achieving as healthy a balance as possible. Many of us take an antibiotic for a bug and consider the job done. That is really just the first step. Like strip mining, the gastrointestinal ecology must be restored or it will remain a barren interior environment, unable to provide nourishment for the other areas of the body.

Here is a list of nutrients and their use in decreasing intestinal permeability. This treatment for intestinal permeability is somewhat non-specific. This simple kind of protocol is used while we are waiting for the results from the lab work to be returned.

◆ *Fiber.* Permavite contains an insoluble fiber, cellulose, which seems to decrease and clear toxins. In powder form, it mixes well with water and has a mild flavor. The general recommendation is to use this prior to two meals a day.

It is specifically formulated for intestinal permeability, based on observations made by Dr. Leo Galland that different kinds of fiber affect intestinal permeability. He found that insoluble fibers reduce intestinal permeability and that the soluble fibers tended to increase it. So this formula is based on the insoluble cellulose and has other components in it to soothe and heal the GI tract. Cellulose products available in drugstores include Citracel and Fiber-Con. Permavite contains specific added nutrients and is available from Allergy Research Group.

◆ *Quercetin* is a bioflavonoid that is very useful in some kinds of food allergy sensitivities. This can be a helpful component in dealing with intestinal permeability.

◆ *Enzymes and enzyme stimulants* provide digestive support using either digestive enzymes to promote thorough digestion or glandular products to stimulate the body's own enzyme production. A related but stronger product is Proteozyme, an excellent quality digestive enzyme product from Germany (available through Smart Basics). There are vegetarian equivalents to these products; Interplexus has such a product, which is called Polyzyme. Since many of these plant-based products are made from mold fermentation, it's important to monitor your response.

◆ *Bioflavonoids* aid in strengthening the gastric mucosa and also help settle or reduce liver reactivity due to allergies.

◆ *N-acetyl cysteine (NAC)* is also important in reestablishing normal flora because it helps decrease the toxicity of abnormal bacteria while the person is rebuilding normal flora.

REDUCING INFLAMMATION

This part of the protocol adds components that may help with inflammatory tendencies. These nutrients may have a beneficial impact on inflammation at sites remote from the GI tract.

Inflammation can show up in a couple of ways. One is the actual perception and symptoms of inflammation, such as burning and irritation. There are many other conditions that do not produce a strong sense of inflammation but still involve reactions—diarrhea or cramping, gas and bloating, or spasms (as in irritable bowel syndrome). Inflammation can also take a form called subclinical inflammation, which doesn't show up on testing or even on an endoscopic exam, but which produces symptoms, for example, in response to certain foods.

◆ *Peptide products* can have a settling effect on inflammatory processes. Cytolog is a peptide extracted from colostrum made by Allergy Research Group.

◆ *Magnesium* is available in a number of different forms. There are some kinds of lab work that can delineate specific magnesium compounds appropriate for each person's individual chemistry. Two labs highly respected for their metabolic profiles include Vitamin Diagnostics and Body-Bio Corporation. Some of the more easily assimilated forms of magnesium are magnesium citrate, magnesium glycinate, magnesium fumerate, magnesium aspertate, and magnesium malate. These are usually well tolerated and well absorbed.

◆ *MSM, a therapeutic form of sulfur,* is a way to deliver sulfur to the system in a soluble form. Methyl-sulfonyl-methane is now widely available. It is sometimes used to supplement treatment for *H. pylori* and many practitioners in the field of nutritional medicine have specific regimens for its use.

◆ *Digestive enzymes* often minimize inflammation, but if the gut is inflamed, they occasionally worsen the condition. The most trouble-free brands that I have seen are the German products such as Proteozyme and Wobenzyme, available from MarcoPharma. Also check with your compounding pharmacy.

ESSENTIAL FATTY ACIDS

These essential (in other words necessary) fats have been found to decrease gut inflammation and leaky gut (hyperpermeability). Essential fatty acids are very powerful regulators of our chemistry, toning down inflammatory processes in the body triggered by the prostaglandins. This means that having sufficient levels of the right essential fatty acids may moderate inflammation. When you are supplementing with these nutrients, consider these factors:

♦ *Individual variations are the rule and not the exception.* The guidelines and suggestions here are extremely general. To ensure that you are getting the right combination you might invest in testing, such as the red blood cell membrane fatty acid test offered through BodyBio Corporation in New Jersey. This type of testing tells exactly which nutrients are and which are not there and allows extremely precise fatty acid supplementation.

♦ *Absorption and digestion of the essential fatty acids is often complicated by damage to the GI tract.* The villi, the finger-like structure of the small intestine, have the job of absorbing fatty acids. If there have been long-term GI problems, the villi are often damaged. For instance, a gluten sensitivity that has gone undiagnosed and unchecked can destroy so many of the villi that a person may be operating with only 10 percent of the total villi. The impact of this damage on their capacity to assimilate fatty acids, especially the long-chain fatty acids, may be 10 percent or less. In that case, taking supplements may provide very little benefit, in spite of a great nutritional need for them.

♦ *Fatty acids most often supplemented are the omega-3s and the omega-6s.* The omega-3s are extracted from cold-water fish and dark green plants (the foods of our ancestors). They are also available in soy, walnuts, and flaxseed oil. Many people tend to be low in the omega-3s. Omega-3s are known to have a beneficial effect on the brain and the nervous system, and deficiencies are characterized by excessively dry skin. Cod-liver oil is the traditional supplementary source of omega-3s.

Omega-6 fatty acids are found in vegetable oils such as corn and safflower oil (as well as flaxseed oil), so most Americans get enought omega-6s. But about 15 percent of the population are unable to fully break down omega-6s, perhaps due to a genetic defect. They benefit from supplements rich in omega-6 that are already partially metabolized, such as evening primrose oil, or borage oil that supply a form of fatty acids called GLA (gamma linolic acid).

There are two tricky aspects to these supplements that makes nutritional testing the most ideal way to supplement them. First, they compete with each other. Dr. Leo Galland points out that feeding fish oil to a person who needs GLA may actually increase their omega-6 deficit (*Power Healing,* Random House, 1998). People whose dryness does not respond to omega-3s may have a need for omega-6s.

Omega-6 fatty acids are important in toning down inflammation, so this supplement is very relevant to many people with GI conditions. But too much omega-6s can cause inflammation through the buildup of arachidonic acid in the body. So be sure to moderate your intake of red meat, dairy products, egg yolks, and shellfish, especially if you are taking an omega-6 supplement.

There is believed to be an optimum ratio between the two oils, which is usually one part omega-3 to four parts of omega-6. This is the baseline. Flaxseed oil happens to contain that ratio inherently, which is one of the things that is so attractive about it. You are just taking one product. On the other hand, if you are one of the people with a need for the GLA form of omega-6, you will need borage or primrose oil and may find that your health improves significantly with this addition. There is no way to be certain which will work best on a case-by-case basis prior to using them. Body Bio Laboratory provides special testing of individual requirements for fatty acids.

The Strategy: Strengthening

JERRY STINE

This is a more intensive rebuilding program for people who have had long-term chronic conditions or strong indications of environmental illness. It is aimed at improving overall strength and reducing some of the gastrointestinal-based metabolic stresses for those with GI conditions or illnesses that result from hyperpermeability, such as asthma, allergies, chronic fatigue, or joint problems.

This protocol is to strengthen people who have a sense of feeling debilitated or physically stressed. It is an important preparation for an aggressive eradication program, particularly in the treatment of parasites. That is the major point of strengthening.

OBJECTIVES OF STRENGTHENING

The primary goals of the strengthening program are to reduce stress on the GI tract and on the liver. Stress can be reduced by cutting exposure to food allergens and dealing gently with overgrowths of candida or whatever kind of overgrowth shows up in testing. When we talk about gently, we mean *not* using harsh or fast-acting substances. We are also talking about supporting the liver detoxification systems as completely as possible. But all of this is done very carefully. There is always the slow buildup of each nutrient used and very careful attention to the diet in terms of any food that could be problematic because of allergies or because of starch/carbohydrate or wheat/gluten sensitivities.

WHEN TO USE THIS

Use this program if you are frequently fatigued, highly stressed, sensitive, or feeling brittle; this protocol can be helpful if you have multiple symptoms in multiple areas. A good way to screen for this is to note the scores on your metabolic screening questionnaire (see Chapter 1); any indication of sensitivity to perfumes and chemicals or strong reactions to foods and drugs is a sign to proceed carefully.

Promote change gradually. Protocols should not be too complicated. Supplements must be introduced at very low doses and built up to the optimal doses gradually. The main consideration here is attention to detail and taking the time to work through this. A strengthening protocol can take a month to arrive at full doses of all the products. That is not at all unusual. Then it is usually maintained for at least another month to make sure that the body has "cooled off" as much as it can from whatever stresses are coming from the GI tract.

WHAT TO EAT FOR STRENGTHENING

In these kinds of protocols, the choice of foods in the program are absolutely critical. I strongly encourage testing to determine allergies. Foods can be problematic in a number of ways.

With an overgrowth of bacteria or yeast, avoid diets high in sweet and starchy foods (carbohydrates) because they tend to encourage the "bad bugs" and people notice that they feel worse after eating these foods. Some parasites also thrive on simple carbohydrates, and you can help to minimize your condition by selecting what you eat carefully. That means getting a book that gives the carbohydrate content of foods, becoming an avid label reader, and monitoring your reactions to what you eat. Helpful books include *40-30-30 Fat Burning Nutrition* by Joyce Daoust and *The Zone* by Barry Sears.

There are other kinds of sensitivities that accompany inflammation or ulcers, which may mean that foods with lots of fiber may cause pain or spasms. Each person and each response to every food is individual. And it often changes from day to day as well.

Allergies can have disastrous effects on the gut and be significant factors in conditions as serious as Crohn's disease. A respected nutrition journal published photos of the inside of the digestive tract during the intake of milk by an allergic person: The image was like a tiny little explosion inside the gut.

Foods that show up as allergenic in testing or that are a problem in any way should be carefully avoided for at least a month. It is sometimes viewed as a hardship, but this is absolutely essential at this stage. This stress on the body from allergenic or high carbohydrate foods (which might stimulate yeast or some bacterial overgrowth) must be really avoided. You need to be supported in sticking to this—enlist the help of those you love, and avoid those who sabotage your efforts to get well.

Supplements to Heal Leaky Gut
JEFFRY ANDERSON, M.D., and MICHAEL ROSENBAUM, M.D.

When the integrity of the GI lining is impaired, undigested food particles and toxins can be absorbed much more easily.

Major nutrients that can be useful in healing leaky gut include:

IMMUNE SUPPORT

♦ *Colostrum* (freeze-dried from goat's or cow's milk) is a rich source of secretory IgA and other immuno-globulins to replace deficient gut immunity.

♦ *Lactoferrin* is an immune complex derived from molecules found in the milk of lactating mammals: both colostrum and lactoferrin act as major immune barriers against the invasion of pathogenic bacteria, viruses, and parasites. Lactoferrin is a potent natural antibiotic.

♦ *Thymus extracts* stimulate and enhance the immune response both in the gut lining as well as generally throughout the body. One is Thymic Longevity Compound from Econugenics. Probably the strongest (and most expensive) is Nat Cell Thymus from Allergy Research Group. This contains frozen liquid thymic growth peptides from fetal and juvenile bovine thymus.

NUTRIENTS FROM PROTEIN—AMINO ACIDS AND PEPTIDES

♦ *L-glutamine (amino acid)* is the preferred fuel of the cells lining the mucosa of the small intestine. It's an important building block for the production of normal intestinal mucus, it's required for adequate production of SIgA, and to maintain normal intestinal permeability following injury or infection. Lining cells in the small intestines (enterocytes) need to be fed with glutamine and the large intestine lining cells (colonocytes) require butyrate, which is metabolized by beneficial flora in the gut.

◆ *NAC.* In addition to its benefits as a natural chelator and potent antioxidant, NAC (N-acetyl cysteine) is also a potent detoxifier and enhances the detoxification of toxins produced by pathogenic bacteria. It rebuilds immune function by stimulating cellular immunity in the gut lining and directly increases macrophage and lymphocyte or white blood cell function in the gut lining. NAC also helps replenish intracellular glutathione. Again, NAC is important in reestablishing normal flora because it helps decrease the toxicity of abnormal bacteria while the normal flora is being reestablished.

◆ *Seacure* is composed of peptides, which are the building blocks of protein, extracted from predigested whitefish. Many of the small peptides contained appear to duplicate growth factors. So the effect that you get on the GI tract far exceeds the six small capsules a day. You don't get that much protein—only three grams of protein a day, but the effect on conditions like irritable bowel syndrome can sometimes be very profound. These particular peptides appear to act as growth factors to help to heal the lining of the GI tract.

PROTECTIVE AND SOOTHING NUTRIENTS

◆ *Vitamin A* is essential for production of protective antibodies (secretory IgA) and to maintain the integrity of the GI mucosa.

◆ *Zinc* is necessary for growth and wound healing, and it's rapidly depleted in the body. It is much more necessary in cells that have a rapid turnover. Zinc is especially relevant for the lining cells of the GI tract, which are replaced about every four days. So zinc is critical when it comes to the lining of the GI tract.

Among its many functions, zinc also increases the release of vitamin A from the liver. If you are zinc deficient, you may actually have enough vitamin A in the liver and be unable to make use of it. Vitamin A is responsible for the integrity of the cells lining all the mucosal surfaces of the body, including the entire respiratory tract and the entire digestive tract.

♦ *MSM, a form of the mineral sulfur*, enhances the body chemistry probably by raising glutathione levels in all the cells. This helps to prevent oxidative stress throughout the GI tract. It is supposed to prevent pathogens—bacteria, yeast, and parasites—from adhering to the bowel wall, so that the body can flush them out much more easily.

♦ *N-acetyl-glucosamine (NAG)* is essential for the secretion of the protective mucous lining of the gut (the glycocalyx).

♦ *Quercetin* is one of the bioflavonoids, which are especially helpful in food allergy/sensitivity and leaky gut, as well as inflammatory processes in the gut lining.

♦ *Epithelial growth factors* can be particularly helpful in healing the GI lining cells. They are found in several widely different sources: peptides (from protein), glandular extracts, deglycerated licorice, and in stevia, the natural sweetener. They have been used to treat all kinds of intestinal disorders, including colitis, Crohn's disease, and irritable bowel syndrome.

VITAMIN B COMPLEX

Phosphatidal choline supports normal barrier functions by repairing and maintaining the integrity of cell membranes and tight junctions, which helps to diminish leaky gut and sustain normal permeability.

FATTY ACIDS

The butyrates are short-chain fatty acids that are important for the lower portion of the intestinal tract, particularly the colon. The major role of the colon is to reabsorb water and maintain electrolyte balance in the body. Butyrates are the preferred food of the colon lining cells. Our primary source is from the beneficial bacteria, so when there is an overgrowth and dysbiosis, butyrate levels drop. Butyrates are available as a supplement from a number of manufacturers.

HERBS THAT MEND THE MUCOSA

These herbs are specific for healing leaky gut and damaged gut mucosa. Some of these botanicals also enhance detoxification. Part of the process of rebuilding the lining is the ability to repair.

◆ *Olive extract* is a natural antibiotic that tends to have antibacterial, antifungal, and antiparasitic effects on undesirable flora; the active constituent is oleuropein.

◆ *Silymarin* is an exceptionally healing herb extracted from the milk thistle weed and has a potent anti-inflammatory effect on the GI lining. It also has a direct antioxidant effect.

◆ *Ginkgo biloba extract,* which we usually consider a mild mental stimulant, has also been found to protect cell membranes from free radical damage. It has an anti-inflammatory effect as well.

◆ *Licorice root* (whole licorice root) is a herb that has profound anti-inflammatory effects on the gut lining.

◆ *Deglycerated licorice* has had the glycerin removed. So it is called deglycyrrhizinated licorice, or DGL. That form of licorice is also very soothing to the upper GI tract and may help to promote healing and get rid of leaky gut. It's useful in decreasing inflammation related to gut permeability and therefore stabilizing to the gut barrier function.

◆ *Slippery elm* has a soothing effect on inflamed gastrointestinal lining.

◆ *Stinging nettle* has an antihistamine effect that tends to reduce allergic inflammation.

COMMENT ON SUPPLEMENTS

All of these supplements may have bearing on healing. It depends on the particular case—each person has his or her own individual issues. There are other considerations here that we have not discussed, including the possibility of trace element imbalances or the presence of toxic metals like lead and mercury. Those possibilities have to be explored. This is part of the history-taking process—to identify all of the issues that must be dealt with to help people increase their metabolic resilience and to decrease their metabolic stress.

A Review of Treatment Strategies

LEN SAPUTO, M.D.

1. Correct, or at least improve, the underlying disease condition whenever possible.

2. Eliminate the known triggers of leaky gut: NSAIDs (nonsteroidal

anti-inflammatories), alcohol overconsumption, infections, parasites, malabsorption, malnutrition, and allergic triggers.

3. Provide nutritional support.

4. Avoid or minimize toxic exposures.

5. Provide liver support based on the status of liver function and detoxification.

6. Supplement with "permeability factor" nutrients (the combination of L-glutamine, glucosamine, GLA, gamma oryzanol, phosphatidal choline).

7. Support with the Four Rs: remove, replace, restore, repair—based on the studies of Dr. Jeffrey Bland, a respected biochemical researcher who has provided much of the ground-breaking analysis in this field.

8. Insure adequate exercise, rest, stress reduction, and balance of body, mind, and spirit.

9. Be very careful about antibiotic usage.

10. It's important to assess GI function in order to manage GI conditions.

11. Whenever we detect leaky gut syndrome, we must also assess and manage the liver, beginning with a liver detoxification profile as the basis for understanding the situation.

12. Enhancing immune function is vital.

13. Screening with stool and intestinal permeability testing is a reasonable step in assessing chronic conditions and essential in the seriously ill.

14. Ideal nutrition is critically important, but unless the GI tract is functioning ideally, much of this value is lost.

26

Detoxing from Toxins

JEFFRY ANDERSON, M.D., AND JERRY STINE

❖

Stored toxins can continue to cause damage to cells, tissues, and organs, creating inflammation and dysfunction even after the day-to-day exposures are eliminated. Although the external sources may be removed, the toxins remain in the body until they are cleared. To fully detox, it's essential to support two specific processes:

- *Detoxication,* the internal processes of the liver by which toxins are eliminated from the body
- *Detoxification* enhancing the release of toxins from the tissue through the use of specific therapies, including sauna, exercise, and nutrient support

SOURCES OF TOXINS

The gut is the source of much of the toxicity in the body because a good deal of what goes through the gut is absorbed, whether by design, accident, or pathology. Leaky gut can cause absorption of material that clearly should not be absorbed.

The first category of toxins are actually produced within the body (endotoxins) in the gut through impaired digestion and abnormal bacteria or yeast overgrowth, which leads to:

- Fermentation and putrefaction by-products from overgrowth and poorly digested food
- The presence of parasites and their toxic by-products
- Constipation

These processes lead to a certain amount of internally generated toxins, which will be absorbed by the body before they are eliminated and will eventually be stored in tissues and cells.

The second category of toxins are contaminants that are ingested not by design, but primarily because of contaminated food or water. This category includes food additives, pesticides, agricultural contaminants in meats and dairy products, and heavy metals in fish. Water may contain chemicals and their by-products, pesticides, and heavy metals as well.

A third category are the toxins recycling through the body. Toxins intended for discharge may accidentally be released back into the body. When the process works as it is meant to, toxins are bound to special transport molecules (conjugates) in the liver as part of the detoxification process. Conjugated toxins are then secreted into the bile and on to the GI tract, where they are further bound to the stool for final disposal from the body.

Certain harmful bacteria secrete an enzyme that unbinds toxins and chemicals from the stool, and they are reabsorbed again. Some of the toxins will be disassociated from the binding site, re-released into the system, and reabsorbed back into the liver and general circulation.

Toxins absorbed on the skin or through the lungs can also damage the GI tract and contaminate the cells and tissues.

So the starting point is the gut. If the gut is toxic and toxins are absorbed, they all go through the liver. Ideally, the liver will be able to detoxify them or at least diminish their toxicity by changing them into less toxic substances, to be excreted in urine or feces.

If the liver is overburdened due to a chronic or persistent toxic overload, then a bottleneck effect can occur that may eventually reach a level beyond the capacity of the liver to handle. The liver detox machinery can become stressed and compromised. The overburdened liver will make every effort to do its job but may actually create an additional toxic load—more free radicals and even more toxic intermediate metabolites. If they can't be excreted, the body must store them. Internally generated toxins and especially ingested chemicals and pesticides will be stored in fat. Heavy metals will be stored in protein tissue such as muscle, bone, and cartilage.

The increasing accumulation can cause widespread cellular damage. You must begin detoxing by starting with first things first, which is the gut. Make sure that you are not constipated, that you don't have putrefaction, and that you don't have an overgrowth of yeast or bacteria and their toxic by-products. Clean out. Get rid of bad bugs and put in the beneficial flora by taking probiotics (acidophilus and bifidus).

Once you have begun to clear the GI tract, you can start addressing the liver and body detox issues.

When you improve the GI tract environment, you take the stress off the liver because the burden of toxins is decreased. And there is less stress on the immune structures in the gut (the lymph tissue) as putrefaction drops and overgrowths decrease. Then there is less need for a constant high level defense effort and everything in the body just starts to work better. But the essential point is this: you can't deal with the downstream problems (symptoms in the body) until you have treated the upstream problem (malfunctions in the gut).

LIVER SUPPORT

Liver support refers to the general activity of supporting detoxification mechanisms within the liver, and reducing detoxification stress. There are several key issues here: facilitating the detoxification mechanisms, encouraging recovery and healing in the liver, and reducing stress in the liver.

Reducing liver stress means reducing intestinal permeability and minimizing the intake of any substance that will be a toxic burden on the liver. The objective of enhancing detoxification chemistry in the liver is to supply those nutrients or herbal products that seem to reinforce the liver detoxification mechanisms. The goal is to help the liver regenerate and rebuild, and that involves supplying nutrients essential to that process. Luckily, the liver has rather phenomenal regeneration capabilities.

This program is potentially useful to anyone who has a chemical sensitivity, a food allergy, or chronic GI problems. Checking with the doctor is the first step, as with any illness. These situations and quite a number of others, especially chronic degenerative conditions, will benefit from the liver protocol support.

The most important way to support the liver is to reduce or stop the liver's exposure to increased amounts of toxic materials. Another major component of detox is to supply the specialized nutrients for the GI tract and the liver—those specifically necessary for healing the digestive tract, and other nutrients specifically useful for facilitating liver function and recovery. Improving the liver's ability to detoxify both toxins generated in the body (endotoxins absorbed from the gut, from metabolic processes) and those from external sources is crucial.

Overloading the detoxification mechanisms in the liver is of concern for several reasons, because it also causes changes in the internal metabolic environment of the liver and interferes with the liver's role in key metabolic processes, including regulation of fat, carbohydrate, and protein metabolism.

At this point, the body begins to deplete key nutrients, including vitamin C and the amino acid glutathione. If we don't have vitamin C, we can't recycle glutathione. Glutathione is extremely important. When our liver is under stress, we use glutathione in lavish amounts. So the body may be using up precious key nutrients. And this can create a kind of a deficiency condition in the body.

If first-pass detoxification fails, metabolic junk begins to circulate throughout the system, some of which activates the immune response. Allergies and autoimmunity can develop. Direct toxicity can occur from some of the chemicals in foods (both natural and man-made chemicals).

During Phase 1 Liver Detox, biotransformation of the toxins occurs, transforming them into chemical forms that may be even more highly toxic. The only way to deal with the toxicity is to give the body tremendous support with antioxidant factors to compensate for the overstimulation of Phase 1, which typically occurs in anyone experiencing toxic overload. These factors include: glutathione, NAC, and alpha-lipoic acid, as well as vitamin E (preferably mixed tocopherols) and the anthocyanins (a family of antioxidants from plant sources).

Specific Nutrients

SUPPORT FOR PHASE 1 DETOXICATION: Antioxidants tend to be protective against damage from an overstressed Phase 1 detox pathway, which generates a large number of free radicals.

Antioxidant support includes glutathione, NAC (N-acetyl-cysteine), alpha lipoic acid, selenium, alpha- and beta-carotene, vitamins B_2, C, and E, anthocyanins, and riboflavin.

SUPPORT FOR PHASE 2 DETOXICATION: This includes glutathione, NAC, alpha lipoic acid, glycine, L-glutamine, L-taurine, L-cysteine, glutamic acid, aspartic acid, and a form of organic sulfur—MSM (methyl-sulfonyl-methane).

Both Phase 1 and 2 processes depend on a number of critical enzymes. Various B vitamins and minerals are required as essential catalysts for these enzymes to function. These include manganese, zinc, copper, B_3 (niacin), B_6, and folic acid. Broad-based nutritional supplementation is recommended. Required doses of the nutrients are quite varied from one individual to another. Working with exposures requires assessing individual needs on a case-by-case basis.

DETOXIFYING CHEMICALS AND HEAVY METALS

The elimination of toxins involves stimulating the release of fat and toxins stored in the fat cells. Most chemical toxins and pollutants like pesticides and solvents are stored in body fat (as opposed to heavy metals, which are not). Removing these toxins involves mobilizing them out of body fat to make them available for excretion.

This is done through a combination of therapies, by raising the body temperature through saunas (depuration therapy) and/or sustained aerobic exercise. These mechanisms gradually cause the body to break down fat and release the chemicals into the circulation so they can be detoxified and eliminated. This can be compared to melting lard under low heat in a saucepan. Basically you are melting solid fat to make it liquid. The stored chemicals are bound to fat and to a degree can be driven out of fat by increasing the temperature. This is analogous to increasing the evaporation of alcohol if you heat it. The chemicals tend to be volatile, which means that they change from a liquid to a gaseous state through the application of temperature. If the body temperature is raised in a sustained way, the fat cells tend to break down, discharge the fat, and so release the chemicals.

Heavy metals are not stored in fat, so they are not amenable to elimination by this method. They must be pulled out of the body by molecular magnets. This is called chelating. Heavy metals are bound to protein complexes of the body, such as muscles, tendons, and bone. To encourage the release of heavy metals, you can use chelating agents such as vitamins and also specific chelating drugs. The majority of chemical toxins are solvents and pesticides and are basically bound to body fat.

Detoxification is a complex and challenging procedure that should be carried out under medical supervision. Everything we have listed here has potential problems. Aerobic exercise challenges the cardiovascular system. The use of saunas raises the body temperature and can cause dehydration if done incorrectly. It can also cause the loss of body fluids and electrolytes. *None* of these therapies should be done without medical supervision. This is extremely important because if the chemicals are being released into the body, you don't want them to cause further injury. You don't want them to recirculate and cause additional secondary damage.

Detoxing Cells and Tissues: Sauna Therapy

Sauna therapy is highly useful to bake toxins out of the body because they're stored in fat. The object is to burn fat—that is, break down fat cells, as discussed above. So the toxins stored in the fat are released and mobilized for elimination through liver detoxification as well as directly through the lungs and skin. This can be accomplished with aerobic exercise, saunas, or a low carbohydrate diet, or a combination of these strategies. (See also Chapter 31 on personalizing a diet low in starches and sugars.)

- ◆ You may want to join a health club with a sauna or build one yourself.
- ◆ If you have chronic fatigue and are unable to exercise, use the sauna longer.

The protocol usually involves twenty minutes of mild aerobic exercise, a dose of niacin, and then a sauna. The process quite naturally encourages the body to expel the toxins from the fat cells. The ideal temperature is 140° to 150°F. It's important to start slowly—as little as five to ten minutes each day or every other day. The time is gradually increased as tolerated.

Niacin (vitamin B_3) should be started in small amounts of 50 to 100 mg per dose (one to three doses a day) and gradually increased to a maximum of 1,500 mg total. Niacin (B_3) flush can be eliminated by taking one baby aspirin twice a day for those who tolerate aspirin. This eliminates the flush completely.

Some people experience liver inflammation from higher doses of niacin (B_3), and many people can experience worsening of their condition if detoxification is too aggressive. Toxins can be mobilized more rapidly than the liver can handle, stimulated by too much sauna, too much exercise, or too restrictive a diet. For this reason, medical monitoring is rigorously advised!

NUTRITIONAL SUPPLEMENTS TO BE USED WITH SAUNA THERAPY

- ◆ *B vitamins*, especially niacin—up to 1,000 to 1,500 mg per day can be used. Medical monitoring is required. This would be taken two hours before entering the sauna.

◆ *Minerals:* Potassium, magnesium and a mixture of trace minerals, including copper, zinc, selenium, manganese, chromium, iodine, and boron.

◆ *Salts that make the body more alkaline:* Sodium bicarbonate, potassium bicarbonate, calcium carbonate; 1 to 3 grams are generally taken one to two hours before or after the sauna depending on the individual's needs.

MISCELLANEOUS NUTRIENTS

◆ *Alpha-keto-glutarate,* 75 mg three times a day. This helps the detoxification pathways to operate more efficiently.

◆ *Activated charcoal,* 1 to 3 teaspoons a day for no more than three days per week.

◆ *Bentonite clay in colloidal suspension:* 1 to 3 tablespoons a day for not more than three days a week. Both bentonite and activated charcoal bind toxins to be eliminated in stool. However, they also bind essential nutrients and must be restricted.

◆ *Polyunsaturated vegetable oils,* including olive, saffron, safflower, corn, walnut, or avocado oils or a mixture of these oils. The polyunsaturated vegetable oils help prevent the recirculation or reabsorption of fat-bound chemicals in the GI tract. They also serve to replace the eliminated chemically contaminated fat in the body that has resulted from the sauna therapy.

◆ *Herbs:* Botanicals can be used to support the liver's detoxification pathways and protect the liver from damage during detox and the breakdown and release of toxins. Useful herbal remedies include milk thistle seed extract (silymarin), red clover, dandelion, goldenseal root or Oregon grape root, curcumin extract from turmeric, and ginger.

Detoxing Cells and Tissues: Aerobic Exercises

Aerobic exercise can be highly beneficial. Even walking is helpful—just do what you can do. (Also, see Chapter 43 on gentle exercise.)

Foods That Heal

Antioxidant-rich foods tend to protect all organs and tissues as well as the GI tract. These factors buffer cells against oxygen or free radical damage generated by pollutants. Antioxidants also aid the cell in repairing damaged structures such as cell membranes and restoring cellular function, including detoxification. These nutrients include the carotenoids and vitamins A, C, and E. Antioxidants come in many different molecular or chemical forms and are present in extremely diverse sources of plants or foods. They are far too numerous to list. The most common ones are the ones we have suggested.

Vegetables

◆ *Green leafy vegetables:* Rich in vitamin A, carotenoids including alpha- and beta-carotene, lycopenes, and lutein. Kale, collard greens, dandelion greens, chard, beet greens

◆ *Yellow-orange vegetables:* Also high in carotenoids and other plant-based nutrient factors (therefore called phytonutrients). Carrots, yams, squash

◆ *Cruciferous vegetables:* red cabbage, broccoli, Brussels sprouts

◆ *Tomatoes (cooked) and beets:* rich in lycopenes and anthocyanins, which are both types of nutrients with a protective antioxidant effect

A liquid diet can be used for a short period to give the gut a rest. Another helpful strategy during detox is to simplify the diet, which reduces the GI load.

Fruits

Each antioxidant has a subtly different biochemistry. For example, vitamin C is a pure water-soluble antioxidant that protects certain tissues and structures vulnerable to oxidative damage, whereas other antioxidants are fat-soluble and protect structures like the fatty layer of the cell membrane against oxidative damage. These include vitamin E and glycolic acid, which is found in citrus fruits, grapes, plums, red currants, blueberries, and raisins.

Antioxidant Supplements

People with high susceptibility to toxic damage probably require supplements of antioxidants and cellular protective agents in addition to food sources. Antioxidants work much more efficiently if they are taken in combination, and they seem to be more effective when they are present with other factors in fresh foods that may act as synergists or enhancers of the antioxidant function. This is why it is important to get at least a large part of your cellular protection and antioxidant factors from fresh foods—vitamins (including antioxidants), minerals, and other nutrients.

Protein and Amino Acids

It is also important to have a balance of amino acids from your diet from a wide variety of protein foods, including nuts, seeds, legumes, dairy products, eggs, fish, and meats and poultry, depending on your diet. Obviously some of those things do not apply for vegetarians. But the wider the variety of protein foods you consume, the more balanced your amino acid pool will be for the body to use for cellular repair and protection. Many of the most important chelating and antioxidant amino acids (for example, glutathione and NAC) are found in both vegetable and animal protein foods.

People also need digestive enzymes that can help break down the protein into amino acids (protolytic enzymes) as well as peptides for absorption. People with a significant problem probably need amino acid supplements. The first step is a supplement that has all the essential and nonessential amino acids in balance (basically determined by measuring normal people's amino acid profiles). This will include all the amino acids we are talking about in the list, which are antioxidant, cellular protective, or chelating. These often provide some benefit.

Amino acid supplements can be tailored in a much more individualized program, but that requires professional testing and guidance. The simplest way to do this without having to test is to get health food store supplements that have 25 to 30 amino acids in them. They will contain the most important ones listed. One good basic amino acid supplement is Formula 2 by Scientific Consulting, which is patterned after the amino acid content of human breast milk. It is obtained from doctors rather than through health food stores. Another is Integrated Health, available at some health food stores.

Nutritional Supplements

These individual nutrients are now generally available in most all health food shelves.

◆ *Amino acids:* N-acetyl-cystine, glutathione, methionine, taurine (all act as both natural chelators, as well as antioxidants)

◆ *Vitamins:* Alpha-lipoic acid, vitamin B complex, vitamins C and

E, mixed carotenoids, anthocyanins and pro-anthocyanins (which are powerful antioxidants)

♦ *Fatty acids:* Omega 3 and 6 and 9 oils, all essential fatty acids (found in primrose, flax, and fish oils)

Chelators

Foods with a high chelating value will help to draw metals from the body. Natural accumulators of heavy metals include eggs, beans, and other legumes and the herb cilantro. Amino acid supplements that act as natural chelators include N-acetyl-cystine, glutathione, methionine, and taurine (they are also antioxidants). A good approach is to eat a wide variety of good-quality organic food protein sources, preferably from vegetables and animals. People vary tremendously in their specific needs for certain amino acids and in their pattern of amino acid deficiencies and requirements. Individual requirements for nutrients can be determined by laboratory analysis.

If there is a clear-cut problem with heavy metal toxicity or pollutant damage, a person may also need supplements. The more complex the problems of pollutant damage and gastrointestinal dysfunction, the more complex the treatment. There are nutritionally based physicians who have many tools to help individuals find the right solutions. This often requires laboratory work and individualized supplement programs. But if you want to get started on something on your own without doing any damage or missing too many factors, you can eat a balanced diet of these foods and take enzymes to help with the breakdown and assimilation.

Pharmaceutical Chelators

If the heavy metal toxicity is serious, an environmental physician should be consulted. Such a physician may consider treating with a pharmaceutical heavy metal chelating drug, such as DMSA, DMPS, and penicillamine.

27

Detox from Damaging Habits

ELSON HAAS, M.D.

❖

If you have digestive illness, you'll want to pay particular attention to toxins that may irritate or upset your digestive tract from the regular use of sugar, nicotine, alcohol, caffeine, or chemicals—what I call SNACCs. There is value in taking breaks from these kinds of habits to reassess your health and how you feel. You can't truly tell what effect these SNACCs are having until you take a little vacation from them. Research shows that all these substances can upset the digestive tract, and I notice that in my patients. Digestion most always improves when they let go of damaging habits.

These habits can initiate or aggravate many digestive problems:

♦ *Sugar* supports the infestation and overgrowth of the bad bugs—yeast, certain bacteria, and parasites.

♦ *Nicotine* can cause increased acid production, exposing the body to adverse effects.

♦ *Alcohol* is a direct irritant to the gastrointestinal mucosa. It commonly causes gastritis, liver damage, and all kinds of inflammatory problems in the GI tract.

♦ *Caffeine* also increases acid production. It is an irritant and can cause gastritis and ulcers.

♦ *Chemicals* include a wide variety of food additives and pesticides that can act as irritants to the gut. Over-the-counter medications, especially NSAIDs, are direct irritants to the gastrointestinal mucosa. Unfortunately, NSAIDs can also promote gastritis and ulcers.

If you have any of these habits, you don't want them to become burdensome or addictive. You want to occasionally take a breath, take a break, take a vacation so you can clearly assess whether these are adverse influences in your life. And the only way to do that is to not do them. That means avoiding them. All of these substance abuses, so common in modern-day cultures, can act as insidious poisons when used consistently over the years. The incidence of chronic, debilitating disease is steadily growing, often linked to these long-term habits. They are also prime contributors to poor health in our aging years.

Clearing substance abuse is the first step to restoring health. If you have a problem in your body, correcting your lifestyle may significantly cut your exposure or eliminate the cause. This is an integrated approach to medicine. Another important aspect of integrated medicine involves the way we look at problems. From the Western point of view, problems of the body become "What can I take to make this go away?" But we need to ask basic questions about our health: "Why is this present in my body? Are there things that I can change? Are there things that I can do or not do that will relieve me of this problem?" Then we have a better understanding of the major influences on our health. When I stopped smoking and drinking coffee, I no longer had acid reflux.

There's a great quote: "There are no diseases, only mistakes in living." That is the core of this philosophy. I address each of these substances fully with ways to clear them in my book *The Detox Diet: The How-to and When-to Guide for Cleansing the Body of Toxic Substances*.

SUGAR

There are many problems associated with sugar abuse:

♦ *Allergies and sensitivities* may be increased by high sugar intake.

♦ *Diabetes* is the end result of insulin burnout and a depleted pancreas, which alters sugar metabolism.

♦ *Low blood sugar (hypoglycemia)* is associated with excessive sugar intake and linked to chronic fatigue, mood changes, and depression.

♦ *Obesity* can occur due to too much insulin or its effects on other hormones; this is discussed in books such as *The Zone*.

♦ *Altered immune responses*—sugar may trigger inflammation in the gut or immune suppression, as well as a temporary drop in the level of our white blood cells.

♦ *An overgrowth of yeasts, certain bacteria, or parasites,* the fermentation of food, and infection by any of these microbes; sugar is one of the favored foods of yeasts and some bacteria.

Often people have the strongest emotional resistance to the idea of getting off sugar. But physically, it's probably the easiest! In the beginning, it may be hard just to take the first step, mostly because of the emotional and mental attachment that people have to sugar. Sweets may serve as a comfort to us, linked to feelings such as "I want my sweets. Mama, tell me everything is going to be okay." What I find working with people to get rid of their habits is this: Once they get through their first few days, they come to realize that they are no longer subject to those cravings and begin to feel clearer and more alive. Some people go through a couple of days of irritability and lost sleep, but they typically steady out quite soon. Then they find they are not so run by sugar. It's almost like a bad relationship, when they are finally free of it and begin to feel better. Often, a week or two later, they say that their moods are steadier, their energy is better, and they don't have those disturbing highs and lows. So people can see the actual difference as they progress from week to week.

What Drives Cravings for Sweets?

A couple of other important factors contribute to sugar cravings. Imbalances in flora and the overgrowth of yeast or parasites need to be addressed because they seem to drive people's cravings for sugar. Yeasts and many bacteria thrive on sugar and they also ferment sugars and starches, which generate gas, bloating, and other toxins. These toxic by-products may be absorbed into the bloodstream and affect mood, energy, and physical symptoms. Not enough protein in the diet can also cause sugar cravings. People typically have a diet that is too high in starches and sugars, especially refined carbohydrates. By improving protein quality and by creating a more alkaline diet, sugar cravings begin to decline. Eating more greens, grains, and proteins (both animal and beans), with less refined flour, cheese, and heavier food, they start to feel more balanced.

Key Nutrients

There are probably three or four key nutritional supplements that can help us with sugar cravings and addictions. One is chromium, which is the important mineral for glucose metabolism, as part of glucose tolerance factor, and it helps the body handle sugars better. L-glutamine seems to support the brain and to reduce cravings for sugar and alcohol. Vitamin B complex and vitamin C minimize the stress from the body's transition. Drinking lots of water to stay hydrated usually reduces cravings. Treat yourself to spring water or imported mineral water, lemon water (hot or cold), or herb tea (hot or iced).

NICOTINE

There are many problems associated with nicotine abuse. Nicotine is known to be an irritant, and has been found to inflame or aggravate existing inflammation of the delicate stomach lining—the gastric mucosa. Most of the research on nicotine has looked at smoking in general. A research review by the State University of New York found smokers are more likely to develop:

♦ *Reflux conditions* due to reduced saliva production and loss of muscle tone at the gastro-esophageal sphincter.

♦ *Gastric and duodenal ulcers* that have a slower rate of healing with a higher rate of relapse. Other research shows smoking to be one of three major risk factors for ulcers. A Norwegian study found the risk of perforated ulcers among smokers to be ten times normal.

♦ *H. pylori* infection and its complications, namely gastritis and ulcers.

♦ *Impaired stomach functions*—decreased blood flow, mucus and bicarb secretions.

♦ *More free radical production,* which leads to inflammation and disease.

♦ *Less responsiveness to medication.*

Nicotine also increases cancer risk. Numerous kinds of cancer are linked with smoking, as we see in the media. Lung cancer is of course the most common. However, gastrointestinal cancers may also be increased in smokers and tobacco chewers. These cancers include:

♦ Smokers have more than double the incidence of *stomach cancer* over nonsmokers (International Agency for Research on Cancer, Lyon).

♦ *Colorectal cancer* risk can be doubled for men over 50 who smoke (Finnish study).

The most promising information came out of the Finnish study of over 56,000 people. Researchers found that men over 50 who quit for ten years reduced their cancer risk to that of nonsmokers! So that tells us that it's never too late to lower your disease risks by making healthy changes.

Smoking is one of the most difficult habits to stop. It's hard because it's so deeply addictive and tied into other lifestyle habits—drinking coffee or alcohol, talking on the phone, or a variety of work activities. It even becomes associated with our breathing; to keep breathing without nicotine is like being in a constant state of withdrawal for days or weeks. For the average person, it takes about a week to begin feeling better. Nicotine patches help, but mind-set is still the key. You have to be really determined to quit.

The research shows some benefit from nicotine patches or gum, although some nicotine continues to circulate in the body. Still, the nicotine in a patch is less than you would get from smoking, and many patches are designed to be used in stages, decreasing the nicotine as the body becomes more accustomed to doing without it.

Many of the serious problems from nicotine take twenty, thirty, or forty years to develop. Although it can take as long as a year to overcome the addiction to nicotine, the benefits to digestion and health are clear. The body is relatively forgiving of these addictive substances day to day, but on a long-term basis, there is often a big price to pay in health and life.

ALCOHOL

The continued use of alcohol over the years is very destructive to most of the components of the digestive tract. Alcohol can cause major gastrointestinal problems including varicose veins in the esophagus (called esophageal varices); gastritis and ulcers; inflammation all the way through the digestive tract; cirrhosis and liver damage; and compromise of the pancreas's insulin production. So alcohol is a really important issue for anyone with gastrointestinal problems. Most people who are habitual drinkers eventually develop GI problems over time. Alcohol is likely the most damaging irritant of the common addictive substances.

Most people who just have a drink or two a day usually have no problem stopping. They may go through a mini-withdrawal for a day or two, and then usually they're fine.

Casual alcohol use commonly serves as a transition from daytime and work into the evening's relaxation. People want to loosen up. However, there are many better ways to accomplish this: working out after work, yoga, a hot shower or a soak in the tub, or taking a walk. Most any of these activities can help make that transition to a more relaxed state. The solution doesn't need to be an artificial substance to relax you.

People with GI symptoms should more seriously consider giving up that drink or two a day. If you have digestive illness, try taking a break from alcohol for two or three weeks to see if it makes a difference in how you feel. The whole point of removing irritants such as alcohol is to see if it helps you feel better. Some people will need a few weeks to see any significant results. They might see some change right away, but other benefits may take longer to experience.

Many of the changes in lifestyle habits we make require us to notice how we feel from week to week, rather than from hour to hour or day to day. If we give something up for three weeks, we'll notice benefits that we don't usually see in just three days. And in three months, we should see even greater improvement. Changes can be progressive. If someone diets and loses 10 pounds in two weeks, then resumes their old diet and gains it back, that makes no sense—it doesn't really help them. But a person who stays on that diet could lose 30 pounds over 60 days. Giving up alcohol is a good beginning for any lifestyle improvement. It can help us begin to lose extra weight, lower the stress and irritation on our digestive tract, and allow us to be more connected and genuine with our true feelings.

CAFFEINE

The research on caffeine and digestive problems is sparse. However, caffeine does seem to be connected with a number of GI conditions, including indigestion, stomach ulcers, and cancer. In general, caffeine's adverse effects on the body are from its actions as:

♦ *An irritant.* One of the problems is that the acids in coffee are irritating. And research has confirmed that patients with indigestion were more likely to experience their symptoms after drinking coffee. There are links with stomach ulcers as well, and clearly it aggravates gastritis and ulcer conditions and the pain from them.

♦ *An intensifier.* A number of studies have found that caffeine intensified the effects of medications or other chemical habits, perhaps by its effects on body chemistry and the liver's many functions. Researchers noticed this relationship in a study that found caffeine worsened gastric ulcers when used in combination with nicotine.

♦ *A carcinogen.* Studies have linked high levels of coffee consumption to increased incidence of pancreas and bladder cancer.

♦ *Acidic.* Coffee can tend to make the body more acidic and stimulate acid secretions. Because it's a diuretic, it causes the loss of calcium, magnesium, and potassium, which are more alkaline. As we lose more of the minerals, our body chemistry shifts toward acidity, and this makes us more prone to inflammatory conditions.

Caffeine tends to promote headaches, irritability, and ultimately fatigue. It makes people more tense, so there is increased tension throughout the system, including the GI tract. People tend to skip meals and replace them with coffee (and a pastry or a cigarette) to boost their energy. For example, a lot of people don't eat breakfast and then drink a couple of cups of coffee throughout the morning. This can have an adverse effect on the gut because we're taking in irritants, but we don't have any food or much digestive juice to dilute the coffee and make it less toxic to protect the stomach.

To break the coffee habit, most people just need to go through a brief period with a headache and some irritability, and that can generally be handled quite well. Usually by the third day, they are pretty clear and their energy begins to feel more balanced.

The detox process can be smoothed with a little aspirin or ibuprofen for the headache. Then the challenge is to get our own natural energy cycles back in sync. Coffee gives us a boost when we need it, as if by magic. But here, too, there's a price. This energy comes from the release of our deep stores of glycogen from the liver and the stimulation of adrenal and liver function.

If we become fatigued a little, this is an opportunity to find other ways to support our energy, either with herbal teas, the blue-green algaes, or a wholesome snack, such as almonds or sunflower seeds. Many people have better energy if they make a fruit smoothie with some protein powder. Then they get some carbohydrate and a few fructose calories, as well as the protein nourishment. Adrenal function is also important. The adrenals are key for sugar metabolism and for dealing with stress.

One of the primary questions is this: Wouldn't it be nice to feel what your own natural energy and natural cycles are? People who take in caffeine daily and then use relaxants later in the day to slow them down don't really know what their own rhythm and potential are. This awareness becomes healing.

CHEMICALS AND DRUGS

Chemicals come in a wide variety of forms. There are chemicals in food (such as additives and pesticides), over-the-counter medications, and prescription drugs, not to mention street or recreational drugs. Many drugs have damaging effects and side effects, including problems related to digestive health, because chemicals tend to:

♦ *Act as irritants and carcinogens, especially additives and pesticides.* Pesticide residues on food can be irritants; some pesticides and food additives also have carcinogenic potential, such as the by-products of nitrates (the nitrosamines). Consuming the cleanest possible water and food, organic whenever possible, will minimize these irritants.

♦ *Cause leaky gut syndrome.* NSAIDs (nonsteroidal anti-inflammatory drugs) are well-documented irritants and triggers of leaky gut syndrome, a problem that leads to malabsorption.

Since there are tens of thousands of drugs, both over-the-counter and prescription, you can imagine the possibilities for gastrointestinal complications from drug use, overuse, and abuse. Check with your doctor and/or your pharmacist to be sure the medication you are taking or are considering doesn't have harmful side effects for your GI tract.

The medical literature shows that damage to the GI tract can also result from recreational drug use, primarily from crack cocaine, but occasionally from overuse of other street drugs as well. A couple major concerns include:

♦ *Stomach and intestinal ulcers as related to smoking crack cocaine.* This link was reported in many studies, from hospitals in Los Angeles, Brooklyn, and the Bronx.

♦ *Ischemic colitis and GI hemorrhaging* were seen in hospitals in the Bronx and London, as well as Michigan and Ontario.

The liver is important because it must detoxify most of the chemical substances we take in from our environment, our food, and our medication choices. And irritation can be caused in the gastrointestinal tract directly from the drugs.

When we make good choices in what we eat and minimize harmful habits, we give our digestive system the best chance for optimum health. Ideally, as natural medicine comes more into mainstream thinking and practice, it will increase the use of reliable substitutes and natural therapeutics that have less potential for damage to our inner health.

Elson Haas, M.D., is the medical director of the Preventive Medical Center of Marin, an integrated health care facility, which he founded in 1984. A graduate of the University of Michigan Medical School, Dr. Haas has practiced medicine in a variety of clinical and hospital settings in the San Francisco Bay Area. He is the author of a number of highly successful books: *Staying Healthy with Nutrition* (a 1,200-page resource book on nutrition), *A Diet for All Seasons*, *The Detox Diet*, and *The Staying Healthy Shopper's Guide* (all from Celestial Arts Press). His bestseller, *Staying Healthy with the Seasons*, offers the perspectives of both Eastern and Western medicine and nutrition.

Dr. Haas provides specialized health programs incorporating lifestyle counseling and natural therapies within his family practice. In conjunction with his work as an author and speaker, he gives workshops and presentations on integrated medicine, nutrition, and detoxification. He can be reached through the Preventive Medical Center at 415-472-2343 or by e-mail at EMHaas@sonic.net.

28

Rebalance Lifestyle

ELSON HAAS, M.D.

❖

Our health is a by-product of our life—our genes and constitutional state, our upbringing and the habits we develop, our diets, our stresses and how we deal with them, our illnesses and how we treat them. All of this and more affects our level of health.

How we live—our lifestyle choices—is the key to long-term health, quality of life, and vitality in our later years. The five keys to good health and disease prevention are:

1. *Diet*—what we eat and how, our intake habits
2. *Exercise*—stretching and working our body regularly to keep it flexible and strong
3. *Sleep*—adequate rest and sleep (and dream time) for each of us, crucial to recharging our batteries, healing many problems, keeping our moods balanced and staying healthy
4. *Stress management*—learning to deal with life's ups and downs
5. *Attitude*—keeping a positive outlook so that we treat ourselves and others with the life-supporting respect and care we deserve

NOURISHING YOUR BODY

EAT WHOLE, NATURAL FOODS. My nutritional message in my personal life, my practice, and my books has been to turn back to a nature-based diet for greater vitality and health. Eat closer to the earth's food sources—from the gardens, orchards, and farmer's markets. Move away from the boxed and canned foods and the refined and chemical-ized cuisine. Focus on fresh fruits and vegetables, whole grains and legumes, nuts and seeds. Limit animal-based foods and refined/processed foods. This basic approach, emphasizing grains and vegetables, can greatly improve health, both in our immediate future and over the years.

AVOID TOXICITY AND DEFICIENCY. Another key understanding about nutrition is the concept of toxicity versus deficiency. The basic premise is that when we get out of balance from a nutritional point of view, we have toxicity, which means we have too much coming in that we can't handle. Toxic congestion can lead to all the chronic inflammatory degenerative problems. They're caused by too much intake of the things that the body doesn't process well—overconsumption of animal fat, excess chemicals, too many SNACCs—sugar, nicotine, alcohol, caffeine, and chemicals. We need periods of cleansing and letting go of these abusive habits to improve our health. These temptations/habits are potentially harmful to us. At the other extreme is deficiency or depletion, which occurs when we are not getting enough of the things that we need. In this case we need improved nourishment to rebalance our body.

MINIMIZE PROCESSED FOODS. So when we eat a diet that is high in processed foods and low in all the fresh things and whole grains, we're getting toxins. But we're not getting enough nutrients. So we may have a chronic problem of imbalance, as a result of both excess toxins and not enough nutrients. That can result in what I call obese malnutrition, which is common in our culture. Our bodies are craving nutrients, but as long as we're eating out of habit, we're not really meeting the basic needs of our bodies. If we just have steak and potatoes or coffee and doughnuts when we're hungry, we aren't really providing what our bodies are calling for, which is nutrient-rich food. One of the ways that you lighten up and become healthier and more vital is to get rid of foods that are high in calories and low in nutrients and to begin consuming foods that are high in nutrients and low in calories, such as fruits and vegetables, whole grains, beans, fish, and poultry, which are basically healthier source foods.

EXERCISE

EXERCISE FREQUENTLY. Our exercise program must be frequent (at least three to four times a week), consistent over the years, and balanced, which is very important. A balanced exercise program should include regular stretching for flexibility, weight work for building tone and strength, and aerobics for endurance and stamina. Exercising regularly will improve body function and health as well as attitude. It is one of our best stress managers, relaxers, and mood elevators.

BUILD STRENGTH GRADUALLY. We should exercise realistically at our current level of physical strength and endurance so that we can progress consistently and avoid injury. If we are just beginning and not in great shape, we can start slowly and build as our stamina and strength improve. If we have been working out regularly and are already fit, then it is beneficial to periodically evaluate our state and progress and make appropriate changes to exercise at our full potential, whatever that might be. If you have days when you don't feel well enough to walk in the hills or ride a bicycle, there are also quiet healing exercises you can do.

SLEEP

GET ENOUGH DEEP SLEEP. Sleep offers life's balance for all of our activity, on the physical, mental, and emotional level. Like breathing fresh air, drinking good quality water, and eating a nourishing diet, our nightly quality sleep is crucial to our well-being. There are many stages of sleep important to our body's recharging process, and although we all do not regularly recollect our dreams, we need to sleep deeply enough to go into that theta wave, REM (rapid eye movement), dream sleep. If we are not sleeping well, apply the other principles of preventive medicine, such as eating well and avoiding stimulants, exercising regularly earlier in the day, and managing stress. And we don't have to turn to medications for sleep because there are many natural remedies that can help, such as calcium and magnesium, l-tryptophan (back again), and herbal relaxers, including valerian root and kava kava.

GET ENOUGH SLEEP. Sometimes when we don't sleep well enough, it may be that we can't digest well—both food and life experiences. In terms of sleep, we're just not current. We may have too many things we are thinking about, too many things we should have done, too many things we want to do. Then there are frustrations with our jobs, with relationships, or with money. All these things are stressors, which can also interfere with the quality of our sleep.

CHANGE YOUR ENVIRONMENT. If you sense that you're not getting enough sleep, consider all possible factors: Is your bedroom too stuffy or cold? Is your bed too hard or too soft? Do you have allergies that would be improved by hypoallergenic bedding or pillows? Are you

Relax and Recharge

❖

Breathing Easy

When you wake up in the morning, there are two simple exercises you can do. First, take five to ten minutes to lie on your back, close your eyes, place either hand just below your navel on your lower abdomen and the other hand over your heart. And as you breathe in slowly, bring your breath down into your lower hand and slowly let it fill your abdomen and then your chest. And then as you breathe out, go in reverse and end by contracting your lower abdomen.

This is a way that you can start to exercise with your abdominal muscles and intestinal tract. As you breathe in, you say in your mind that you are breathing in relaxation, healing, and energy—whatever you wish.

Letting Go

As you breathe out, you tell yourself you are releasing worries, fears, disease, or whatever you want to say. And at the same time, you are just letting your body relax on the bed or floor and you are taking time to relax and recharge your body. Also let your mind relax, just breathing in this and breathing out that. Don't think about anything that may be troubling to you.

Some people report that the deep abdominal breathing can almost immediately create a positive shift in how they feel, in the quality of their consciousness and attitude. Relaxed deep breathing seems to make a fundamental and instant difference in the way they experience things.

Gentle Massage

After you do some relaxed breathing, start some gentle awakening in your digestive tract through a little self-massage. Start in the area around your navel. Slowly massage your colon. Work all the way around the outside of your abdomen. If you are looking down, it would be clockwise. You slowly massage the tissue. If it doesn't hurt, press a bit more firmly. Do that half a dozen to a dozen times. Breathe in between each time you go around. Go a little deeper with your massage as you breathe out. If you feel a tight area in your colon, you can massage that a little more. Self-massage is a way to support peristaltic activity. A lot of people with chronic digestive problems, especially those with a sluggish digestive tract, just don't have good peristaltic activity. You can stimulate that a little bit. Many people find that they can then get up and use the bathroom.

using an electric or synthetic blanket that overstimulates you? Are there pleasing routines that would enhance your sleep, such as meditation, warm milk before bed (if you tolerate dairy), or reading something relaxing before you fall asleep?

CHANGE YOUR PATTERNS. Do you sense that you need more sleep?

Try a variety of sleeping patterns. You can do this spontaneously, using your intuition to guide you. You can also explore your sleep habits systematically. For a week, try going to bed half an hour earlier each day. If this is helpful, of course continue. Or you may find that you're still not getting enough rest. Healing chronic illness places a tremendous demand on the body, a requirement sometimes best met by extra sleep. If this is the case, for the second week, add an additional half hour. Continue this pattern weekly in increments until you find yourself waking naturally, without an alarm clock, well-rested and refreshed.

COPING WITH STRESS

We have known for some time that worry and stress can affect the health of the digestive tract. Managing stress is a key element in minimizing health risk and enjoying life. Stresses are our body/mind responses to our personal experiences, and we are individual in the issues to which we respond and react. There are so many illnesses and diseases that are generated or worsened by stress that it is imperative that each of us develop skills to deal with mental and physical demands and emotional challenges. Managing stress is important because it encourages a more relaxed and healthier mind and body. If you look at stress in terms of lifestyle, we don't grow up in a society that supports or educates us on dealing with the typical stresses that we have.

Exercise, sports, outdoor activities, and especially internal disciplines like yoga or tai chi are all extremely valuable in dealing with both daily and long-term stress.

Simple relaxation techniques. We are so oriented toward action that we probably don't put enough emphasis on learning how to just be. We're not really trained in relaxation exercises and meditation and doing stretching, breathing, and other things that unwind the body so we can let go of the mind-body stresses we tend to perpetuate.

Meditation is another very effective way to clear our mind of chatter and restore inner balance. Daily meditation can gradually shift our self-image and quiet some of the harsh inner voices we carry with us from our childhood.

Body work and massage therapy. When we're exposed to a conflict or challenging situation, we tend to internalize a lot of emotional baggage. When we have little episodes that we didn't fully resolve, they get stored in our minds as images and thoughts, but they are also stored in our bodies. Frustrations or anxieties that aren't completely resolved or healed can cause tension, muscle tightness, and even pain. Body work and massage therapy can help.

Water therapy baths and showers, saunas, and swimming. Water is therapeutic. It is so cleansing, flowing, relaxing, and supporting. We are mostly water, so in a sense we are connecting with our dominant element. Hot water has the added benefit of soothing and relaxing tight tissues and muscles.

Coping skills: There is value in having a whole repertoire of constructive ways to cope with stressful situations. This involves refining our abilities in conflict resolution and good communication, and being able to read ourselves and others.

Emotional and spiritual nourishment. We may also crave nourishment on a more fundamental human level—the need for affection, intimacy, giving to others, and spiritual experience.

Spending time in nature is a wonderful stress reducer.

I believe that one of the greatest problems of modern day life is the *indigestion of life.* Most of us do not have enough personal time to digest and assimilate our daily experiences—work, relationships, and food—that we consume in rapid-fire fashion throughout our day-to-day existence. This leads to the implosion of energy and the suppression and potential explosion of emotions or bodily symptoms. These are our body's attempt to convey the messages that we don't have time to receive and incorporate. It can be helpful if we take time to quiet ourselves, to breathe and listen, to experience and enjoy. The concept is to take the time to relax and assimilate our experiences, just as we would an excellent meal. To become current with our life makes us ready for new creativity and experiences. This can lead us to more optimal health.

ATTITUDE

◆ *Staying positive and motivated to experience life,* unafraid to handle challenges or deal with uncomfortable emotions, is also crucial to health.

◆ *Begin with a personal assessment.* Our personal well-being is ultimately up to each of us. We can begin by assessing our health and lifestyle. We want to make changes that matter: changes that will provide more energy, improve our overall health, and increase longevity. Lifestyle medicine is the highest art of healing for each of us.

◆ *Use supportive self-talk to maintain a positive inner dialogue.* The way we talk to ourselves *can* make a difference in the decisions we make. If we use positive self-talk every time we start to have a negative thought, we can begin to shift our habits. Learning to think positively about our self is often a first step in loving ourselves and making healthy lifestyle changes to improve our overall well-being.

◆ *We may need therapy to help us cope in some situations.* We can't just change overnight by using positive self-talk alone. Sometimes these problems are more deep-seated and need to be addressed in therapy or with a counselor who can help uproot the psychological weeds that may be undermining personal habits.

My goal is to remind you that you hold much of the power over your health. What really matters is how you live—what you do, what you eat, and what you think and feel. Take hold and do what you can to be vital and healthy. It is really worth it! Be well.

As a doctor, I believe that the most important thing I can do is encourage my patients and readers to make personal changes in their lifestyle—diet, exercise, proper sleep, stress management, and attitude. Attitude underlies the whole pattern of how we take care of ourselves. I feel I have accomplished something useful if I can get people to change their attitude and encourage them to care for their body.

29

Renew Immunity—A Checklist

MICHAEL ROSENBAUM, M.D.

❖

Key Influences on Your Immune System
- Genetics in general
- Inherited allergies
- Nutrition
- Stress
- Age
- The integrity of the gut lining
- The health of the microflora
- The presence of infection in the gut or anywhere in the body

SUPPORT YOUR ANTIBODIES

- *Any kind of infection, even the flu, can lower your stores of antibodies* (our precious secretory IgA). An infection anywhere in the body, even a tooth abscess, can affect the gut by increasing stress and reducing the SIgA .

- *Stress reduces antibody levels.* Any kind of stress can do this. Two German studies indicate that mental relaxation procedures, such as meditation or biofeedback, can lead to increased secretion of SIgA, in comparison with a vigilant task. To promote this positive effect, stress reduction, moderate exercise such as yoga, tai chi, or Qigong, meditation, or any kind of mental relaxation are very important for a healthy digestive tract.

- *Poor diet and low nutrient levels generally also lower immune protection.* It's been shown that children in third world countries who have protein calorie malnutrition (PCM) have lower antibody levels and therefore frequently get diarrhea conditions because they're lacking the SIgA to protect them against diarrhea. Once you get diarrhea, you lose even more lining in the gut, and it becomes a vicious cycle.

◆ *Antibody levels decrease with age.* It seems that there are many more things that reduce secretory IgA than easily increase it, so you really have to be on guard. Research has found that nutrition can actually affect the way your genetic makeup is expressed. Good nutrition can tip the balance toward health.

◆ *Vitamin A in particular is critical in replenishing the lining of the gut* and maintaining the integrity of the mucosa. Unfortunately, lack of vitamin A happens to be the most common vitamin deficiency in the entire world. Other nutrients that increase SIgA include zinc taken with vitamin A, colostrum (for people who are not dairy intolerant), and probably L-glutamine.

30

The Basics

THE TEAM

Food needs and tolerances are very individual. Here are some foods known to be good for your health, and special concerns that may come up for people with digestive illness. The strategy is simple:

◆ Choose foods close to their natural state, source, and season.
◆ Select foods that are free of additives and pollutants.
◆ Whenever possible, use organically grown fruits and vegetables.
◆ Plan meals around freshly cooked and, if tolerated, raw foods.
◆ Minimize your use of packaged, boxed, and canned products.

FOODS AND FLUIDS

Water

BENEFITS: Spring water is the best. Other good sources include bottled water that's well filtered, using a method such as carbon-block or reverse osmosis. Use bottled or filtered water in cooking, to make herb teas, and to dilute fresh fruit or vegetable juices (about half and half).

CONCERNS: Never drink tap water unless you know it's from a top quality source. Tap water is considered a major source of parasitic infection, according to doctors and the news media!

Easy Ways to Eat an Alkaline Diet

Consider adding a green salad at least once a day and also at least one cooked green vegetable a day. In addition, try a tablespoon of liquid chlorophyll a day, choosing one of the tasty brands such as DeSoussa's or World Organics. These three simple additions will help to keep your system more alkaline over the course of the day. This can encourage good digestion and minimize toxicity.

Vegetables

BENEFITS: These are the basic staple of this diet. Eat all the raw watery vegetables or juices your body can handle. Heavier vegetables (such as broccoli and peas) are best steamed or stir-fried in very little cooking oil, but they can also be taken raw when tolerated. Starchy vegetables (potatoes, yams, and other roots) should be baked or steamed until soft. (Monitor for tolerance to starches.) Cruciferous vegetables (broccoli, cabbage, cauliflower, and Brussels sprouts) are very health-promoting. Sea vegetables (like those used as side dishes in traditional Japanese cooking) include dulse, hijiki, wakame, and nori. They are excellent sources of minerals.

CONCERNS: Some people with inflammatory conditions find that they can't handle the fiber of raw foods or salads, and in some cases, even cooked vegetables. In these situations, experiment to find what you can handle, by trying juiced raw vegetables, soft or puréed cooked vegetables. One of the benefits of vegetables is their alkalinity. If you find you must limit vegetables, supplement with liquid chlorophyll such as DeSoussa's.

The Glycemic Index

Foods that are low on the glycemic index tend to cause low insulin production. For example, oatmeal is low on the glycemic index. Wheat triggers more insulin than rice or oatmeal. Potatoes, starchy breads, and sweets all require a huge dump of insulin. This is a stress best avoided.

Whole Grains

BENEFITS: A secondary staple of this diet, grains provide valuable starch, fiber, minerals, and vitamins. Use whole grains only and flours made from whole grains. Brown rice, cracked wheat, buckwheat, barley, and oats are just a few of the many grains available from your natural food supplier. These can be prepared plain, baked into breads of many kinds, or made into different kinds of pastas.

CONCERNS: Whole grains are usually an excellent staple. But some people with digestive disorders can't tolerate grains, especially wheat and other grains containing gluten. Others can't tolerate starches or sweeteners (carbohydrates). This is especially true of those who have GI infections or bacterial overgrowth.

Legumes

BENEFITS: Legumes are another secondary staple. Beans and peas are excellent sources of protein, complex carbohydrate, and fiber. They can be eaten as a main course in various modifications of traditional "beans and rice" dishes. Soybean tofu is an excellent and versatile source of protein. Beans are also good chelators, substances that help to clear the body of toxins.

CONCERNS: Beans and soy products tend to be harder to digest and are known to cause flatulence in some, but all recommendations are individual. The product Beano is helpful to some people. Beans are also high in starch, so they don't work for people who are carbohydrate-intolerant because of overgrowth.

Lean Meats

BENEFITS: Another secondary staple, lean meats can supplement protein in the diet. In any case, they should be lean. The best are fish or fowl rather than beef or pork, which tend to be higher in fat. Roast, broil, or bake. Take care not to brown. Remove the skin from fowl, because it's very high in fat. Those who choose to be vegetarian can do fine with added legumes and other vegetable sources of protein.

CONCERNS: Meats are best obtained from "organic" suppliers. It is important that food preparers, especially at home, learn to protect food from prolonged exposure to temperatures that permit bacterial overgrowth. Keep foods cold until you cook them, then hot until they're eaten.

Eggs

BENEFITS: Eggs should be restricted to those from free-ranging birds fed organic foods. They are best soft-boiled or poached because frying will increase detrimental oxidation of fats. The best eggs are those from clean environments, as free of salmonella as possible. Eggs are high in lecithin (a precursor of cell membranes), and contain beta-carotene, the entire B complex, essential amino acids, and minerals such as sulfur and chromium.

CONCERNS: It is probably best to limit their use to several times a week. Be sure they're well cooked to avoid problems from salmonella.

Fruits

BENEFITS: Fresh, seasonal, and unprocessed are best. Take in limited quantity. They tend to promote good regularity. Best taken without other foods, in the morning as breakfast or as a mid-morning or mid-afternoon snack. That is, when you eat fruit, eat just fruit. This is because fruits are digested more quickly than meat or grains and they move through the digestive tract more rapidly. If fruits are eaten alone, it will minimize fermentation due to slow motility.

CONCERNS: Dried fruits should be used only occasionally and with caution because they are very concentrated sweets and are often chemically treated, typically with sulfur, which tends to promote allergies. People who are carbohydrate intolerant due to GI overgrowth may crave fruits and sweets, and find they are gas-producing. In that case, it's best to leave them alone or minimize them.

Nuts and Seeds

BENEFITS: Whole, untreated, good quality nuts and seeds can be a great snack or even part of a substantial quick meal. They can be added to various vegetable and grain dishes for flavor and added protein. They are high in fat, however, so use nuts and nut butters in moderation. Keep nuts and nut butters in the refrigerator after opening.

CONCERNS: Watch out for rancidity. When nuts and seeds are hulled (especially if they are broken), they become more susceptible to oxidation, which is what makes them rancid. If there's any hint of a funny taste, discard them, because rancid fats are a major source of free radicals. If you're concerned about heart disease, you might want to use peanut butter sparingly. It seems to have an unidentified substance that contributes to heart disease. Peanuts often contain a low level of mold called aflatoxin, known to cause cancer; the amount of aflatoxins allowed is regulated by the government, but this is still a reason to monitor your response and moderate your intake.

Oils

BENEFITS: These are an important part of the diet. The body needs about two tablespoons a day of a good quality oil rich in the essential fatty acids. The best oil to use on a daily basis is canola oil or olive oil (rich in monounsaturated fats) as a condiment and in salad dressings. Fresh flaxseed oil is a superb source of essential fatty acids. One tablespoon can be taken as a daily supplement. Additional vitamin E should be taken with it—about 400 IUs a day. Don't cut out fats altogether—your body needs fats to make hormones, cell walls, and the myelin that coats and protects your nerves.

CONCERNS: Purchase natural oils, rather than hydrogenated ones. For the same reason, it's best to use natural butter rather than margarine products. The basic rule, however, is that the diet should be low in fat overall. Aim for about 20 percent of total calories.

Fermented Foods

BENEFITS: These are an excellent source of trace nutrients and friendly bacteria for some. They include modest amounts of good quality live-culture low-fat yogurt, miso paste for broths, and health food store sauerkraut.

CONCERNS: Like everything else, response is individual. People with candida overgrowth or GI infection tend to have more problems tolerating fermented products.

Sweeteners

BENEFITS: These are best used very sparingly. Raw honey, Canadian maple syrup, and stevia are probably the best.

CONCERNS: For people with carbohydrate intolerance, stevia may be the only option. Any sweetener, no matter how pure, provides food for bad bugs. Monitor your response.

Salt

BENEFITS: Requirements are highly individual. Vegetarians have a higher requirement because they get less naturally in their diet. Best used very sparingly. Good sources include sea salt, sesame salt (a mix of sea salt and sesame seeds), Bragg's Liquid Aminos, and natural soy sauce. Some of the low salt products and salt substitutes are quite decent, such as Vege-Sal, Spike, and Mrs. Dashes.

CONCERNS: Many people are virtually addicted to large amounts of salt and salty foods. This can contribute to high blood pressure and may be a factor in other degenerative conditions. Moderation in all things—base your use on your health needs.

Spices

There are almost countless herbs and spices that can be used to add flavor and medicinal effects to our foods. Choose nonirritating, natural, and organic herbs and spices whenever possible. Some spices probably have antimicrobial benefits. But for people with inflammation, strong spices must be moderated or avoided.

Vitamin and Mineral Supplements

Best to use natural sources rather than synthetic. A plan for your optimal supplements can be worked out with your nutritionally oriented practitioner. In addition, seek advice on specific health conditions, but continue to monitor your reactions to what you eat, since no one can totally predict your own unique responses.

INCLUDE BENEFICIAL FLORA IN YOUR DIET

The first consideration is to be sure one is not dairy intolerant. In some intermittent allergies, yogurt can be tolerated every fourth or every seventh day. If not, supplements are available containing *L. acidophilus* and bifidobacteria without any added components of milk. These foods and products can be quite helpful:

- Following antibiotic therapy
- Following illness
- Following digestive upsets
- In response to stress
- Before and during long distance travel

FOODS AND FLUIDS TO AVOID OR MINIMIZE

Canned or Bottled Drinks and Sodas

Apart from mineral waters, these drinks tend to be high in sugar and low in nutrients. Carbonated beverages are high in phosphoric acid, which contributes to the demineralization of bone (osteoporosis). Alcoholic beverages are to be avoided, except for those who want to add one or two glasses of wine to their daily health regimen. The research on this is still mixed, so use moderation.

Even bottled fruit juices have been processed in bottling and are nowhere near as nutritious as fresh fruits. In addition, juices are too sweet for your body—they require a blast of insulin to metabolize, which puts a real stress on your pancreas. A good way to deal with this is to eat fruit rather than drink juice. A pint of orange juice, for example, contains the juice of ten oranges. We would almost never sit down and eat ten oranges, but we think nothing of drinking a pint of juice.

BETTER OPTIONS: Spring or mineral water, fruit juice cut half and half with water, lemon water (hot or cold), or herb tea (hot or iced).

Sugar and Other Sweets

Humans naturally like sweets. But in nature, sugar is present in small quantities in various foods, mainly fruits. Concentrated sweets imbalance the metabolism, accelerate aging, contribute to atherosclerosis, and can hasten the onset of diabetes. They also encourage the overgrowth of bad bugs.

BETTER OPTIONS: Sweets also seem to drive a craving for more sweets. You can cut those cravings by drinking more water and other wholesome liquids. Cravings can also be minimized by taking a little extra vitamin C or an anticandida herb such as Nutribiotic (grapefruit seed extract with artemisia).

Hydrogenated Fats

These altered fats can have damaging effects on the body and are best avoided. They're found in soft margarines; many other processed foods contain them because they are inexpensive and have a long shelf life. However, this is another good reason to avoid processed foods.

BETTER OPTIONS: Monounsaturated oils such as canola or olive oil (try Bertolli's Light), and for some people, butter (such as sweet butter) or ghee (clarified butter, used in East Indian cooking).

Caffeine

Minimize coffee. Decaf may be acceptable in small amounts, although there is some evidence that even decaffeinated coffee may be bad for your health. Also minimize black tea, caffeinated soft drinks, chocolate, and over-the-counter medicines like No Doz, which are the major sources of caffeine. It is best to get your "energy" by other means. Try a grain-based coffee substitute like Caffix or Pero, but don't expect them to taste like your normal cup of java.

BETTER OPTIONS: Consider how you use coffee. If you use it for a morning pick-me-up, consider adding some form of protein to your breakfast, perhaps a smoothie with protein powder. Carry snacks with a little protein (like nuts) for later in the day. If it's just a beverage, try switching over to spring or mineral waters. If it's social, go out for tea (herb or green teas).

Canned Foods

With the exception of quality tomato products that can be used in moderation, canned foods are to be generally avoided. They have been heat-treated and tend to be low in nutrients. Furthermore, they often contain trace contaminants from processing. Commercial canned foods are also typically very high in salt. Like everything else, practice moderation.

BETTER OPTIONS: Develop a routine that allows you the few minutes to quickly cook fresh vegetables (steamed or sauted in the wok). Most vegetables take less than ten minutes. Consider investing in a mini-food processor to cut prep time.

White Flour Products

These include breads, pastries, and pastas. White flour, even when "fortified," is low in nutrients and thus provides only empty calories. The high starch content of the flour tends to promote yeast and bacterial overgrowth.

BETTER OPTIONS: Whole grain breads, especially low-yeast breads such as whole wheat pita bread and whole grain tortillas.

Processed and Luncheon Meats

These often have many additives, altered fats, and high salt content. The preservatives nitrate and nitrite are of special concern because in the body they may become nitrosamines, known to cause cancer.

BETTER OPTIONS: Read labels. Some deli meats are nitrate free.

Fried Foods

Frying uses heat levels that damage many nutrients and changes the structure of the fats, making them unhealthy for the heart. It is best to avoid fried foods altogether.

BETTER OPTIONS: Try oven-baked potatoes! They're astonishingly good. Stir-frying vegetables in a small amount of a good quality oil and water is okay because they will cook at temperatures that are more like steaming.

Browned Foods

Avoid all browning of foods. Browned proteins are aged protein. The brown stuff contains toxic and carcinogenic compounds created by the process of browning. This is true of meats, vegetables, and starches.

Dairy Products

There seem to be several issues with dairy products. Sort through the concerns and see which ones affect you. Some people lack the enzyme lactase and therefore can't handle lactose, the natural sugar in milk sugar. For these people, supplementing the enzyme or using acidophilus milk products may solve the problem. Others are sensitive to milk protein (especially casein), and that can be more difficult to overcome. Nonorganic dairy products may also contain pesticide residues from feeds, drugs given to the cows (such as hormones), and bacterial and chemical contaminants from processing.

BETTER OPTIONS: Organic whole milk is now more readily available, and for those who tolerate dairy can be a decent food. Of these, plain yogurt, plain kefir, and butter can provide significant nutrients. As always, tolerance is totally individual. Calcium is the only nutrient you are likely to miss if you find you must cut out dairy products.

Low-fat cheeses (lactose free) such as Swiss, sharp cheddar, Edam, and Jarlsberg are lactose free, and used in moderation are a good source of protein. Goat cheese can also be a quality food. Blood type and heredity are important factors in dairy tolerance. Check *Eat Right 4 Your Type* (D'Adamo. G. P. Putnam's, 1996) for information on the genetic aspect of your food tolerances.

Fast Foods

There is a huge industry producing fast and convenience foods that are typically highly processed, devitalized, and calorie-rich goodies. Avoid these foods or keep them to a bare minimum. We now believe they contribute to the huge problem of obesity in the United States.

BETTER OPTIONS: If you're on the road and don't have many choices, remember that some of the major fast food chains now offer salads with grilled chicken or feta cheese, pita pockets, and even decent vegetarian burgers.

Junk Foods

These are another side of the fast food category, especially sweet and salty munchies. They add empty calories, altered fats, and sometimes harmful additives to the diet. Since many of them are sweet or starchy, they tend to encourage the bad bugs. Cut your cravings with the strategies listed under "Sugar and Other Sweets" above.

PRESERVATIVES: These chemicals add shelf life to packaged convenience products. They are added to virtually all processed foods and are another reason to avoid packaged, bottled, and canned processed foods. There's a lot of research available about the concerns. For more information, browse Ruth Winter's book *Food Additives* (Three Rivers Press, 1994).

Alcoholic Beverages

Extreme moderation is needed. It depends on your genetic heritage. If you come from a teetotaling family, alcohol may not be for you; some people just can't metabolize alcohol. But the research shows that for others, alcohol in moderation can be beneficial. For example, the Mediterranean tradition of red wine turns out to offer benefit for the heart, not only because of the helpful bioflavonoids, but also because it contains anthocyanins, the red-pigmented nutrients.

HOW TO ADAPT TO THIS DIET

Take it in stages. It will depend on where your diet is now and how fast you want to move. It is best to expect that it may take you quite some time to make all of these changes you want in your diet. And generally make one change at a time so you can tell what's working and what isn't.

Cut out the elements worst for your health first.

1. Cut out tobacco, sugar, and junk foods. Sometimes that's all you have to do. You may find you don't need other changes.

2. After getting used to that, check your response to dairy and wheat. These are the two foods most likely to cause digestive allergies. In addition, check for sensitivity to corn and citrus.

3. Begin phasing out processed foods and white flour products.

4. Work to refine your program to fit to the needs of your own unique body and chemistry.

What to Do When Eating Out

Simply choose menu items you know you can tolerate. Don't worry about blowing it once in a while. It isn't what you do now and then that counts, as much as what you do day in and day out. What if you get serious cravings? Don't try to bully yourself into accepting this way of eating.

Reason with yourself. Give yourself a vacation meal now and then (say, every Saturday night at first) when you can eat anything your little heart desires for that one meal. Call it your freak-out dinner. After a while, as your body adapts to eating well, you'll find that you don't really need such meals that often. But even then, an occasional freak out will help you be less obnoxious to your friends and family.

Food Combining

The basic idea here is that every food has a specific condition for optimal digestion. For example, fruits need very little digestion in the stomach and can pass through quickly. On the other hand, proteins require a more prolonged time in the acid environment of the stomach for best digestion. Starches are mostly digested in the small intestine.

♦ Fruits are best eaten alone—that is, without any other food in the stomach.

♦ Proteins or starches are combined with vegetables. Using this system, a meal would not typically contain both a large amount of starch and a large amount of meat. For example, fish might be served with a big salad. Rice would be served with cooked vegetables. An Oriental dish might contain meat in small quantities with the rice, but not a large portion.

♦ Try this system and see if you find your meals more digestible. If so, it becomes quite easy to integrate into meal preparation and actually seems to make planning a little easier.

Eating in Time with Your Biorhythm

The body has many natural rhythms. They range from long cycles like yearly hormone production peaks to the very rapid cycles of the brain waves. In terms of food consumption, the most important rhythm is the daily cycle.

Another natural rhythm to keep in mind is the breath cycle. You will get the most out of what you eat if you breathe well. Make sure to stop to breathe between bites. Don't be in a big rush to finish your meal. If you are in a hurry or under time pressure, take juice rather than solid food: you'll find it more digestible.

A final natural rhythm to tune in to is the annual cycle. Many foods have a season when they are available fresh locally. The body tends naturally to eat more heavily in the winter and more lightly in the summer. You may also want to consider engaging in an annual cleansing diet or brief juice fast to help rebalance the excesses of your preceding year. This can contribute greatly to your health.

Eat Right for Your Type

Consider your genetics, the physical heritage from your ancestors. We can't change genetics overnight. The implications are that it can be helpful to eat as our ancestors did. This approach also makes an argument for eating whole foods rather than refined, since that's what our ancestors ate. Check out Dr. Peter D'Adamo's book *Eat Right 4 Your Type* (Putnam's, 1996).

Acid-Alkaline Balance

Excessive acidic waste in our body can stimulate a variety of problems, including chronic infections, difficulties with incomplete digestion, and allergies. One way to counter that is to make your diet more alkaline. The Japanese, for example, have structured their diet to be alkaline. They also drink alkaline water to overcome other sources of acidity. One helpful approach is to shift our habits by finding more alkaline substitutes for foods we enjoy.

BENEFITS: Not overconsuming pasta and bread can be helpful in this regard. Rice, millet, and tofu are much more alkaline than wheat. We may choose to eat more rice and less pasta. We may want to change to green teas and herb teas. Bitter greens tend to be very healthy for the gallbladder and pancreas. And again, try adding a green salad at least once a day, at least one cooked green vegetable, and a tablespoon of liquid chlorophyll.

CONCERNS: Meat, tomatoes, and wheat are more acidic. Coffee and black tea are also acid-producing. There are so many variables in our diets that push us toward acidity that we almost have to do something every day as a counterbalance. The key here, as in most things, is balance.

31

The Ideal Diet

RICHARD KUNIN, M.D.

This diet has only one rule: Find the ideal balance of starch and sweets. It is not a prescription for what to eat, but a method of discovering your own most ideal diet. The key is finding the right amount of starches and sweets (carbohydrates) for your unique body and chemistry. Eating a diet targeted to this balance point can make an enormous difference in how you feel.

It's simply a matter of eating a low-starch diet for two or three days and then adding starches back into your diet gradually until you find your own ideal balance. That's all there is to it.

Finding your ideal intake of starches and sugars is the logic behind this approach. Here are the key ideas.

♦ Starches and natural sugars are essential to our energy and our body's repair.
♦ Our bodies have a minimum requirement.
♦ But we may be tempted to overdo sweet and starchy foods.

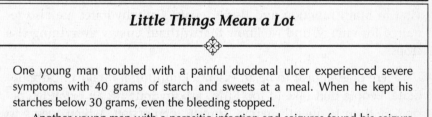

Little Things Mean a Lot

One young man troubled with a painful duodenal ulcer experienced severe symptoms with 40 grams of starch and sweets at a meal. When he kept his starches below 30 grams, even the bleeding stopped.

Another young man with a parasitic infection and seizures found his seizure activity doubled at 55 grams of carbohydrates. He was able to remain free of major seizures as long as he kept his carbs around 25 grams at a meal.

♦ Our requirement for carbohydrates is unique to our own body and situation.

♦ If we have a yeast or a microbial infection, we may actually crave highly sweet or starchy foods, not because our body really needs them, but because the microbes need them to survive.

YOUR BASIC DAILY REQUIREMENTS

The basic fuels that your body needs to function come in three forms: carbohydrates, protein, and fats. They are all essential to each of us, but the need varies from one person to another.

♦ *Carbohydrates are our primary energy source, like the fuel in a car's engine.* We know carbohydraates as sweet foods (such as fruits and desserts) and starches (potatoes, bread, and rice).

♦ *Proteins are the raw materials used to build our body* (in foods such as steak, chicken, fish, eggs, cottage cheese, and tofu). Without protein to create and repair our physical structure (bone, muscle, and even hormones), we can't exist, like a car without a frame. Our protein requirements can generally be predicted, averaging about 1 gram for every 2 pounds of body weight.

♦ *Fats are as essential for lubricating our bodies.* Typically, fats are derived from animals (butter, lard, and marbling in meat) and from vegetables (olive, flaxseed, and corn oils). Our body's daily need for essential fats is believed to be satisfied by about a tablespoon of flaxseed or cod-liver oil daily.

♦ *In contrast, our carbohydrate requirements are highly individual.* Our body stores only enough carbohydrates to last us a day. We can't accumulate them the way we do fats and protein. Fortunately, our body can literally manufacture carbohydrates from fats and protein, to assure a continuous supply. This is important, because carbohydrates are vital to brain function and tissue repair. Carbohydrates are also required for energy, and we know that without energy everything else stops.

There does appear to be an essential minimum intake of carbohydrate. People that take in too little carbohydrate for an extended period of time frequently report chronic depression, which seems to dissolve when their starch intake is raised to the level that meets their need. Other reactions to low carbohydrate intake include lethargy, headache, insomnia, and fatigue; people report that it's difficult to be highly active when they're on a diet too low in starch and sugars. Interestingly, similar symptoms occur when we take in too much. Finding the balance point is the answer.

The research indicates that we also can consume too many carbohydrates. Our requirement for carbohydrate is unique to each of us, and so is our ability to tolerate and metabolize carbohydrates. This explains why some people are able to consume junk foods without consequence, while others find them highly destructive.

The short-term effects of too much carbohydrate can be dramatic. Someone with unstable blood sugar from diabetes or hypoglycemia may experience low energy, dizziness, or mental confusion after consuming a high carbohydrate meal. Our own individual response to starches and sweets is based on our unique biochemistry, genetic make-up, current health status (level of exercise, fluid intake, overall diet and more), and the possible presence of an illness.

WHY DO WE HAVE CRAVINGS?

Sweets are a potent attractant, so basic to our nature that even newborns are calmed by the taste of sugar. This suggests a link to the endorphin system and justifies the assumption that the same system plays a part in the addictive aspect of sugar. Extensive research has confirmed this. It may also explain the frequency with which we observe people eating sweets to reduce emotional pain.

Overconsumption may also be related to the abundant availability of refined sugar and starch in our modern diet. The addictive potential of carbohydrates is heightened by refining it; simple starches and sweets tend to drive our appetite rather than satisfy it. Most of us have probably said, "I can't believe I ate the whole thing." In contrast, complex carbohydrates tend to drive hunger less. (Probably fewer people binge on brown rice than on cake and cookies.)

From the beginning of human existence, our ancestors ate whole foods—plants, meat, nuts, roots, and fruits in season. The farmers that followed the hunters ate whole grains and plants, as well as meat. Finely milled grains—refined starches—were available only to the very rich on a regular basis, and historically they were the ones with degenerative disease. In the twentieth century, automated machinery for milling came into widespread use. Refined wheat, rice, and cane sugar became widely available. Now, refined carbohydrates are the staples of many industrial societies. We find refined starches in white bread, crackers, croissants, doughnuts, cakes, and cookies; sweeteners such as sugar, fructose, and corn sweetener in ice cream, candy, juices, and sodas; and as unsuspected additives in everyday foods such as ketchup, frozen vegetables, and prepared meats.

WHY DOES IT MATTER?

High carbohydrate diets have been found to contribute to serious illness, including adrenal exhaustion; allergies; atherosclerosis; bacterial overgrowth; chronic fatigue; deficiencies of copper, chromium, and vanadium; dental problems and tooth decay; depression, anxiety, and mood disorders; diabetes, digestive fermentation and putrefaction; headaches; heart disease; hypoglycemia (low blood sugar); over-stimulation of the immune system and immune suppression; insulin overproduction, insufficiency, or resistance; increased intestinal permeability; neurological problems and seizures; obesity; parasitic infection; sleep disorders; and yeast infections.

For someone with a microbial infection, carbohydrates may cause immediate problems. We know from research that carbohydrates are the preferred food of yeasts, small gut bacteria, and certain microscopic parasites that thrive on starches. As a result, people with this problem may experience insatiable cravings for sweets and starches.

Symptoms can include bloating, gas, lethargy, gastric pain, sleepiness, difficulty in concentrating, or anxiety. These symptoms can occur after almost every meal unless the cycle is broken by changing the content of the diet. When sugars and starches feed destructive yeasts or microorganisms in the gut, toxic by-products may be created: These toxins must be filtered out by the liver and detoxified. This may overwhelm and even damage the liver. When the liver is unable to totally transform the toxins, they can circulate throughout the body as destructive substances.

Dr. Leo Galland, an internist who specializes in these problems, finds that "almost all patients with an overgrowth of small gut bacteria have a history of carbohydrate intolerance, with bloating. Digestion and elimination tend to be altered and fatigue is almost always present. These patients have already tried to follow a healthy diet and found that their health has gotten worse since increasing the carbohydrates."

If you are taking in too many carbohydrates, this new way of eating can make a big difference. Patients have told me that this diet changed their life.

What level of carbohydrate is the most ideal? It is a question of individual differences and balance. And a question of what is right for you. Finding your own individual level is the key.

A KEY TO SELF-KNOWLEDGE: KETONES

Ketones can provide clues in determining your ideal diet. Measuring your ketones can provide a baseline for the Listen-to-Your-Body Diet. Ketones are mild acids, a kind of reserve fuel that is released when burning fat under conditions of starvation, for survival. Ketosis is the state that exists when the body is burning stored fats. Ketosis is easy to determine: It can be measured with a simple drugstore kit that detects the chemical presence of ketones in the urine. A supply of keto sticks can be purchased at any pharmacy. The strips change color depending on the presence of ketones in the urine.

HOW TO DO THE LISTEN-TO-YOUR-BODY DIET

The whole process is very simple: Eat a diet very low in carbohydrates for two days (consisting of chicken, fish, or meat with a salad). Do not remain on this initial diet for more than five days without informed medical supervision. The point at which your body begins burning stored fats is ketosis. The day after you reach ketosis, begin adding back carbohydrates.

Continue increasing your carbohydrates day by day. Notice and record the changes in your mood and energy. Keep a record of your emotions, your energy and activity level, and your carbohydrate increase.

HOW TO BEGIN: THE CAVEMAN DIET

In the first stage it's not necessary to track the amounts of protein or fat to any precise degree. The goal is to limit carbohydrates to specific levels, to observe your body's response, and to note your symptom patterns.

If you have been tracking symptoms or keeping a food log, this information can serve as a baseline against which to compare the responses you'll have throughout the stages of the new diet exploration.

The Week

❖

Day 1. Caveman diet (high protein, low starch)
Day 2. Caveman diet (high protein, low starch)
Day 3. Add vegetables
Day 4. Add starches
Day 5. Add fruits
Day 6. Optional: add sweets if desired

    The changes you will observe in yourself may be enormous. It's usually easy to identify your optimal day, the day when you feel effortlessly at your best.

---

1. For one week before starting the diet, take a complete vitamin and mineral supplement daily. This is simply nutrient insurance.

2. The first two days of the trial diet, eat only average portions of the following:
   - *Protein foods*—1 serving per meal
   Eggs (any style)
   Fish or shellfish
   Chicken or turkey
   Meat of any kind, unbreaded: lamb, pork, beef (hamburgers without the buns)
   - *Vegetables*
   Two leafy green salads a day, with dressing of one tablespoon of oil and vinegar or lemon. Normal portions of salad would provide about 6 grams of carbohydrate per serving, totaling 12 a day.
   - *Liquids*
   Water or unsweetened herb tea are the only beverages allowed.

3. On the third day, add 6 additional grams of carbohydrate at every meal.
   - Choose from the following:
   One cup of milk or yogurt (12 grams)
   Three slices of tomato (6 grams)
   Half an avocado (6 grams)
   - At breakfast: Have 12 grams total carbohydrate at breakfast
   - At lunch: Have 18 grams total (salad of 6 grams, plus 12 more grams)

♦ At dinner: Have 24 grams total, (salad, plus 18 more grams carbohydrates)
Watch how you feel and respond; keep a simple diary to track mood swings.

4. On the fourth day, add more carbohydrates. Breakfast 36 grams, lunch 48 grams, dinner 60. Add three portions from the following starches (or from other comparable food that you tolerate):

Slice of bread (preferably whole grain) (12 grams)
Rice, ¼ cup after cooking (12 grams)
A potato, ½ large, baked or boiled (12 grams)

5. On the fifth day, add an additional 36 grams in the form of juices and fresh fruit—by adding 12 grams per meal. Breakfast 72 grams, lunch 84, dinner 96.

Fruit juice, 4-ounce glass (12 grams)
Vegetable juice, 8-ounce glass (12 grams)
Fresh fruit, ½ of any (banana, orange, apple, etc.) (12 grams)

6. On the sixth day, you have the option of testing your response to sugar. Double your previous daily carbohydrate intake and observe your reaction to refined sugar or corn sweetener, with three portions from the following:

Candy bar (24 grams)
Cake or pie (36 grams per slice)
Ice cream (36 grams per two scoops)

Since this part of the test is optional, as a test of your reactions, eat as much as you feel like—or none at all. You are now somewhat over 200 grams, still only two-thirds of the carbohydrates in the average American diet.

Are there cautions for this one-week test diet? Anyone with kidney trouble, irregular heart rate, or heart disease should be prepared to raise their blood sugar in the first few days of the program, by eating fruit or taking a drink of fruit juice if they get too hungry or feel light-headed. This is also true for anyone, however healthy, who feels unusually uncomfortable. The quick relief of symptoms with only a glass of juice will demonstrate the powerful effects of diet.

You can also use this simplified diet as a chance to monitor allergic sensitivities.

Once you have completed the trial diet, resume whatever diet you prefer, but think back over the previous six days. Review your food log and responses. You should be able to clearly identify the day when you experienced optimal energy and well-being. Note your symptoms and their intensity at various levels of carbohydrate intake. Remember, your responses are unique to your own body chemistry and also your diagnosis.

You may find you're unable to tolerate carbohydrates, even at relatively low levels. What else can be eaten? Check the diagnosis section in the back of the book. Also, purchase a book that reviews the content of common foods and begin experimenting to discover your tolerance. You might also look over a diet low on the glycemic index, like Joyce Daoust's *40-30-30 Fat Burning Nutrition* or *The Zone* by Barry Sears.

A feeling of well-being and decreased symptoms are the goals of the Listen-to-Your-Body Diet. At best, the diet can provide a feeling of lightness and more energy, rather than the sense of being bloated and too full. There are also positive psychological benefits: improved clear-headedness, focus, alertness, better moods. For sufferers of dysbiosis, a real decrease in symptoms can result.

STAYING AT YOUR BEST

The best way to test your sense of well-being is to stay at your optimal level of carbohydrates for a few days, then increase or decrease starches and sweets and see what changes. The Listen-to-Your-Body Diet is personalized, basic nutrition. To continue it into the second and third month and beyond, one need only remember what happened in that first week. There is no need for drastic change, just the process of observing and honoring your body's requirements. The result is a small change that can make a big difference in healing and feeling your best.

However, a word of caution. Make an effort to create your diet from choices of fresh, wholesome, nutritious food, to be sure that you stay well nourished. Our cravings can result from foods low in nutrients. Many people appear to overeat in a desperate search for nutrients that are difficult to get in the American diet: calcium, magnesium, chromium, selenium, copper, zinc, manganese, and vitamins, particularly folic acid, pantothenic acid, and pyridoxine.

The Listen-to-Your-Body Diet can be thoroughly explored in one or two weeks. This is usually enough time to monitor a variety of foods and food balances and their effects on your symptoms and well-being. This process will confirm your ideal level.

A diet moderate in carbohydrates can provide a chance to recover. This is the author's observation based on long-term follow-up. Frequently, people are able to increase their intake of carbohydrates somewhat over time. Many people who were carbohydrate intolerant eventually are able to consume up to a hundred grams or so a day. Most do just fine unless they have a bad day or week, in which case they cut back their carbohydrates to a much lower level. The Listen-to-Your-Body Diet provides a method for putting yourself back in balance.

Our response to carbohydrates will vary, depending on our mood, the climate, how much exercise we are getting, and whether we have an infection. Another major factor is whether the original problem has been eradicated. Has the initiating cause been totally, successfully resolved or not?

This may remain a complex issue, even after the balance point is determined, but at least the individual has a tool that is in his or her own control. This is an educational method, an empowering approach to increase our awareness of our own response to starches and sugars. Once we have calibrated our carbohydrates, this same approach can be used to balance out our intake of proteins and fats.

Learn to read the signals from your body and your symptoms. Your self-knowledge will provide a useful tool for reducing symptoms. The resulting feeling of well-being will be your motivation to maintain your ideal carbohydrate level. Be sure to listen to your body.

32

First Aid for Inflammation

PAUL LYNN, M.D.

❖

Suppose you have a case of immediate severe stomach distress, with or without diarrhea, caused by:

- ◆ Flu (a viral influenza)
- ◆ An acute food poisoning from a pathogen such as salmonella or shigella bacteria
- ◆ Food irritation or sensitivity that causes diarrhea (without any obvious pathogens)

If there's a fever, it is usually an infection that is bacterial or viral. Bacterial infections can also develop without a very high fever.

Nutrition can be used to soothe and heal inflammation. There are a number of simple but potent healers that include slippery elm, flax-seed, L-glutamine, and protein peptides (Seacure). These four nutrients can be used in a variety of combinations, based on your general symptoms.

In all these cases, the first important thing to do is to make an appointment to see the doctor as soon as possible. If you are very ill, go to an emergency room or acute-care medical center. While you are waiting to be seen, you can also take the L-glutamine and Seacure. They will not interfere with the medications, but they will make the work of the antibiotics or the antiparasitic therapies easier. The L-glutamine does not compete with medication; it is one of the building blocks of protein, which your body uses to repair tissue. For this kind of intense episode, consider taking 1,000 mg of L-glutamine and one capsule of Seacure every hour until the doctor is seen, and keep taking the preparations [at a lower dose] even after beginning the medication. Once the symptoms of diarrhea recede, cut down on the

L-glutamine. When there is no inflammation present, L-glutamine can be constipating. So discontinue the L-glutamine once the diarrhea has stopped.

Strong and healthy cell walls shield against the invasion of pathogens. If you have an infection (whether it be viral, bacterial, or parasitic), and you take preparations like L-glutamine, that can help repair the intestinal lining so it is less susceptible to future infections. This means the organisms will not present as much of a problem, even in parasitic infections. Research has found that when there is exposure to pathogens, the chances of getting sick are related to our tissue resistance to infections as much as to the degree of exposure.

For chronic, long-term conditions (with pain, diarrhea, and cramping), consider taking one L-glutamine and one Seacure twice a day, on an ongoing basis. That would keep an inflammatory diarrhea-like syndrome under control until there is a more definitive way to address it. Just that much will strengthen the lining and tissue of the intestinal tract, making it a less welcoming host to either allergenic or chronic infectious problems.

For inflammation and constipation as a chronic condition, consider taking the Seacure, but not the L-glutamine. But in addition, try taking flaxseed on a daily basis. It's the seeds, whole or powdered, that have a beneficial effect; flaxseed oil is not really that useful as an anti-inflammatory for the intestinal tract. If flaxseed causes a problem, try capsules of slippery elm. These plants reduce inflammation through a mucous-like quality they develop when they're combined with liquid.

The flaxseed acts like a poultice to draw out inflammation and provide very gentle roughage that will allow more regular bowel movements. Typical doses would be two tablespoons of flaxseed a day. Slippery elm does the same thing, but it may be just a little less potent. One could take a few more capsules of slippery elm—anywhere from 500 mg a day to 3,000 mg a day (one to six capsules a day) or four to six capsules of Seacure. Always begin with one capsule per day and build up gradually by adding one capsule each day.

Chronic constipation and inflammation do not constitute an immediate, medically acute situation, but it is essential to address this type of condition. If you have chronic constipation, seek medical help even if you are using the nutrients. Many doctors will prescribe the use of a stool softener. If someone with this condition does not seek medical care, the risk here is that constipation could develop into fecal impaction. This might require seeing a doctor in the emergency room to have the impacted material in the lower colon removed manually.

Don't neglect your body while waiting for the nutrients to work. If a condition of chronic constipation has been going on for more than two weeks, it is essential to seek medical care to address the underlying condition, regardless of taking nutrients. These techniques should not be used as a way to avoid the doctor. We say this as both a disclaimer and to inform you of the importance of tending to either extreme diarrhea or constipation. These suggestions on first aid are meant to be just that—first aid, and not a substitute for medical care.

FLAXSEED

Use the whole seed, taking a typical dose of two tablespoons a day. There are several easy ways to prepare it, depending on your needs. If your inflammation is mild, just use two tablespoons a day sprinkled over foods to provide a tasty nut-like flavor. The seeds will become a gel as you digest them, creating a soothing effect in the digestive tract. Another good way to take flax is to prepare the seeds as a cereal by simply pouring an equal amount of boiling water over 2 to 4 tablespoons of the seeds and letting them stand covered for five minutes. This produces a pleasantly flavored dish with the consistency of cooked cereal.

Flaxseeds provide fiber and essential fatty acids. People who find they are still sensitive to the seeds will want to try them ground as a complement to other foods, over salads or cooked rice, or added to their morning smoothie. This can be an effective remedy for constipation and some kinds of inflammation. Flaxseed can also be used to counter the effects of drugs or nutrients that tend to be constipating. For example, some people tend to get constipated when they take L-glutamine. If this happens, the flaxseeds can be taken as a complement to the L-glutamine.

L-GLUTAMINE

This amino acid (from protein) works in a different way by strengthening the muscular and mucosal part of the intestinal lining. If you have a mild ongoing chronic inflammatory disease or condition, then taking low doses of L-glutamine (500 mg twice a day) may be sufficient to control the inflammation and clear that vague sense of intestinal ache. L-glutamine can also be specifically useful for leaky gut syndrome. L-glutamine and Seacure can be used together or separately. I usually use them together in the beginning. The Seacure and the

L-glutamine are then taken in combination until you become stabilized. Then see if you can get by with just L-glutamine.

L-glutamine helps to repair the mucosal lining and restore muscular function while discouraging diarrhea. It can be exceptionally useful
in cases of food poisoning or infection through its action to slow diarrhea. In general, it slows down transit time by restoring mucosal function. Most people tolerate and need high doses when having food
poisoning or infections. However, remember there are always rare individual sensitivities. Monitor your own unique response whenever
you take any substance. When food poisoning occurs, such an acute
situation calls for L-glutamine, taken every two hours until the problem is corrected. It even helps both with viral stomach flu and dysentery caused by bacteria. L-glutamine is also a good nutrient for the
nervous system. It is relaxing because it produces glycine, so it is a
useful anti-stress nutrient.

The Role of L-glutamine During Infection

If you have an acute inflammatory reaction or infection anywhere in
the body, your system will draw L-glutamine out of the muscles and
put it into the blood so it can be used for repair. That's what makes
you feel as if your muscles are weak during a fever or acute illness.
When you take the L-glutamine by mouth, your body doesn't have to
pull this nutrient out of the muscle tissue. So taking L-glutamine can
help you retain a certain sense of muscular stability during the intense
acute phase of a cold or flu, which makes you feel stronger and better.
It minimizes that sick feeling. L-glutamine also has a multifaceted action when addressing the inflammatory processes of the GI tract.

In modern medicine, L-glutamine is given intravenously after intestinal surgery in order to quickly repair the tissue. In most cases, any
condition that tends to tear up the delicate lining of the GI tract will
probably benefit from L-glutamine.

PEPTIDES

Peptides are the building blocks that make up protein, composed of
specific combinations of amino acids. There is a product now available
that is a combination of peptides and individual amino acids; it's called
Seacure. It can be used for conditions of irritable bowel syndrome when
no infection is present or detectable. When there's infection, I rely
more on high doses of L-glutamine along with Seacure. The combina-

tion works very well. Seacure's mechanism is to speed up repair of the mucosal lining that has been damaged through irritation or infection. It helps heal very quickly. You can take from three to twelve capsules a day, but typically six to eight capsules a day is the dose.

Doctors report that Seacure is quite useful for the treatment of irritable bowel and leaky gut syndromes. People with leaky gut syndrome may have any of a number of symptoms. Leaky gut can be viewed as an early stage or low-grade level irritable bowel syndrome. These conditions often lead to a susceptibility to food sensitivities. There may be bloating, gas, and pain, or sometimes just pain in the digestive tract without bloating or gas. Other people may have susceptibility to candida and other pathogens, which can be accompanied by fuzzy-headedness or drowsiness after eating.

These conditions also sometimes cause susceptibility to constipation or loose stools. Flaxseed can be used when there is constipation and L-glutamine can be used for diarrhea. Seacure can be used when there is an acute circumstance of inflammation without infection. Using L-glutamine and Seacure can often allow you to regain control very quickly. In some cases, just taking one of each twice a day, ongoing, may be enough to manage irritable and leaky gut syndromes. Many people are maintained quite well on two to four L-glutamine and Seacure per day. It doesn't take a lot to support the body's ongoing maintenance.

CHLOROPHYLL

The other component of this anti-inflammatory program is to include the daily use of liquid chlorophyll to detoxify the GI tract and restore normal acid-alkaline balance. Chlorella, a freshwater algae, also works quite well, but it causes diarrhea in a few people. I never get a complaint about liquid chlorophyll, and it's a day-to-day detoxifying agent that is pleasant tasting. Using liquid chlorophyll on a daily basis can reduce everything from rectal burning or itching to skin rashes and general complaints related to toxicity. Two popular brands are DeSoussa's and World Organics. Use either one ounce of liquid chlorophyll or 1,000 mg of chlorella every day to keep your body more alkaline.

Minimizing toxins in the body. The nutrients that tend to reduce toxicity in the body are liquid chlorophyll, chlorella, and flaxseeds. Flaxseeds can draw inflammation and toxicity out of the body. In herbal medicine, flaxseed is often used as a poultice on the skin, for example, to draw out a boil. If you use it on a sprained ankle, it will draw out the inflammation. Similarly in the digestive tract, another valuable part of anti-inflammatory treatment is reducing toxicity on a day-to-day basis. It's hard for some people to find a diet that won't cause some level of sensitivity or toxicity.

SLIPPERY ELM

This is an herb you can buy at the health food store. It's another alternative to flaxseed. Some people just don't like taking the seeds. You can buy slippery elm in 500 mg capsules, and typical use is one to four per day. Slippery elm reduces inflammation and irritation just about equally to flaxseed in the small and large intestines. But it doesn't help constipation the way flaxseeds do, nor does it provide the nourishing omega-3 fatty acids. It does provide fiber, and it's a strong anti-inflammatory herb. Slippery elm works quite well for people with loose stools or inflammatory stomach (in contrast to conditions that only involve the intestines). This can be helpful because many forms of fiber, such as wheat bran, have a tendency to be harsh. For highly sensitive people, even psyllium is too irritating.

Slippery elm has even less potential to irritate than flaxseed, which is fairly mild. Slippery elm can relieve the irritability related to the gastritis. (Flaxseed tends to work better further down the intestine.) In contrast, flaxseed doesn't work particularly well for the stomach if there is gastritis. Chlorophyll is also reported to benefit gastritis.

MSM

Another nutrient that is beneficial for stomach inflammation is MSM. If it's clear that food sensitivities are a major part of the problem, try using 1,000 mg of MSM twice a day. Some people use up to two grams twice a day for food sensitivities. Continue it for up to about a month to see if it is working. MSM can also relieve gastritis and stomach ulcers quite dramatically and sometimes very quickly. I'd say that probably 75 percent of my patients who have taken MSM four times a day get a remission and a healing of their symptoms, with the ability to come off medications over time. Don't stop your prescription medication for ulcers or irritable bowel syndrome without consulting with the doctor who wrote them! Let them know of your improvement, and then work together on a plan to gradually end them.

THE ROLE OF ALLERGIES IN GI CONDITIONS

If you have an obvious problem with intestines or intestinal health, you should eliminate dairy, wheat, and of course sugar. I'm not even saying all gluten—just wheat, dairy, and sugar. These three foods tend to be the three excesses in our diet that generate disease in our intestinal tract. They account for many digestive problems. Eliminating these foods alone can potentially remove the stress from the GI tract.

Wheat and dairy can be reintroduced after one to three weeks and monitored to note any sensitivity. I find that more people can tolerate grains such as oatmeal and rye. Perhaps this is because they don't eat these as much, and gluten in small amounts doesn't cause problems as often.

◆ However, people with conditions such as celiac disease may be totally gluten intolerant. For them, it is essential to absolutely avoid all foods and products containing gluten. Gluten sensitivity can be confirmed through testing.

◆ Butter is often an exception to a diet with no dairy. Some people can eat butter, which seems to be more digestible than milk or cream. Others are totally dairy-intolerant.

◆ Sugar is another story. It typically causes fermentation.

If people can eliminate the foods that trigger sensitivities and keep their GI tract tuned with the supplements I have discussed, this can resolve a lot of problems with inflammation.

PAUL LYNN, M.D., is director of the San Francisco Preventive Medical Center and has been involved in integrative medicine since 1971. A graduate of Louisiana State School of Medicine, he trained at Charity Hospital in New Orleans. He spent several years in Europe and India immersed in the study of natural medicine, and has also studied natural therapy under the pioneers Drs. John Christopher and Bernard Jensen. His work includes a focus on healing through diet, nutrients such as amino acids and peptides, and immune enhancement. Dr. Lynn's current contributions include innovative work in the use of low-dose natural hormone therapy.

Dr. Lynn is available for consultation at the San Francisco Preventive Medical Center, 415-566-1000.

33

Nutrients for Repair

RICHARD KUNIN, M.D.

❖

There are simple rules. You've got to eat—that's the first rule. But you'd like to eat healthy, and that's the second rule. And the third rule is to eat in balance with the needs of your own body. That's a high goal. And that's what orthomolecular medicine—also called nutritional medicine—is all about. If you ask for it, physicians will soon be providing it. The technology and the knowledge are here. But there is a need for more doctors trained in this field, in response to growing public interest.

HEALTHY OR NOT SO HEALTHY

In health, there is always a genetic component and an environmental component. The environmental component consists of the good things that nourish us (air, water, and nutrients) and the bad things we all must deal with (pollutants and other physical and mental stressors). We accept the need and value of adapting to stressors, but we would rather avoid and remove pollution. As a rule, stressors are inevitable, whereas pollution is largely unnecessary.

When all is well, we are hardly aware of our body and least of all our digestive system, except for the pleasures of taste, texture, and the fulfillment of appetite. The rest is automatic until something goes wrong.

When things go wrong, it's useful to focus on the key nutrients. Nutrients are the raw materials used in the thousands of manufacturing processes of your body; they're an integral part of this big complex system. They're key because if they're depleted, nothing works right. If you look at the things that go wrong most often, you get some idea of why things can malfunction in the digestive machinery—the intestinal tract—and fail to heal. Repair is actually quite rapid in the gastrointestinal environment, which regenerates every four days or so. This suggests the possibility of rapid healing if all the right raw materials are in place. So theoretically, an insult could begin to heal itself in as little as four days if the right nutrients are available to the system.

For example, vitamin E serves as a vital backup if protective antioxidant levels in the cells are reduced, which is likely to happen whenever you have any illness at all. These deficiencies may not look so obvious under everyday conditions, but they really matter when you're sick. If you have chronic illness, every one of these nutrients probably should be reviewed. This is key.

When you are chronically ill, a lack of any one of these nutrients could be *the* cause. In fact, we're saying that these factors should all be considered because they work in an interrelated way. Many have essential functions throughout the body and turn up in the most surprising places. If any one component is missing, it may short-circuit an entire process.

HOW NUTRITION SUPPORTS YOUR DIGESTION

In discussing optimal nutrients for intestinal health, we must think about the health of the entire body first and then the specific organs of the intestinal system. The functioning of each organ in our digestive tract provides evidence of the health condition within.

How do we determine our needs? First there is the old-fashioned way, the art of medicine based on the doctor's knowledge and acumen. Physical examination provides valuable clues. But equally important, we now have specific laboratory tests that identify the blood levels and tissue levels of vitamins, minerals, and other nutrients. And it's now easier to find a doctor who is familiar with these tests and employs them in orthomolecular or nutritional medicine.

ORAL SYMPTOMS

The Gums

The gums, teeth, and mucous membranes all reflect nutritional status. When your gums are bleeding, you've got trouble. And that trouble is likely to affect your entire digestive tract because it means your connective tissues are weakened. So if you see bleeding gums, think *folic acid*. Not unimportant because folic acid deficiency also implies the accumulation of homocysteine, a natural biochemical by-product in the body that can become toxic when the levels are too high. This in turn suggests an increased risk of heart attacks and strokes, and bleeding gums are a known predictor of coronary risk. Of course *vitamin C* is also important for healthy gums, but folic acid is the more common, chronic deficiency.

The Tongue and Mouth

Dental and periodontal infections can cause trouble. They are quite serious because they can become a reservoir of pathogenic bacteria or organisms that can (1) cause secondary abscesses throughout the body, particularly in the brain, kidneys, or heart valves, (2) act as a constant drain on your immune reserves, and (3) wear out the jawbones, which causes tooth loss. Folic acid, for example, is also one of the important nutrients here.

The condition of the tongue is a clue to vitamin deficiencies, sinus infections, and immune status (a coated tongue can be caused by yeast overgrowth). Yeast/fungi and other organisms can move up the esophagus from the stomach, gallbladder, and bile ducts, especially if there is weak stomach acid. The first sign of AIDS is often thrush, a yeast overgrowth on the tongue, due to immune suppression. This can also occur in pregnancy, because of the immune-suppressing effect of the pregnancy hormone progesterone. Diabetics are susceptible to thrush, perhaps as a result of high sugar levels, and probably immune suppression as well. Generally, the most common cause of inflamed gums is the presence of resistant bacteria, often induced by mercury in dental amalgams. Other oral symptoms that reflect nutritional status:

- ◆ *Vitamin B_2 deficiency:* magenta tongue
- ◆ *Vitamin B_3 deficiency:* cracked lips, pigmented hands, diarrhea, mental confusion
- ◆ B_{12} deficiency: smooth tongue, beef red

Mucous Membranes in the Nose, Throat, Esophagus, and Intestinal Lining

Vitamin A deficiency can complicate inflammation and make it more difficult to heal any mucous membrane area, including the lining of the GI tract. In order to have normal production of mucus, there must be sufficient vitamin A. The active form of vitamin A is called retinol. This is not the same as carotene, but under healthy conditions carotene can be oxidized into vitamin A, and therein lies some confusion. The conversion is often very inefficient, particularly in people coping with illness, the very ones who need it most. In this case, the solution is to provide vitamin A directly through a vitamin pill or cod-liver oil.

The Esophagus

Constriction of the lower esophagus (achalasia) often seems to cause regurgitation, burning under the breastbone, and a lump in the throat. Most often associated with deficient folic acid, but also B$_6$, magnesium, and vitamin A deficiencies.

THE STOMACH

Symptoms: Indigestion (dyspepsia, belching, bloating), nausea, and pain in the upper area of the abdomen, especially on the right, are common. (Left side pain is associated with the colon.) When we eat, the stomach responds immediately, secreting acid even before we begin chewing or swallowing. It tells us right away what's going on in our body. Most people don't attend much to their body's messages. I encourage you to increase your mindfulness of how your body is working and the things you do that make it work better.

Heartburn is one of the key symptoms of the stomach. What does heartburn mean? Hyperacidity, but also that the tissue defenses aren't working so well. Why aren't they working well? There is often a diet connection—for example, a *selenium* deficiency. It is believed that the incidence of gastric cancer in the United States has dropped about 80 percent in this century since Dr. Kellogg invented whole grain breakfast cereals in about 1910. By eating these regularly, people have been getting better quality grains, not just white bread. That little extra selenium in whole grain cereal is enough to lower the rate of stomach cancer. And there is *copper*. Copper deficiency is associated with hyperacidity. Why? Because copper is necessary to the cell hormones that regulate acidity (called prostaglandins). Vitamin A is another important nutrient in the stomach, key in the production of protective mucus.

When Your Stomach Won't Empty

Delayed emptying often involves the function of the pylorus, the muscular ring that holds the contents of the stomach until food is sufficiently digested to be moved on to the duodenum. The pylorus opens when acidity declines to the quality of vinegar, about pH 4. Hyperacidity delays emptying. When that occurs, the stomach can become locked up and may hold the food for as long as three hours after eating—it's semi-disabling to have this experience.

The first thing you can try is buffered vitamin C (calcium-magnesium ascorbate). The classic treatment is Alka-Seltzer Gold, which is sodium bicarbonate without aspirin. The other is Pepto-Bismol— essentially the mineral bismuth. Pepto-Bismol is especially indicated if there's an ulcer infection, caused by the bacteria *H. pylori*. Omega-6 fatty acids such as those contained in cod-liver oil are another dietary factor in some cases.

Eating too many sweets also affects the production of mucus by binding copper, which increases gastric acid and decreases the formation of protective mucous in the stomach, setting the stage for gastritis or ulcers.

DEFICIENCIES THAT CAN AFFECT THE STOMACH
- Copper deficiency: hyperacidity, indigestion/dyspepsia
- Zinc excess: stimulates hyperacidity and often provokes indigestion/dyspepsia
- Selenium deficiency: Chronic indigestion, increased risk of gastric cancer
- Taurine deficiency (usually secondary to homocysteine excess): gallstones, pain in the abdomen, intolerance of fat.

THE PANCREAS

Pancreatitis can cause abdominal and back pain and is associated with poor digestion as well. Antioxidant supplements are protective.

Water is important. Do you know how much in the way of pancreatic secretions you produce in a day? More than two quarts! So if you don't drink two quarts, how much pancreatic juice can you make? How much saliva? It's true that some liquids are reabsorbed and recycled in our system, in the colon for example. But suppose you've got diarrhea. What happens to the level of liquids in your body? Clearly the body is at risk for dehydration when pancreatitis occurs, especially if diarrhea prevents the reabsorption of water.

Vitamin D is an endocrine activator. Since the glands of the pancreas must produce digestive enzymes, and these pancreatic secretions depend on vitamin D, you can see how important it is. In addition, when there's a prediabetic state, there's an increased vulnerability to infection. Diabetes is also a vitamin D–related condition, in another aspect of its functions. So a strong case can be made for the importance of vitamin D.

THE SMALL INTESTINE (DUODENUM, JEJUNUM, AND ILEUM)

If you're looking for a symptom reflecting the condition of the small intestine, watch for abdominal bloating after meals, about 30 minutes to an hour later. Stomach symptoms are fairly immediate, and that makes diagnosing the upper intestine a bit easier. In contrast, second-guessing the colon is more complicated. Sometimes the peristaltic rush after meals focuses attention on large bowel irritation, spasm, or gassiness. But identifying the cause of these symptoms is challenging; colonic gas is a remnant of food eaten hours or days before.

Simple sugars and sweets are hard on the gut because they are a readily available food for opportunistic flora, especially yeasts, fungi, bacteria, and certain invasive parasites. A broad variety of sweeteners are added to most commercial processed and restaurant food, including corn sweetener, fructose corn syrup, cane sugar, brown sugar, honey, molasses, turbinado sugar, fruit juices, fruit concentrates such as apple or pear, as well as highly sweet dried fruits—raisins, dates, apricots, banana chips, and prunes. Minimize sweets to maintain a GI environment hospitable to beneficial flora, rather than encouraging the "bad bugs."

Vitamin A

The gut is the barrier between your precious self and the rest of the universe out there that wants to destroy you, wants to turn you back into a pile of molecules. And between your cells and that sanctuary which your body must defend daily (your digestive tract) lies a miracle substance called mucus. Mucus is the barrier. It's antioxidant, antibacterial, and a decoy all at once. It acts like flypaper, catching the bacteria and carrying them out of your digestive tract in stools. The protective effect of this intestinal barrier is limited by the quality of your mucus and of your defending antibodies—secretory IgA. Both require vitamin A.

Yet vitamin A is deficient in one of five people to begin with. And if you don't eat the right foods or you don't make enough vitamin A from carotene, you can predict the outcome. Trouble. Again, here's where a single multivitamin or a daily teaspoon of cod-liver oil makes a big difference—by producing extra retinol, or vitamin A.

Maintaining the gut is a big job. No question about it. You have both a big surface and a high metabolic rate in the intestinal tract. Vitamin A is used in proportion to the surface involved and the metabolic rate. Vitamin A is a major factor in the growth and healing process of the GI tract—especially because the gut is constantly regenerating its lining, a two-to-four-day process (judging by serial biopsies during fasting). This puts a huge demand on certain nutrients that have to do with DNA synthesis. One of the premier nutrients is vitamin A, with folic acid and vitamin B_{12} close behind.

There are three major sources of vitamin A in nature and they are: butter, eggs, and liver. I often recommend cod-liver oil, which contains 1,250 IU per gram or 5,000 IU per teaspoon. Make sure you get good quality fish oil that's been assayed for pesticides and peroxides. Vegetables do not produce vitamin A. Rather, they produce carotene, which is a source of vitamin A, but not always a reliable one. In the case of intestinal disease, diabetes, hypothyroidism, or the presence of toxic metals or chemicals (which inactivate important enzymes), the metabolism of carotene into retinol is likely to be weakened. Exposure to toxins increases the need for vitamin A, but at the same time it decreases our ability to process it. One research study found that exposure to the highly toxic chemical dioxin caused a decrease in liver stores of vitamin A by 50 percent in just one hour!

Vitamin A also stands out because of its role in detoxification. Infections and pollutants take their toll on vitamin A, and when it's depleted, nothing heals well. Your whole healing apparatus starts to malfunction. This is a practical thing. When disease lingers or is chronic, consider that problems occur not only from how bad the disease is, but also how insidious the depletion of nutrients is, and the general state of your immunity.

Vitamin A is a little essay all by itself, because of its interactions. For example, if you have inadequate protein, you run into the problem of insufficient transport proteins for vitamin A. If vitamin A lacks the binding protein, it doesn't get to the tissues where it is supposed to go. But for the transport protein to work, you must have zinc. Vitamin A also requires thyroid, but thyroid itself requires selenium, etc. These are all depletable factors. That's why these nutrients are so important. You are not as likely to recover unless you also replenish your deficient nutrients.

The Vitamin B Complex

All the B vitamins have to do with the bowel because the gut is essentially a gigantic energy machine. Most of the micronutrients are actively transported into the bloodstream, which requires energy. It takes energy to make energy. The amino acid *carnitine* guarantees that this process will happen, so the energy will get to where it can be used. Once it is there, the B vitamins are important in the activity of the engine of the cell, the mitochondria.

Niacin, for example: one of the cardinal symptoms of niacin deficiency is chronic diarrhea.

Pantothenic acid (B_5) deficiency also results in sluggish motility and gas. This nutrient is so important for motility, it is used after abdominal surgery to get the bowel moving again.

Folic acid is of major importance because it is involved at every level in dental, liver, and intestinal aspects. Folic acid is protective when yeast and parasites are present. And it's important for healing as well as resistance. When there's irritation of the upper duodenum due to wheat/gluten sensitivity or microscopic parasites such as giardia, folic acid isn't well digested. This is important. In these cases, we do best to supplement with folic acid. The folic acid in vitamins is actually better absorbed than the folic acid in food, which has to be digested. This is an important consideration and explains why nutrients in vitamin form can be so important for people with digestive illness. But the point is that without the folic acid, the healing mechanism is hampered and the process of inflammation can become chronic.

In order for your body to use folic acid, it requires T3, activated thyroid. Selenium and trace minerals are essential to this process. Thus, supplemental selenium helps to correct the folic acid problem and improves immune resistance and healing of all kinds of GI problems.

Vitamin B_{12} is basically the same except B_{12} is absorbed in the terminal ileum (very farthest end of the small intestine, where it joins the large intestine), whereas folic acid absorption is mostly in the duodenum (the first portion of the small intestine, adjoining the stomach). B_{12}, folic acid, and vitamin A are particularly important to the healing of the GI tract and digestive enzyme production. Nutritional status can be seriously compromised if they are deficient.

When the cecum-colon valve leaks back into the small bowel, bad bugs can migrate back up into the small intestine, which inevitably means an alteration of the transport proteins for B_{12}. So a B_{12} deficiency can occur not only at the stomach end of the small intestine, but at the ileum. Ileitis or ileocolitis leads to B_{12} problems, and the undigested food now goes on into the colon.

Vitamins C, D, and E

Vitamin C is important for controlling inflammation and for immune resistance. Without vitamin C, you encounter immune suppression. The intestinal tract is not only a digestive organ, but also an immune organ. It must resist the onslaught of infectious agents in food at every meal. The first thing that goes wrong when there's a deficiency of vitamin C is the possibility of a chronic infection in the gut wall. It doesn't always show up as diarrhea, but if you are deficient in vitamin C, the local immune cells in the gut are hampered too. The results are a digestive tract that is leaky, bloated, sore, malabsorbing, toxic, and digesting poorly.

We take vitamin C for granted because it has become so available in this country, but this kind of depletion still needs to be considered. Especially since people who are sick use up their vitamin C and B complex. So they need even more than usual amounts.

Vitamin D works at the intestinal level for the absorption of calcium. A vicious cycle can occur. Without adequate vitamin D, calcium is not absorbed, and then the function of all the glands of the body are diminished and the whole digestive process is ultimately compromised. This causes poor blood sugar regulation. So the lack of digestive abilities makes you more vulnerable to malabsorption, and then the body operates at a suboptimal level.

And then there's vitamin E. Antioxidant support is strongly dependent on vitamin E as a backup when the cellular antioxidants are compromised, which is likely to happen whenever you have an inflammatory condition. The antioxidants *inside* the cells are proteins.

They are made by the cells, but they require amino acids (cysteine especially) and minerals (selenium, zinc, copper, manganese), all of which are often deficient.

Essential Fatty Acids

Essential fatty acids assure that there's the right amount of moisture in the cell by regulating hydration. You don't want your cells to become shrunken or dehydrated, nor do you want them to be swollen with edema. The essential fatty acids also regulate calcium metabolism and the calcium traffic of the cell wall. They turn on inflammatory and anti-inflammatory defenses at the cell level (through prostaglandins and their products).

Because fatty acids are part of all cell membranes, they affect all cell activities. Deficiencies can cause almost any symptom: if you run short, the skin gets dry, the bladder cannot hold urine, bowels become irregular, hair falls out, skin itches, nerves get raw, and so forth. So the fatty acids are extremely important but confusing, in that deficiency can cause constipation on the one hand and diarrhea on the other. It is a paradox.

There are omega-3 fatty acids (such as flaxseed oil) and the omega-6s (like fish oil). Both classes are important. By and large, the omega-6s build up your resistance to infection. The omega-3 pathway provides anti-inflammatory nutrients (EPA and DHA), but at the expense of decreased resistance to infection. If you don't get enough omega-3s, the body can become pro-inflammatory.

Symptoms of an omega-6 fatty acid deficiency includes thinning of hair, dry skin, and increased susceptibility to infection. In mild cases, you may see only the dandruff or eczema as it spreads across the face and the neck. Some people have claimed that fatty liver and anemia goes with it, too. An omega-3 deficiency, on the other hand, is more often associated with neurological problems, increased allergies, and inflammatory symptoms.

Other Nutrients

Glutamine and carnitine are amino acids specifically beneficial to the lining of the gut. Glutamine is an amino acid. Carnitine is a specialized amino product. It is a potential factor in support for the engine of the cell (the mitochondria), which converts fats into energy. To get the full energy out of any cell, particularly the high energy cells of the gut that make all these secretions, you must have every cell working. Carnitine and glutamine nourish the digestive tract, so it can enhance nourishment of the rest of your system.

In summary, the most important factors include vitamin A, short-chain fatty acids, carnitine, glutamine (the amino acid most prevalent in the digestive tract), and nucleic acid precursors, such as glycine (the metabolic by-product of glutamine in most people), and folic acid.

Of the nutrients that promote the production of antibody defenses (SIgA), vitamin A and zinc are most essential. B_{12}, folic acid, B_6, and the amino acids are all source materials required for competent GI defenses.

Glucosamine and other sugar aminos are found in aloe, a favorite treatment for digestive disorders. (Sugar aminos are also called glyco-proteins or lectins.) They bind and dispose of undesirable microbes that otherwise bind to *you*. This is how aloe enhances your body defenses.

THE COLON

Food for Flora—FOS (fructo-oligosaccharides) are nonabsorbable carbo-hydrates often added to probiotic supplements of acidophilus and bi-fidus to support the growth of the friendly flora. There are pros and cons to this approach. The good news is that some of its sugars will break down into nutrients that both nourish the gut and feed the flora; these are acetate and especially butyrate. However, some sugars also ferment to lactic acid, which is an irritant in the colon. So for people who are lactose intolerant or especially sensitive, it is probably a better idea to get probiotics without the FOS. On the other hand, for those who have headache and lethargy, signs of ammonia intoxica-tion, FOS can help promote fermentation—which uses up excess am-monia and thus cures headache and fatigue in some people. Monitor your response.

Short-chain fatty acids, such as butyrate, are the preferred fuel for cells in the lining of the colon. People who are depleted in butyrates have higher risk for chronic colitis and eventually cancer. You've read that butyrates are actually made by the friendly flora. While this is true, the friendly flora must have the raw materials to work with. Both starches and proteins are the source from which fatty acids are made by the flora. If these are not sufficient, there are straightforward ways of getting them from fats: They're found in butter and cream. Some cases of bowel irregularity or diarrhea resolve quickly by simply increasing fat intake. For those who are totally dairy intolerant, butyrates are now also available in supplement form.

NUTRITIONAL DEFICIENCIES THAT RELATE TO THE COLON

- All the B vitamins working together, and particularly
  —Vitamin B_1 deficiency: constipation, flatulence
  —Vitamin B_5 (pantothenic acid): flatulence, sluggish motility
  —Vitamin B_6 deficiency: irritable bowel, prediabetic conditions, high blood sugar
- Thyroid deficiency: constipation, irregularity, excess gas
- Carnitine deficiency: gas, chronic bowel irregularity, fatigue
- Glutamine: gas, chronic bowel irregularity, fatigue
- Excess lactose (milk sugar): gas, constipation, narrow stools, hemorrhoids
- Excess fruit sugars (disaccharides): gas, constipation, narrow stools
- Calcium deficiency: unformed stools, increased risk of colon cancer
- Iron excess: constipation, abdominal cramps, black stools

THE LIVER

The liver is the chemical factory and detoxifier of the body. Large meals, especially high intake of animal protein, can overload the liver. The liver is the most vulnerable organ in the body to damage by homocysteine, a metabolic by-product that can increase just from too much animal protein in a meal. Although homocysteine occurs naturally in the body, high levels also put us at risk for heart attack and stroke. The most protective nutrients in this cycle are folic acid, B_{12}, B_6, choline, and betaine (TMG). These nutrients are crucial in protecting the liver from homocysteine. Fortunately, this nutritional protection is afforded by nutrients in diets adequate in fruits and vegetables (sources of folic acid, antioxidants, choline, betaine) and animal protein (B_{12}, choline). The liver also stores vitamin B_{12}, usually enough for a few years, so it is almost always available unless you happen to be on a strict vegetarian diet. If so, be sure to have your levels checked and take a B_{12} supplement, preferably the sublingual form.

In addition to the dangers of high homocysteine, there are many toxic substances and free radicals. Inflammation and toxic products from dysbiosis often produce free radicals that can reach the heart and cause inflammation there. Glutathione, a nutrient that acts as cellular defense, is a peptide manufactured by the cell from glycine (a form of glutamine), glutamic acid, and cysteine. To supply the cell with these raw materials, be sure to get enough of the sulfurous vegetables such as the mustard family: cauliflower, broccoli, Brussels sprouts, or animal proteins, such as fish, fowl, meat, milk, and eggs. These are the best sources of methionine, from which cysteine is derived.

Methionine is also reused for a number of other essential functions, involving protein synthesis and methylation. Without it, your body cannot produce choline, carnitine, creatine, adrenaline, or inactive histamine. However, every time you eat animal protein, you dump a load of methionine on the liver and the liver converts some of it into homocysteine, which is toxic, especially in the case of deficient folic acid, B_{12}, B_6, and betaine; if these vitamins are deficient, then liver damage is more likely to occur.

Betaine (TMG) is especially protective. If everything else fails, your body can use the supplemented betaine to rescue you from high homocysteine, recycling it into methionine before it can do any damage.

Vegetarians are less susceptible to this problem than those who eat high protein animal foods because vegetables do not overload the methionine pathways. But vegetarians have their own nutritional challenges. They are at risk for B_{12} deficiency, since only meat has B_{12}. On the other hand, fruits and vegetables are rich in folic acid, antioxidants, choline, and betaine. Of course, the liver also stores vitamin B_{12} in large amounts so that it's almost always available for the first few years on a meatless diet. This fools some people, who don't run into problems until they've been on a meatless diet for several years.

THE ANUS

Bleeding from hemorrhoids, indicated by red blood passing with stools, is also usually a sign of inflammation of the colon or rectum, and the most common causes are lactose intolerance and food allergy. Deficiency of vitamin B_6 has also been implicated. These symptoms need to be related to the doctor in order to make the necessary corrections.

SPECIFIC NUTRIENTS

Fiber is important. Our food often lacks protective fiber. The right kinds of fiber can nourish friendly flora. Fiber also provides a biochemical (phytate) that binds and inactivates excess iron. Some sources of fiber appear to be easier to tolerate than others, particularly for people with GI conditions. Two excellent sources are flaxseed (whole or ground) and rice bran (as part of the grain or as a supplement in foods). Plant-based sources, depending on your tolerance, includes fibrous vegetables such as celery. Wheat and oat bran must be monitored for sensitivity and particularly for delayed reactions to gluten, which is an inseparable part of all the grains in the wheat family.

One way to be sure you get good fiber is to start making your own bread. The dangerous iron and trans-fats would be avoided. However, it's important to minimize fresh yeast in the diet, through a balanced emphasis on grains, beans, nuts, and seeds.

Trans-fats (otherwise known as saturated and partially hydrogenated oils) actually interfere with the cell energy required to produce enzymes, transport food molecules across membranes, and accomplish digestion and absorption. For example, although margarine appears to be a natural oil, the hydrogenation process makes it full of unnatural trans-fats. Research studies show that the energetics of the cell are weakened by 10 percent due to trans-fats. These fats get into the cell membrane and take twice as long to metabolize as normal fat cells. Once in place, they slow down the cell activity, so that the energy of the cell is less efficient.

Vegetable oils also have a big effect on intestinal function. The polyunsaturates include almond, canola, corn, cottonseed, safflower, and sunflower seed oils (most of the sources of oil in the vegetable kingdom except for peanut and olive oils). But there is a surprise. Most vegetable oils turn out to be vulnerable to processing. Extracting with heat or chemicals can cancel out the very health benefits for which they've been touted. The highly processed vegetable oils are subject to oxidative damage which affects human health by promoting damage to the cell wall (the membrane). Fortunately these vegetable oils are more stable if they are cold pressed or expeller pressed. So be sure to get good brands of naturally processed oils, store them in the refrigerator, and use them up within about six weeks.

The drawbacks of processed fats. Background: The U.S. Navy has long had a port of call at Hong Kong. An increase in intestinal complaints, particularly ulcers, has been observed when ships docked there. By contrast, when the same ships and crews docked in Singapore the intestinal complaints dramatically declined. Medical research revealed the reason. When the ships put into Hong Kong, the food was cooked with polyunsaturated fatty acids. When they put into Singapore, they used stable, saturated fats, from coconut oil and palm oil.

The polyunsaturates, when processed, are subject to rancidity and may cause irritation on contact, particularly upper intestinal problems and ulcers. The tropical oils, coconut and palm oils, on the contrary, seem to have a healing and protective effect. Research on tropical oils indicates that although they are saturated fats and some do raise cholesterol, there is no associated increase in adverse health effects. You'll be hearing more about these oils in the future, as new research findings expands the dialogue on good and bad cholesterol and its function in human health.

Flaxseed oil. Protective processing is also important for the ultra-polyunsaturated omega-3 oils such as flaxseed, even more vulnerable than omega-6 oils. They need to be processed and stored in the dark. Reliable brands of flaxseed oil include Spectrum, Flora, Omega Nutrition, and Barlean's.

Blood type can be relevant. Recent research indicates your blood type can actually provide clues to detecting food sensitivities. Your blood type is based on chemical markers called antigens. The immune system tolerates the antigens of your blood type in order to avoid a self-destructive autoimmune condition. Your body also tolerates antigens from outside sources that resemble the constituents of your blood type.

All foods contain antigens (elements that trigger our antibodies), and since we best tolerate foods with antigens compatible to our blood type, this approach can provide valuable clues to overcoming food sensitivity. For some people, it doesn't matter if they eat a food that is different from their own type, particularly if it's taken in moderation. But if your body is combating any kind of illness, you don't want to waste precious immune energy.

The most important thing is to deal with the major factors. Learn to read food labels, avoid the foods that don't really nourish you, and change the other aspects of your situation that you can correct. You can't fix it all, but if you make good choices about the things within your control, you will most likely begin to see encouraging improvement.

34

The Role of Hormones in Healing

PAUL LYNN, M.D.

❖

Digestive problems are often accompanied by allergies and fatigue. People with these concerns say they're tired quite a bit, they have allergies more than average, and they have achy muscles. Some of these symptoms may relate to an underlying medical problem. Your doctor might call it adrenal insufficiency syndrome or subclinical adrenal hypocorticoidism. Basically, the problem may be low level exhaustion—the exhaustion of the adrenal glands from continually battling problems in the digestive tract and other physical and mental stresses.

Supplementing low hormone levels can definitely be worth doing. Doctors who use hormone therapy find that when even low levels are supplemented, improved blood levels of hormones translate directly into improved adrenal function.

WHAT IS NORMAL?

When medical labs report the results for hormone levels, there is a very wide range that is considered normal. The labs determine their normal range through statistics, rather than by comparing hormone levels with actual patient symptoms in a medical setting. One key to whether low or low-normal hormone levels should be supplemented is whether a chronic health condition is also present. Long-term illness can challenge adrenal function and may persist longer if the adrenals are compromised. In many cases, these situations can be improved through the use of hormone supplements.

It's also important to consider individual response in evaluating the lab results. In addition to the issue of what constitutes a normal test result, there is the consideration of biochemical individuality. It's

---

When the Complaint Is Fatigue and the Lab Test Comes Back Normal

❖

Do you have just enough energy to make it through the day? It could be a case of adrenal exhaustion. This problem is often not picked up in blood tests!

When doctors check the status of the adrenal glands, many people test in the normal range. The natural cortisone level (also called cortisol) wouldn't necessarily be low in terms of the standards given by the labs. Part of the confusion comes in because people with adrenal insufficiency often test in the low to normal range.

For example, the normal range for DHEA is 90 to 430. If someone tests with a DHEA level of 125, the lab report would indicate normal. And their doctor would probably say, "The test came back normal." But the person being tested may be struggling and exhausted most of the time.

---

a fact that we're all a little unique in every aspect of our functioning. For example, think about the size and shape of the hands of everyone in your family; usually there is an enormous range in size, shape, structure, strength, and dexterity. In the same way, we each have patterns in our body chemistry that are a little unique. So levels that are perfectly normal for one person may not be for another.

ENCOURAGING HEALING WITH DHEA

If your adrenal hormones are low, your immune system will not be able to function at full capacity and you may find you're more susceptible to certain conditions such as food allergies, for example. There

HORMONE LEVELS

Hormone	Normal Range (statistically determined by medical labs)	Adequate Range (observed in medical practice by doctors)
DHEA	90 to 430	Higher than 175
Cortisone	4 to 12	Higher than 6
Progesterone	1 to 25	Higher than 5

are several ways in which a hormone such as DHEA can affect your ability to heal from a chronic illness.

Using DHEA to Improve General Functioning

Raising hormone levels closer to the middle of the normal range has been found to improve overall functioning. It can alleviate the sense of physical exhaustion. A greater tolerance for exercise often occurs, which in turn improves muscle tone and function. There also tend to be improvements in the pain in the knees and lower back that are associated with lower adrenal function. As these improvements progress, the overall functioning of the body is enhanced and you will find yourself more resistant to allergies and common infections.

Promoting Repair

The second way DHEA supports the immune system is by promoting quicker repair. DHEA is a hormone that promotes cell growth. It's an anabolic hormone (one that handles repair and rebuilding), so it also helps the body heal injured tissue. In the intestinal tract, allergies or pathogens can cause major inflammation because the intestinal mucosa is very sensitive. The mucosa is much less durable and resistant than our skin. Whenever there is inflammation or damage from an allergy or an infection, you want it to be healed as quickly as possible so it doesn't become a chronic condition. DHEA helps speed up the repair necessary to make the mucosal tissues in your GI tract whole again. That's a second way in which DHEA can be beneficial to people with the syndromes of poor digestion.

Treating Autoimmune Conditions

DHEA is closely linked to the functioning of the immune system and has been used to treat autoimmune disorders. Stanford and other universities have done quite a bit of clinical testing of DHEA in high doses for people with rheumatoid arthritis and lupus. Much of the research has been done on lupus, an autoimmune disease believed to have similar features (in terms of the immune system) to irritable bowel syndrome. In both conditions, it is the abnormal overstimulated response by our body that causes most of the injury. It is possible that DHEA can be beneficial in other comparable immune-related conditions.

Supporting the Immune System

Restoring DHEA levels also restores some of the functions of the immune system. It enhances the ability to create white cells to fight infection by bacteria or parasites. It also helps maintain the levels of antibodies such as secretory IgA that protect against invaders and allergens. So DHEA directly supports immune activity.

Providing Energy for Coping

Supplementing DHEA can also improve a person's psychogical outlook, expecially if hormone levels are really low. By the time I see patients, they have often had these problems for years and they are understandably frustrated and discouraged. They may be coping with chronic indigestion and abdominal pain, or alternating diarrhea and constipation. Chronic conditions of this type can depress our hormone function in a number of ways.

If the adrenal hormones are burdened too much for too long, adrenal exhaustion can result. That has been known since the original studies on the stress syndrome by Hans Selye in the 1930s. With chronic illness, we're looking at a situation that may compromise function without bringing on total exhaustion. In these situations, when we test for adrenal hormone levels, the results will often be in the low-normal range as I suggested earlier. But despite hormone levels that *look* normal, actual adrenal function can still be very depressed and the person may really be struggling to maintain.

Brightening Mental Outlook

In some cases of adrenal depression, people feel so discouraged that they do not want to take the steps that would probably help them. They may have made many false attempts at improvements over the years. Although they're not so discouraged that they don't come into the office, they feel too discouraged to trying anything new. Part of this pattern of thinking is typically related to low adrenal function. A person may feel overwhelmed all the time as a state of being. That in itself makes immune function worse. That is another indirect but important way that DHEA can promote the healing process.

In these situations, DHEA can help to brighten the outlook. People are then in a better position to look for new therapies that would benefit them. They have the mental energy to try new approaches. When

DHEA levels rise, the psychological outlook gets brighter, probably through improved supply of the neurotransmitters, and the person is more willing to take on a therapy program to help himself.

LOW DOSE THERAPY WITH CORTISONE

Cortisone's main functions are antiviral and anti-inflammatory. Synthetic cortisone is given routinely by doctors as a medication under the generic name prednisone. It is important for people to know that when doctors say cortisone, they usually mean prednisone. They have begun to use those words synonymously, but they are very different compounds. I use only cortisone, since it is identical to what our body produces. Prednisone is not.

When you measure the cortisone level in the blood, the labs will label it cortisol. It is the same substance.

Using Cortisone to Address Inflammation and Viral Conditions

I have used cortisone as a compound for people with irritable bowel syndrome with some good effect in some cases. It doesn't always help, but often it does. It usually helps people who have a low or low-normal level of cortisone, as I have mentioned before. In this case, the cortisone certainly works as an anti-inflammatory in the intestinal tract, and cortisone itself shows the qualities of helping viral conditions quite effectively as well. It probably helps remove some of the viral components of the immune suppression. The book *Safe Uses of Cortisone* by William McKinley Jeffries, M.D., is a helpful reference on the use of cortisone as an antiviral. It helps reduce inflammation from both infections and allergies. Cortisone also contributes to adrenal function.

Low Doses Can Make a Difference

Unusually low doses can provide these benefits. That's an important consideration. The doses for cortisone would be less than 9 mg of hydrocortisone a day. For example, 3 mg might be given once, twice, or three times a day. That is the most you would have to give. Most endocrinologists would consider that such a low dose that it would be considered insignificant, but it's not really. As patients and doctors try it, they will find it very beneficial for conditions such as irritable bowel syndrome.

In conventional therapy, the normal dose for cortisone for someone with arthritis would be between 75 and 150 mg a day. The book *Safe Uses of Cortisone* recommends using up to 20 mg a day. Dr. Jeffries does not give 20 mg a day to everybody, but he considers that to be a safe dose in the low range. In my own medical practice, I have found that people respond well to even lower doses, and usually doses as high as 20 mg a day are not really necessary. I give the 20 mg dose to people acutely ill with irritable bowel syndrome, but that is a very rare circumstance.

The cortisone typically doesn't have a positive effect unless a person's blood level is on the low side of normal. The usual low-dose treatment with 3 mg once, twice, or three times a day is an effective dose that is extremely safe. The use of low-dose hormone therapy opens up a whole exciting new arena in medical treatment.

Low Doses Mimic the Body's Function

My biggest challenge in getting people to try low dose therapy is that they have the impression that such a low dose won't help, or they say, "I've come to a natural doctor and I don't want to take a steroid." But then I explain to them that they will be taking a substance in minute doses that is identical to what is in the body, and that makes people feel comfortable about taking it. Also, I give them Dr. Jeffries' book as a reference.

NATURAL PROGESTERONE

The other hormone that is benefical in healing is natural progesterone. It has frequently been helpful for women with digestive disorders. Gastroenterologists or internists who specialize in digestive conditions typically get a higher number of women than men. In my practice it is probably a four-to-one ratio. In premenopausal women, the hormone levels of progesterone should be checked only during the last week before the menstrual period. If a woman has symptoms of PMS or if her blood level of progesterone is below 5 at that time of the month, she would respond well to taking about 30 mg of natural progesterone from day 12 to the end of her cycle.

Using Progesterone to Deal with Inflammation and Stress

Progesterone is a hormone with both anti-inflammatory and anti-stress properties. I do not know if it directly affects immune function the way DHEA does, although it has been suggested that it does. But it helps patients relax, as a natural kind of relaxant rather than being an anti-anxiety drug. It helps people sleep better and feel more balanced emotionally, in spite of their illness. Relaxation of the stress response is proven to be a strong enhancer of immune function. So that is the third hormone that should be measured in women.

The dosage of DHEA would typically be between 5 mg to 25 mg in men or women (which is very low). It would probably average about half that to get the blood level up sufficiently. People should take it at that level for a few months to see how their immune systems function, providing they have showed signs of low or low-normal levels in their initial blood test.

Testing

I use laboratory testing on blood rather than saliva. At this time, testing on blood tends to be more stable. Blood levels are more reliable. They tend to compare well with the changes observed in the body. I find that the changes in later blood levels reflect the treatment I've given.

Special Considerations About Progesterone

There are three forms of progesterone that I prescribe to my patients for everyday use:

- Skin cream
- Capsules in which the protesterone is contained in oil to protect it from being digested in the stomach
- Tablets that dissolve under the tongue (sublingual)

Unless the progesterone is in one of these three forms, it probably won't be absorbed into the bloodstream for the body to use. Other oral forms are typically digested in the intestinal tract.

Natural vs. Synthetic

All these substances are molecularly identical in composition to the substances in the body. That is the key to their effectiveness in low doses.

Where to Get Hormone Supplements

DHEA is available in most health food stores. Progesterone as a cream is also available in health food stores. Progesterone in the oil-containing capsules or in sublingual tablets is available from specialized compounding pharmacies (see below and also Resources). Cortisone is available by prescription only.

How to Find a Physician Who Uses Low-Dose Hormone Therapy

Check with organizations that provide practitioner referrals, such as the American College for the Advancement of Medicine (ACAM) at 800-532-3688. To locate the nearest specialized compounding pharmacy near you, call the PCCA, Professional Compounding Centers of America in Houston, Texas, at 800-331-2498.

35

Drugs and Nutrition in Combination

TRENT NICHOLS, M.D.

❖

It is important to tailor drug therapy to the needs of the individual. We each have a unique genetic inheritance and nutritional requirements. The stresses and toxic burden of our environment, coupled with our distinct patterns of liver detoxification, will also influence our response. In the context of these factors, drugs and nutrition are currently being used together in highly successful treatment strategies.

THE ESOPHAGUS

Using Nutrients to Complement Drug Therapy

The esophagus is one of the places where drugs and nutrition in combination can be important in healing. Barrett's esophagitis is an inflammation of the esophagus known to be caused by chronic acid reflux. It predisposes people to esophageal cancer in somewhere between 3 and 17 percent of cases. The primary treatment is to block the stomach acid with a proton pump inhibitor. However, in this condition, tissue repair is often overlooked.

Zinc and beta-carotene are typically depleted in such cases, and therefore supplements can make a difference in the course of the condition. Research has shown that 25 mg of beta-carotene, given in combination with the proton pump inhibitor, can increase tissue repair.

Nutritional Factors in the Esophagus

◆ *Alcohol and caffeine should be restricted because they are potent stimulants of acid secretion* and are also known to lower the pressure in the esophageal sphincter.

Using Nutrition to Save an Organ

❖

George had reflux esophagitis. When we biopsied him, the report came back with a diagnosis of Barrett's esophagitis, which meant his acid reflux condition was causing stomach tissue to grow into his lower esophagus. The report also indicated the presence of dysplasia, cells that are often precancerous. We knew we had to act quickly to prevent cancer.

He was put on Prilosec with a proton pump inhibitor to cut back the acid, but when he was endoscoped again, there was no change. At that time, we added specific nutrients to his program—beta-carotene and zinc to assist with healing. We had him make some behavioral changes in his eating habits, making sure that he never ate before going to bed, having smaller meals throughout the day, and eating nothing after about five o'clock in the evening to diminish acid. After another five months, he was checked again by endoscope and we found that he was almost totally healed. There was no Barrett's esophagitis and no dysplasia.

The Other Side of the Story

In contrast, Andy didn't have such good luck with his esophagitis. We requested that he come back to be checked in three months, but he moved out of state and was lost to follow-up. I heard from him about a year later. He had developed cancer from the Barrett's esophagitis, which required that a large portion of his esophagus be removed. Unfortunately, he now has chronic reflux all the time because he no longer has a true esophagus.

♦ *Spicy foods tend to irritate the damaged lining of the esophagus.*

♦ *Fatty foods also can lower the pressure in the esophageal sphincter and should be avoided.* These include fried foods, fatty meats, cream sauces, gravies, butter/margarine, oils, and salad dressings.

THE STOMACH

Using Nutrients in Combination with Drugs to Heal the Stomach

Gastritis with depressed acid production (atrophic gastritis) depletes intrinsic factor, a protein, that is needed for the absorption of vitamin B_{12}. Sometimes in chronic gastritis, acid production is decreased substantially. Since stomach acid performs part of the digestive process, in this condition it needs to be increased by supplementing with an over-the-counter preparation of betaine hydrochloride, usually sold in combination with the enzyme pepsin.

Infections due to *H. pylori* can cause stomach inflammation with or without ulcers. This bacteria has learned to live in the hostile environment of the stomach and to tolerate the hydrochloric acid by developing in a cocoon of ammonia. To get rid of the bugs, you must first temporally get rid of the acid. When you reduce the acid level significantly in the stomach and create a nonacidic environment, the bacteria have trouble adhering to the wall of the stomach.

The mineral bismuth keeps them from adhering and thriving. After eradication of the bacteria, nutrients are needed to encourage mucus production and the growth of new lining cells. These include beta-carotene and vitamins C and E; the minerals zinc, copper, and manganese; and the amino acid N-acetyl cysteine.

Nutritional Factors in Ulcer Conditions

Why do some people get the adherent form of *H. pylori* and have recurrent ulcer disease, while others are cured after one course of therapy? In part it is due to genetics or because they lack the nutrients essential to repair. In other cases, it is due to bacterial resistance to antibiotics.

In parts of Africa and Latin America, almost everyone has *H. pylori* bacteria, but there is very little ulcer disease. Researchers believe this ability to tolerate the bacteria without developing symptoms is promoted by a diet of whole, fresh foods. However, when people with the bacteria immigrate to the United States and begin eating a diet of refined and junk food, they develop all the symptoms of ulcer disease. Refined foods that are high in white flour and sugar are actually lower in essential nutrients. On a diet that is deficient in basic nutrients and fiber (lost in refining), it is much more difficult for the body to repair damage.

When essential nutrients are increased, immunity and healing are improved. Traditional diets of grains, beans, fresh fruits, and vegetables provide enough nutrients to prevent the symptoms of the disease. Fiber is another factor. It's important for good motility. It's also essential because it nourishes the beneficial bacteria that manufacture the fatty acids (the butyrates) that nourish the digestive tract.

When symptoms of ulcer disease are present, it is rational to restrict alcohol and caffeine because they are potent stimulants of acid secretion. Spices such as black pepper and red pepper have also been found to impair ulcer healing.

THE GASTROINTESTINAL TRACT

Drugs and Nutrition in Combination to Save an Organ

Surgery can sometimes be avoided by providing enteral feedings (via a nasogastric tube) or parenteral nutrition (via feedings through the veins) with high caloric content (protein, glucose, and fat). We have seen a number of successes with both methods to save the colon in patients with severe *ulcerative colitis*. In some cases, nutritional therapy was successful even after the condition failed to respond to intravenous prednisone.

The Importance of Nutrition in Coping with Diarrhea

Why do some people have a short-lived diarrhea due to a virus or bacteria from which they recover, and others don't? When the immune

---

Saving an Organ: Ulcerative Colitis

◈

Harry is a man with a high stress job and ulcerative colitis. He owns a large landscaping business, travels throughout the state, and has a hectic life. He's had several severe episodes of ulcerative colitis. The first time this occurred, we thought his entire colon would have to be removed, because he just didn't respond to intravenous prednisone. It wasn't until we started him on intravenous nutrition and a liquid (elemental) diet that we got his albumen high enough to get the drug into his system and get the prednisone into the tissue. Soon he was able to leave the hospital by going home with a central intravenous unit.

In addition to the IV therapy, he continued to take Ensure. Initially he had it pumped in, and later when he could eat again, he used it in place of meals to rest the colon. He continued on oral prednisone for a time after he came off the IV steroids.

Now, every time he starts getting into trouble, he knows just what to do. He starts by reducing the stress. He increases his intake of L-glutamine (to speed healing in the gut lining) and goes on UltraClear Sustain. He calls me and we increase his dose of Asacol, and he checks in for steroids, which aren't usually needed. He has also learned to increase his nutritional support early in the spring and fall to avoid the annual relapse that occurs for so many people with GI conditions.

system is stimulated, many people are able to fight the virus, parasite, or bacteria. Two primary factors in the vitality of the immune system are the nutrients available and the level of stress draining the system.

When people are able to resist illness, it may be because they have replenished the good bacteria such as acidophilus and bifidobacteria and beneficial yeast such as Saccharomyces boulardii. These are the major beneficial bacteria in the GI tract.

Another aspect is the role of nutrients in repair. We need to repair the damaged villi (the finger-like structures that line the small intestine and absorb nutrients from our food). Nutrients important in this repair include vitamins A, B complex, C, and E and minerals such as zinc, copper, and manganese.

Drugs and Nutrition to Treat Irritable Bowel Disease (IBD)

IBD tends to deplete vitamins and minerals due to the associated diarrhea and oxidative stress from inflammation. Zinc, copper, and manganese can stimulate the production of an enzyme vital to the protection of the energy unit of the cell. This powerful antioxidant enzyme, superoxide dismutase, is subject to oxidative stress when there is inflammation.

5-ASA Drugs. One of the cornerstones of IBD drug therapy is the use of 5-ASA drugs. Azulfadine, Dipentum, Asacol, and Pentasa are able to squelch free radicals that occur as by-products of oxidative stress in inflammation.

Manganese deficiency was found to be frequently associated with IBD conditions, in association with the use of 5-ASA drugs, in a study by the author. We also noticed that low levels of manganese typically preceded a relapse. This suggests that replenishing manganese will probably benefit patients when they take 5-ASA medications.

Prednisone, another cornerstone of GI treatment, is used to keep excessive white cells from migrating from the blood into the tissue. These activated white blood cells, called macrophages, release toxic enzymes. The drug also decreases the production of antibodies and immune messenger chemicals in order to minimize inflammation. However, the prednisone must be transported through the bloodstream into the tissue to do its job.

Albumin, a blood protein made by the liver, is needed to transport the prednisone. If malnutrition has depleted the levels of albumin in the body, the prednisone may never reach the tissue. Supplementing with protein is essential in cases of malnutrition, which deplete the production and stores of albumin.

Leaving the Hospital Early: The Role of Parenteral and Enteral Feeding

Patients can sometimes leave the hospital sooner through the use of home nutritional therapy. Parenteral feeding can be given to provide intravenous fluids, using a small portable pump and a special catheter to prevent infection. However, total parenteral nutrition alone (providing nutrition entirely through the vein) can allow the gut to begin to atrophy. It is essential to put some nutrients into the small and large intestine to stimulate hormones such as growth hormone.

We now realize that if critically ill patients in the ICU or after surgery are left on sugar water, they heal much more slowly than if they are started right away on more nutrient-rich enteral nutrition. Parenteral nutrition is used if the gut is unable as yet to tolerate oral feedings.

Enteral nutrition (tube feeding) is provided with a portable pump and a naso-gastric tube; this is typically used for inflammatory bowel conditions. In some cases, this type of nutrition is also enhanced with direct oral intake of a supplement such as Ensure HN or Impact.

UltraClear Sustain is a hypoallergenic rice-based protein that contains essential nutrients to support the growth and repair of the gut lining. The formula is based on research that has identified the most essential nutrients in this rebuilding process, including L-glutamine to nourish the cells, fructo-oligo-saccharides and inulin to support the growth of new flora and decrease ammonia production, as well as probiotics.

Short gut syndrome is known to occur after resection for Crohn's disease or a vascular accident. Short gut syndrome occurs in patients who have had a significant portion of their small intestine removed and require continual parenteral (IV) nutrition. We used to think that they would be on intravenous nutrition forever. We now know that there is a surprising degree of plasticity in the small intestine. As long as you keep feeding the digestive tract and giving it the right sort of stimuli such as growth hormone, with large amounts of glutamine, the small intestine actually grows. This can be a long-term process. The Nutrition Restart Center in Hopkinton, Massachusetts is currently treating patients with this technique.

Saving an Organ: The Small Intestine

We've had many patients with conditions of the small intestine such as Crohn's disease who have been able to avoid surgery. I can honestly say that all my patients who have been able to stop smoking and have followed a nutritional regimen have done very well.

NUTRIENTS FOR THE LIVER

Acute hepatitis and chronic liver disease are often accompanied by nausea, vomiting, and chronic malnutrition. When these symptoms occur, it is essential to control the nausea and vomiting, using intravenous hydration. Secondary therapies that have been found helpful in the author's practice include the use of a liquid enteral diet with vitamin and mineral supplements. Therapeutic acupressure (Acu-Stim) is applied through a portable unit comparable to a TENs (using the P6 point).

Reducing the Side Effects from Medications

Drug reactions occur more frequently when liver detoxification is compromised. This can happen if the nutrients necessary for Phase 1 and 2 processing in the liver are depleted. Phase 2 actually encom-

---

Saving an Organ: The Liver

Sally and Rachel, two nurses, both looked like definite candidates for liver transplants, especially after we saw their biopsies, which came back as chronic biliary cirrhosis. But using nutrition with drug therapy, they were able to heal their livers to the point where the transplants were not necessary. They were on a protocol that included medications plus the herb silymarin, and amino acid support such as NAC (N-acetyl cysteine).

The results have been very encouraging. These were women who had severe, liver biopsy-proven conditions. They have followed their diet, been very careful of what they eat, and avoided exposure to environmental toxins. They also take nutrients and probiotic support regularly and they have been able to avoid transplantation. The combination of diet, herbs, and drugs has definitely been advantageous.

passes six different major detox pathways, each with specific requirements for essential nutrients.

Toxic hepatitis can result from the drug interaction between acetaminophen (Tylenol) and alcohol when taken together by someone unable to perform Phase 2 detoxification. Many drugs are broken down and metabolized in the liver through the same detox pathways, and therefore may deplete the enzymes essential to this process. When this occurs, toxicity can result, because the liver can no longer perform at full capacity. What we call drug side effects can occur when this enzyme system is overextended. At last count, research has identified thirty-five specific drugs that can deplete liver enzymes. The amino acid N-acetyl cysteine under the name Mucomyst is the emergency room treatment for acetaminophen which can cause death due to liver toxicity.

Gilbert's syndrome, which is rather common, is associated with an inherited defect in breaking down blood cells into bilirubin that can result in mild jaundice due to prolonged fasting or viral infections. It was recently discovered that this genetic uniqueness is linked to alterations of specific liver enzymes. Research shows people with this genetic defect tend to be poor detoxifiers, based on functional liver challenges with small doses of Tylenol (acetaminophen). This suggests an unusual susceptibility to toxins. Another study providing nutrient supplements targeted at the flawed enzymes demonstrated improvement in symptoms.

By using supplements or eating certain foods, you can help to stimulate your own liver detoxification. Cruciferous vegetables, particularly broccoli and Brussels sprouts, can provide sulfur and other nutrients essential to liver detoxification.

Nutrients to Support Detoxification

UltraClear is a medical food designed to be used for liver detoxification. It comes in powdered form and contains vitamins, minerals, and amino acids tailored to the needs of liver detoxification. There is also a formula (UltraClear Plus) for people with slow detoxification. Ultra-Clear is used whenever there is a liver detoxification problem, for both liver and non-liver conditions.

We know detoxification patterns are inherited. In addition, many people now have a poor ability to break down toxins, due to the exposure to environmental pollutants. This is also occurring because people are living longer; most people who are older tend to have poor detoxification, just by virtue of a lifetime of requirements placed on the liver.

When multiple drugs are used, magnesium and vitamin B_6 are two of the nutrients that become depleted, affecting the capacity to detoxify and therefore the ability to tolerate medications. Two groups of people who often show these symptoms are those with diabetes and those who overconsume alcohol. These people have unusually high requirements for magnesium and B_6.

Whole foods are not always realistic if someone is severely depleted. Take, for example, sulfur. In someone who is ill, the detoxification process uses up large amounts of sulfur. Sulfur is found in foods that can be fairly difficult to digest, especially during GI illness— vegetables such as onions, garlic, cabbage, Brussels sprouts, and turnips (and also eggs). This is the rationale behind supporting the liver's functions with nutritional supplements.

In some cases, it's difficult to get as much of a particular nutrient as we need. Magnesium, for example, tends to be low in our diet. Our whole society seems to have a very high calcium intake because we eat a lot of dairy foods and many common products are supplemented with calcium. To get enough magnesium in order to create the right calcium-magnesium ratio would require eating about a bushel of spinach a day. Thus the value of supplements.

The Liver-Brain Connection

Ongoing research is being done in conjunction with HealthComm International (Gig Harbor, Washington) and the Institutes for the Achievement of Human Potential (Philadelphia). Work with brain-injured children is highlighting the links between brain function, impaired liver detoxification, and GI integrity. This work builds on a decade of research on the effects of digestive toxins on the brain and nervous system. The research implicates a variety of subtle GI disorders in certain forms of learning disabilities, hyperactivity, and even autism.

Enhancing the Action of a Drug and Saving Money in the Use of Costly Medications

Transplant patients require cyclosporin, a drug that is very expensive. The effectiveness of the drug can be increased and the required dosage

---

A Sample Protocol for Treating Chronic Liver Disease

Diet

- Often protein must be restricted. Nonmeat sources of protein such as vegetable protein contain lower amounts of mercaptan (an amino acid elevated in such cases) and ammonia.
- Salt (sodium) restriction is needed when edema and/or ascites (abdominal fluid) accumulate.
- Fluid restriction is also often necessary with edema and/or ascites.

Medications

- Neomycin (an antibiotic) and/or beta-lactulose (a nonmetabolized sugar) can be given to reduce the ammonia production from bacteria in the gut.
- Spirolactone is a diuretic medication that is useful in treating ascites because it blocks the secretion of aldosterone, a hormone that is overproduced in this condition.

Nutrients to supplement

- Water-soluble vitamins are needed to supplement the metabolism.
- Fat-soluble vitamin deficiency is very common in chronic liver disease, and water-soluble forms of these vitamins (Aquasol A or Aquasol E) should be used while monitoring blood levels to ensure adequate amounts.
- Calcium is often inadequate in these conditions and dietary and/or supplemental calcium up to 1,500 mg per day should be encouraged in those at risk for osteoporosis.
- Zinc deficiency is common in many types of liver disease.
- Magnesium deficiency is due to malabsorption, small bowel disease, or pancreatic insufficiency.
- Specific branched-chain amino acid supplements also appear to be helpful.

Nutrients to be Restricted

- Iron supplementation is often to be avoided because of the dangers of iron overload or because of the Fenton reaction, in which iron can fuel oxidative stress.
- Copper and manganese should be restricted in causes of jaundice because excretion of these minerals is often impaired.

---

reduced by slowing liver metabolism through the use of grapefruit juice. An active ingredient in the juice, naringenin, blocks the activity of one of the liver enzymes, down-regulated liver activity. As a result, less of the drug is needed. Davy Jones, M.D., a Linus Pauling Award recipient of 1997, makes similar use of grapefruit juice with patients to reduce the dose of Viagra, which is a very expensive medication used to treat impotence.

AIDS

For AIDS patients, proper nutrition is extremely important. Now that we have potent protease inhibitors for HIV and treatment for pneumocystis, what is most dangerous to AIDS patients is malnutrition. Mitchell Kaminski, M.D., and Jeffery Bland, Ph.D., have done research on the treatment of the AIDS wasting syndrome as a gastrointestinal disorder.

To restore the destruction from the wasting effects of AIDS, they recommend a nutrient-rich protocol including antioxidants such as vitamins C and E, amino acids such as N-acetyl cysteine and arginine, and minerals including selenium, manganese, zinc, and copper to reduce inflammation. Damage from overly reactive immune responses to inflammation are moderated with CoQ10, essential fatty acids, and lipoic acid. Pepto-Bismol (containing the mineral bismuth) is given to decrease the adherence of cyclosporidia and microsporidia to the intestinal lining and decrease the diarrhea. UltraClear Sustain and extra L-glutamine are also provided as part of this extensive gut repair program.

NUTRITION AS A TOOL POTENTIALLY AS IMPORTANT AS MEDICATIONS

We predict that nutrition will become a tool that any physician or healer will use. Now we tend to think of food as just something that provides calories and satisfies our taste buds. However, we are seeing the distinction between nutrition and medicine blend. The use of specific, carefully chosen nutrients can provide many healing benefits and positive health outcomes, as the new science of nutritional medicine demonstrates.

In the future, with advances in genetics, nutritional science, and bioelectromagnetics, twenty-first century health care will achieve what Thomas Edison predicted.

The Doctor of the future will give no medicines. But will interest his patients in the care of the human frame, in diet and in the causes of disease.
—Thomas Edison

36

Drug Cautions*

LEN SAPUTO, M.D.

❖

We all know that pharmaceutical drugs can add a lot to improve our symptoms, at times can reverse our illness, and can be lifesaving. We value them highly and need them. It is also well known, as mentioned in a recent article in *The Journal of the American Medical Association*, that pharmaceutical drugs are the third leading cause of death in America and lead to over 5 million hospitalizations every year! Only heart disease and cancer result in more deaths.

This paradoxical situation emphasizes the importance of using pharmaceuticals only when the benefits of their use clearly outweigh their possible risks. This requires a value judgment. Often the assessment of a clinical situation and the decision to use or not to use a specific drug can be very difficult. We may not really know what to do. We may not really want to go through the process of exploring nonpharmaceutical alternatives, nor do we really want to take responsibility for the downside of what can happen. We just want to get better and hope that the doctor knows best.

The cells of our body are highly complex, microscopic industrial plants. We know a lot about how they operate biochemically, but this knowledge represents only the tip of the iceberg. The synthetic drugs produced by science and manufacturing and then introduce into our bodies are a unique phenomenon in human history. Nothing quite like them has ever existed in the past. We don't understand fully how they operate and have no idea what they will do to some distant biochemical reaction until some time after they have been in use and a problem develops "out of the blue." This information is sometimes

How Things Go Wrong

Dan developed severe diarrhea at the age of 16, and he was hospitalized for the major dehydration that resulted from the 15 to 20 bowel movements he was having every day. Over the prior three months, he had lost more than 20 pounds, and at 5 feet 10 inches, he now weighed just 130 pounds. His physician did a colonoscopy with biopsies, which confirmed the diagnosis of ulcerative colitis.

Dan was treated with prednisone and Asacol, and his symptoms improved markedly. He began to feel good, gained back about ten pounds, and was having only two to three soft bowel movements a day. Unfortunately, over the following several years, Dan would have a recurrence of the ulcerative colitis symptoms whenever the prednisone was decreased below 10 mg a day. So he and his doctor felt it was essential that he remain on the drug.

However, he began to develop signs of Cushing's disease associated with the overuse of steroids—overweight with a swollen abdomen, yet thin legs and wasting muscles, and weakness with a tendency to bruise easily and heal slowly. He also had chronic indigestion from the prednisone. His physician ordered antacids and Zantac, which controlled his indigestion, but the Cushing-like side effects of the prednisone continued to develop. There was talk of doing a colectomy. Dan knew he was in trouble.

When Dan first came to me, he was depressed and worried that he might never get over his ulcerative colitis. He felt dependent on the drugs, and at the same time feared that they were causing problems that would eventually damage his body in a very serious way. He was right.

Rather than suppressing the symptoms of the ulcerative colitis, we elected to support his digestive tract with the best nutrition possible, and to see if his body could heal itself. He began a program of supplements that included L-glutamine, friendly flora (probiotics), licorice extract, butyrate enemas, anti-yeast herbs, essential fatty acids, antioxidants, and a diet high in nutrients and low in allergens. He was gradually able to decrease the drugs, and within four months, he was off the drugs altogether. For the first time in years, he was having normal bowel movements and yet was no longer on medication. Dan has gained back his confidence and his lost weight, and now has to "diet" to maintain a normal weight!

---

learned the hard way, and a drug is recalled from clinical practice because of serious complications or even death.

This same toxicity is not seen nearly as often when natural therapies (nutraceuticals) are used, such as vitamins, minerals, food extracts, and herbs. Despite the fact that nutraceuticals only occasionally cause serious problems, we read about them in the headlines whenever they do occur. They don't even begin to rival synthetic pharmaceuticals in their magnitude of danger. They are nowhere near the third leading cause of death in America.

One of the major conceptual differences between conventional and nutritional approaches in managing illness is that in mainstream medicine, the treatment is often based on suppressing the symptoms of a disease, and in nutritional medicine it is generally to support the defenses of the body to cure itself of the disease. Working in harmony with the body is much less intrusive to natural biochemical processes and is less likely to result in serious complications from therapy.

Many natural alternatives to synthetic pharmaceuticals are important to consider, especially in people who are ill. Some of the drugs that should be avoided in patients with gastrointestinal disease include NSAIDs, H2 blockers, prolonged antacid therapy, corticosteroid usage, antibiotics, drugs that affect intestinal peristalsis, and artificial fiber.

Nonsteroidal anti-inflammatory drugs (NSAIDs) should rarely, if ever, be used because they are so toxic. It is well documented in the medical literature that each year approximately 15,000 deaths and over 300,000 admissions to hospitals occur from the direct effects of these synthetic pharmaceuticals. Most problems are related to gastritis, ulcers, and gastrointestinal bleeding, though there are also serious kidney and liver abnormalities as well. In addition, there are profound changes in the permeability across the intestinal lining that result in toxic overload to the liver and to the immune system. It has been shown that intestinal bacteria can pass across the intestinal lining and invade the body as a consequence of this increased intestinal permeability. These changes in permeability have been documented to occur after even a single dose of NSAIDs.

H2 blockers such as cimetidine (Tagamet), ranitidine (Zantac), famotidine (Pepcid), and omeprazole (Prilosec) are powerful inhibitors of acid secretion into the stomach. They work wonderfully to relieve our symptoms of indigestion, but there is a price to pay. They all but abolish acid production, and consequently we don't have the necessary acid to digest protein properly or to absorb vitamin B_{12} or various minerals. These medications can also cause other changes that affect the composition of the intestinal microflora.

Deglycrhizinated licorice (DGL) has been shown to be equally effective to Tagamet and Zantac in clinical trials, and it has no effect in changing acid production. What it does do is strengthen the protective mucus layer that lines the stomach, increase the longevity of gastrointestinal cells, improve circulation to the intestinal mucosa, and stimulate the production of secretory antibodies that are shed into the gut. It may even help the body to rid itself of *Helicobacter pylori*, the bacteria thought to be responsible for some ulcer formation in the first place.

Sucralfate (Carafate) is a popular synthetic pharmaceutical that is believed to coat the stomach and form a protective layer that keeps stomach acid from access to the ulcerated tissues. Again, it has been shown to be effective in healing stomach ulcers. However, it is full of aluminum, just like several antacids! It is well documented that aluminum is highly toxic to the nervous system, and it has been shown that there is a significant increase in both blood and urinary levels of aluminum after standard doses of these substances. Aluminum toxicity has been implicated in numerous studies on Alzheimer's disease. Why use something that is toxic when it is just as effective to use a natural remedy that is totally safe?

Corticosteroids (cortisone products) can be lifesaving in patients with certain gastrointestinal problems, and there is a clear place for their usage, especially in Crohn's disease and ulcerative colitis. However, they should be reserved as a last resort. Nutritional support of the gut can be vitally important in preventing the progression of these illnesses. Nutrients such as L-glutamine, probiotics, antioxidants, essential fatty acids, and butyrate frequently promote natural healing and obviate the need for even considering corticosteroids. The very serious effects of steroids can be devastating and have been linked to the development of ulcers, osteoporosis, psychosis, high blood pressure, fluid retention, potassium and magnesium depletion, and more.

Antibiotics similarly are often critical in the management of serious life-threatening bacterial infections. When used appropriately, they are of clear value. However, whenever an antibiotic is taken, there are potentially serious consequences. Maintaining a normal balance of the microflora of the gut is very important in sustaining good health. In the extreme situation, a potentially life-threatening condition called pseudomembranous enterocolitis can develop. This is the result of using antibiotics that kill the normal intestinal microflora and allow the selective overgrowth of highly pathogenic bacteria (*Clostridium difficile*) to dominate. In addition, antibiotics disturb other important aspects of nutrition and GI function.

Pharmaceuticals that "balance" intestinal motility may relieve our abdominal cramping, diarrhea, or dull aching pains, or speed up a sluggish gut, as in esophageal motility disorders. While the symptoms are often improved or relieved, nothing is accomplished regarding the causes of these disorders. In fact, this approach will actually mask the symptoms of the disorder, making us feel like the problem is no longer present. In addition, potential complications may result from the unwanted side effects of the medication.

Occasionally these complications can be lethal, as in the case of a recently withdrawn drug, Posicor, a calcium channel blocker for high blood pressure. When this medication was processed in the liver, it competed with other drugs that used the same two specific CP-450 enzymes; these medications included Propulsid, Mevacor, Hismanal, erythromycin, and others. The result was heart arrhythmias, in a few cases fatal. Drug combinations have become more prolific and more problematic—one of the reasons pharmacists now use computerized drug interaction databases.

Most patients with digestive disorders are labeled as having "irritable bowel syndrome" or "spastic colon." Nearly all of the associated problems can be managed successfully without the use of any synthetic pharmaceuticals by correcting the ecological balance of the intestinal flora (dysbiosis), providing nutritional support for the gut, improving our diets, and eliminating food allergies or intolerances, like gluten sensitivity or lactose intolerance.

We are repeatedly told that we need more fiber in our diets. It is important in preventing constipation, in lowering cholesterol, in adding bulk to the stool, and in detoxification. It is also critically important as a nutrient for those friendly bacteria in our intestinal tracts, vital for the normal function of the digestive tract. So we should be eating fiber—that which is found in food.

When we eat artificial fiber, it may well provide some of the functions that we've discussed, but it cannot function as a nutrient for the bacteria in our intestinal tracts. And many of these artificial fiber products have other "inert" ingredients such as sodium lauryl sulfate, mineral oil, and povidone that are clearly unhealthy for our body chemistry.

So when we are looking for solutions to our health problems, while synthetic pharmaceuticals may save our lives in severe illnesses, because of their ever-present inherent toxicity to the biochemistry of the body, we must beware. Medications have their place, but overuse can be dangerous because of the many potential drug-to-drug interactions and consequent side effects. Another issue is the increased demand drugs place on the the liver for detoxification. It is not prudent to rely on these powerful drugs in situations where it is possible to use natural alternatives that have also been documented to be of equivalent value. We would be wise to use an integrated approach to solving our health care issues that offer safer alternatives when common sense (and our doctor!) tells us they are reasonable choices.

> *Greater than the tread of a mighty army is the power of an idea whose time has come.* —Victor Hugo

37

Benefits of Herbal Therapies

TIMOTHY KUSS, Ph.D.

❖

Since the dawn of time, herbs have been used for their potent healing and recuperative powers. Medicinal plants contain a multitude of active ingredients used by humanity for their healing properties. Aspirin, the most widely used drug in the world, is based on salicylic acid—naturally present in the herb white willow bark.

Herbs help to renew the body, season by season. The healing constituents of herbs supply important ingredients that enhance immunity and optimize health. Medicinal plants have provided the foundation for the modern pharmaceutical industry. In turn, modern science is now validating the efficacy of botanicals in a wide variety of health conditions.

Therapeutic herbs have many benefits. Their primary action is to stimulate (anabolic effect) or soothe (catabolic effect) a given organ or body system. For example, milk thistle stimulates the liver to release toxins and protects the liver against the potentially damaging effects of the toxins themselves. Herbs may also be used to cleanse, build, detoxify, promote tissue repair, improve digestion, stimulate bile flow, regulate hormonal activity and metabolism, fight infection, reduce fever or inflammation, as a diuretic and so forth. With a thorough knowledge of plants, the herbalist has an incredible array of strategies for healing.

Herbs, when used with prudence and good judgment, can assist greatly in correcting many symptoms and disorders. But herbs must be used properly and with discretion. The right herb must be selected for the right reason, at the right time, in the right combination, and for the right duration. A trained herbalist can be a major ally in the pursuit and maintenance of good health.

GENERAL GUIDELINES FOR USING HERBS

1. *Determining dosage:* The physical condition of each individual must be considered in regards to dosage. Age, body size, body strength, and gender should all be considered. A 40-year-old 225-pound man might take three capsules of a particular herb, a 110-pound woman only one.

2. *Sensitivity issues:* Sensitive individuals can experience reactions to certain herbs, especially if introduced at too high a dose. The key principle here is to begin an individual herb *very slowly.* Avoid making any other changes in supplements at that time. I recommend one dose a day for at least three days. Once you've found the herb is well tolerated, the dose can be gradually increased.

3. *Herbs come in many forms:* Botanicals are now available in capsules, tablets, powders, teas, liquid extracts, tinctures, and the whole form of the original plant itself. Preferences tend to be highly individual. Experiment for yourself, buying the smallest quantity possible until you become accustomed to what you like.

For medicinal purposes, your health practitioner may prefer that you take a particular form of a certain herb. For example, St. John's wort standardized extract in 300 mg capsule form offers the most dependable delivery of the active ingredient, hypericin at 0.3%. In comparison, St. John's wort in liquid extract form does not deliver the active hypericin as reliably.

4. *Fresh is best:* Use herbs in their freshest form possible. Freshly picked herbs are delightfully potent and carry the greatest life energy and a higher concentration of enzymes, vitamins and volatile oils; they are generally more effective. In bottled herbs, look for expiration dates and select products from reputable companies.

5. *Strengthen first:* If you have chronic illness or don't feel well, it is important to initially emphasize herbs that are building and sustaining in nature. The body's energies and healing capacity must be increased before a cleansing, detoxification program is begun. Herbs such as fo ti (he shou wu), cayenne, ginger, green tea, and milk thistle help to nourish and revitalize the body's life force.

6. *Time for cleansing:* Once you feel stronger, a cleansing program can be started. Then the life force is sufficient to allow detoxification without overstressing the eliminative organs. Liver, colon and kidney cleanses, as well as parasite detox programs, may be undertaken directly. If a cleansing is undertaken before the body is ready, reactions or a healing crisis may occur.

7. *Acute conditions:* In acute conditions, such as an active bacterial or viral infection, herbs may be taken every three to four hours throughout the day as necessary.

8. *Bowel regularity:* It is vitally important to maintain bowel regularity. Toxins and wastes must be excreted daily to maintain good health. Mild laxative herbs such as aloe vera (capsules or inner leaf), cascara sagrada, or yellow dock may be used to promote a regular elimination pattern.

9. *Congestion:* In Oriental medicine there are thought to be two primary causes for most disease—congestion and depletion. When congestion occurs or depletion or both, blood and lymphatic circulation are disturbed. Signs of congestion include mucus buildup, lymphatic tenderness or swelling, circulatory disorders, cold hands and feet, infection, and inflammation. To clear congestion, it is important to increase circulation. Consider capsicum, cayenne, ginger, ginkgo biloba, ginseng, hawthorn, horse chestnut, rosemary, or watercress. In the beginning of your program, use mild herbs such as burdocks that have both strengthening and cleansing properties.

10. *Timing is everything:* In general, for maximum effect, herbs are best taken between meals, on an empty stomach. However, most may be taken with food as required. In fact, the herbs fennel, ginger, and gentian promote optimal digestion when taken with food. Stimulants such as ginkgo biloba are best taken early in the day to avoid disrupting sleep patterns. Nervines are herbs that tend to relax the body temporarily, such as valerian and skullcap, best taken before bed.

11. *How long is long enough?* Herbs can be used therapeutically or tonically. Therapeutic use is for short periods of one to four weeks at a time. For example, goldenseal and echinacea are used therapeutically, and it is important that they not be taken for more than three weeks at a time.

Tonic herbs can be used for longer periods of time, typically two to six months or longer, to address deep-seated imbalances. Ginseng, milk thistle, and turmeric are often considered tonic herbs. Others such as aloe vera, garlic, and ginger can be taken either as tonics or therapeutic agents. The old rule of thumb is that herbs are used one month for every year the patient has had the condition. Rely on your herbalist or health practitioner for advice in this area.

12. *Rest cycles:* Give the body a rest from the use of a specific herb (or herbs) at certain intervals. In Chinese medicine, herbal blends are used for one- to two-week periods and then usually stopped and alternated with other formulas. In contrast, when the same therapeutic herb is used for many weeks at a time, homeostasis can occur and the herb loses some of its beneficial impact on the body. In the case of antibacterial or antimicrobial herbs, changing the formula may prevent the microbes from becoming adapted to the antiinfective and overgrowing again. Tonic herbs such as milk thistle or dandelion are an exception to this rule and may be taken for many weeks at a time.

13. *Herbs and vitamins:* Herbal medicine is compatible with almost all other forms of treatment. In fact, herbs are usually synergistic with vitamins, especially naturally derived nutrients. Check with your homeopath if you are taking a prescribed remedy.

14. *Herbs and prescription medicines:* Consult with your personal physician or pharmacist on questions of individual compatibility of herbs with prescription medicines. If your doctor has approved the use of an herb in tandem with a drug, whenever possible to minimize interactions, take the herb at a different time of day than the medication. Herbs can also be highly effective following a course of treatment or alternated with drug protocols.

15. *The herbal advantage:* As natural plant-based medicines, herbs are usually quite compatible with the human body. Taken properly, side effects usually do not occur. Herbs can also be quite effective in dealing with the microbial kingdom. The herbal advantage is further magnified when a group of herbs are used together in a combination herbal remedy, and the effect of the active ingredients are exponentially greater.

16. *Gathering herbs:* All plants are best gathered when they are at their peak of growth, usually during the spring and early summer months. The best time to pick herbs is in the early morning hours, after the evaporation of dew and before the sun is high in the sky. The plant's aromatic oils are at their peak at this time. Select plants that are freshly in bloom and that have retained their natural color. Avoid plants sprayed with insecticides.

17. *Quality herbs:* Good choices typically include products labeled organic or wildcrafted (which means the plant was gathered in a natural environment and may be organic). Ask a well-informed staff person in the health food store which companies tend to have the freshest, highest quality herbs. If you use herbs frequently, you may want to order directly from a company that is regarded as a supplier of superior botanical products.

18. *Storing herbs:* Botanicals are delicate and require attentive handling. Heat and direct sunlight quickly destroy the plant's value. Keep your herbs in sealed, clean, airtight, light-proof containers in a cool, dry, dark location. Store herbs away from microwave ovens, computers, televisions, and heat ducts. At airports, hand-check your herbs to avoid x-ray exposure.

19. *Making tea:* When leaves or flowers of a plant are used, pour a cup of boiling water over one teaspoon of the loose herb and let it steep for about ten to twelve minutes; then strain and drink. For roots, seeds, bark, or tough leaves, cover with cold water and bring just to a boil; then simmer for ten to twelve minutes and strain.

20. *Wise counsel:* Different body types can be classified as sensitive or hearty. When a range of dosages are offered, the lower dose is usually appropriate for the sensitive body type, whereas the higher dose is for the more hearty body type.

HERBS TO PROMOTE OPTIMAL DIGESTION

Cardamom (*Elettaria cardamomum*) makes a wonderful, warming, and soothing digestive toner. It is excellent as a tea for indigestion, gas, or colic or to stimulate the appetite.

Chamomile (*Matricaria recutita*) is so popular in Germany many call it "capable of anything." Chamomile is used for many mild gastrointestinal disturbances. It can have anti-spasmodic effects. It also possesses a powerful anti-inflammatory influence on the mucous membranes of the entire GI tract. Chamomile helps prevent and soothe gastritis and mild ulcer-like conditions and speed their healing. It is also used as a mild sedative to calm the nerves and relieve anxiety without impeding normal motor coordination. Chamomile is used for its calming and therapeutic effects.

Gentian (*Gentiana lutea*) is a highly useful bitter tonic herb. Germany's Commission E (scientists who evaluate the safety and effectiveness of herbs) reports that gentian stimulates the taste buds and appetite and increases the flow of saliva and both stomach and bile secretions. Improving these functions may be relevant in cases of dyspepsia, gastritis, heartburn, nausea, jaundice, or diarrhea. Gentian may be taken as a tea or in capsules. It is also available as a tincture (called bitters) sold in health food and liquor stores.

Ginger (*Zingiber officinale*) is known in Asia as the "universal medicine." Research published in *The Lancet* and other prestigious medical journals has validated many of ginger's traditional uses. For example, it was confirmed to be more effective than drugs in treating both motion sickness and nausea. The optimal delivery of active ingredients is best found in the liquid extract, such as New Chapter's Daily Ginger Extract. Ginger in tea form is second best.

Ginger has been found to calm the stomach, improve digestion, lower cholesterol, increase circulation, and enhance overall immune function. These improvements may benefit conditions such as colitis, constipation, irritable bowel, malabsorption, colds, flu, and many other digestive disorders. It tends to amplify the benefits of other herbs and nutrients taken with it. Consider ginger for almost any gastrointestinal complaint. For GI conditions, use the tea or the liquid extract in a glass of pure water.

Fennel (*Foeniculum vulgare*) Hippocrates recommended it to treat infant colic in the third century B.C. Licorice-flavored fennel helps relieve stomachaches and cramps and also flatulence. Chew a few raw fennel seeds immediately following a meal to improve digestion and to reduce gas and bloating.

Neem leaf (*Azadirachta indica*) is a cooling and bitter herb, used in Ayurvedic medicine. Neem has been found to improve digestion, has antifungal properties, and broad antimicrobial properties. This herb stimulates an immune response, which is helpful in treating ulcers and in detoxifying the liver. Neem is usually taken in capsule form or as tea.

Papaya leaf (*carica papaya*) contains papain, a potent protein-digesting enzyme so effective it is the active ingredient in meat tenderizers. Take capsules or tablets or a slice of papaya fruit with or just after protein meals.

Peppermint (*Mentha piperita*) contains volatile oils and other compounds that may settle an upset stomach, absorb gas, improve digestion, and relieve heartburn and colic. Some people find it useful in controlling diarrhea or constipation. It is used in a wide variety of products such as Tums.

Peppermint's essential oils can improve digestive activity by stimulating bile flow. In some, peppermint promotes muscular activity, reduces cramps, and helps relieve headaches caused by poor digestion.

Research shows peppermint has anti-ulcer and anti-inflammatory properties. Peppermint also has antimicrobial characteristics inhibiting a wide range of over thirty different strains of bacteria, viruses, and yeast organisms. Peppermint may be taken in the form of a tea, in a concentrated oil, in tincture, or in enteric-coated capsules.

THERAPEUTIC HERBS FOR INTESTINAL HEALING

Aloe (Aloe, various species) is one of nature's most incredible curative agents. Currently aloe is being used in some hospitals to heal radiation and first- and second-degree burns effectively. Since the skin and the gut lining have some of the same properties, it is understandable that aloe has been found to work wonders there as well.

Aloe helps soothe and heal the stomach and small intestine lining, useful when coping with myriad insults from allergic reactions, celiac disease, gastritis, or ulcers. It can promote bowel regularity as an excellent mild and soothing laxative taken in capsule form at bedtime. To determine the right dose, begin by monitoring your body's response at home on a day off from work. Fresh aloe is rich in mucilaginous polysaccharides, its active component which can be depleted in processing. For best results, use the fresh *inner* gel from a live plant. When using a leaf from your own plant, simply remove the firm outer leaf with a knife so all the toxins are eliminated. Even the gel of the plant near the skin is safe to use. Try one teaspoon of fresh gel in a blender drink. Excellent benefit can also be derived from commercial juice or gel, intended for internal use only. Avoid brands using the *outer* leaf, which is toxic. Aloe concentrated in capsules or tablets is also beneficial, but can be laxative, so time your use judiciously.

Buckthorn bark (*Rhamnus catharticas*) is quite popular in Europe as a laxative and has the same key constituents in cascara sagrada, promoting peristaltic action and intestinal mucous secretions.

Cascara Sagrada (*Rhamnus purshianus*) was called the "sacred bark" by the early Spanish explorers. Cascara is a safe laxative that promotes peristalsis and restores tone to the colon and liver. Begin with just one capsule and use just enough to produce the desired results. Decrease and discontinue dose as your GI function returns to normal. *Note:* Overdose can cause diarrhea or cramping. Not recommended for pregnant or lactating women or for ulcers, irritable bowel syndrome, or for inflammatory conditions in general. *Important:* This herb can cause a sudden unpredictable rapid cleanse, which may occur as much as six hours later. When you begin the herb, try it at home on the weekend and monitor its effects on your system. For laxative use, if cascara is not the right choice for you, consider trying aloe vera in capsule form, taken at bedtime.

Cat's claw (Uncaria, various species) is an Amazonian immune strengthening herb, beneficial to the digestive tract as well. It reputedly has the power to influence deep-seated pathology. Cat's claw is known as the "opener of the way" for its remarkable ability to cleanse the entire intestinal tract and help many different stomach and intestinal disorders. Cat's Claw has been found to relieve swelling and inflammation relevant to the prevention and treatment of ulcers, colitis, irritable bowel, Crohn's disease, and chronic inflammation. Use only cat's claw concentrates for best results, in either liquid extract or capsules. Caution: The liquid is bitter.

Flaxseed is an excellent bulking agent and imparts a very mild laxative effect. Try one to two tablespoons seeds whole or ground sprinkled into a cereal, soup, salad, yogurt, or smoothie. If you have no problems with inflammation, prepare the seeds as cereal by pouring $1/4$ cup of boiling water over $1/4$ cup seeds; cover and steep for five minutes.

Marshmallow root (*Althaea officinalis*): The Roman naturalist Pliny stated, "Whosoever shall take a spoonful of the mallows shall that day be free from all diseases." Marshmallow may be used as a tea, powder, tincture, or in capsules to soothe an upset stomach, ulcer, or any irritation of the GI tract. In lab studies, it has demonstrated biological activity and stimulated macrophage activity. Marshmallow increases function in the GI tract as it nourishes and heals sensitive intestinal mucous membranes.

Slippery elm (*Ulmus rubra*) is a remarkably effective gastrointestinal soother, due to its unusual gelatinous, mucilaginous content. It heals sore and inflamed mucous membranes, including those of the digestive tract. Slippery Elm has been used to address ulcers, diarrhea, and diverticulitis, and to increase stool motility. It may be taken in capsules or prepared like oatmeal, by adding hot water to the powdered bark to make a cereal.

Yellow dock root (*Rumex crispus*) is a nourishing and purifying herb often used in seasonal detoxification cleanses and as a general anti-inflammatory. It is high in organic iron and other minerals, so it has been used in the treatment of anemia. It also has a mildly laxative effect. Use for short periods of time up to eight weeks, in capsules. tea, or liquid extract.

LIVER-PROTECTIVE HERBS

Boldo leaf (*Peumus boldo*) is a South American herb and one of the world's foremost liver and kidney tonics. Boldo is an antioxidant that nourishes the liver, which nourishes the blood, to the benefit of the whole body. Boldo is applied in many liver and digestive disorders, including jaundice, constipation, poor digestion, and gas and bloating. The botanical literature contains references to the use of boldo in cases of hepatitis. The herb may be taken as a tea (one teaspoon per cup) or in capsule form.

Caution: To be safe, pregnant women should avoid boldo.

Dandelion (*Taraxacum officinale*) has centuries of use as excellent nourishment for the liver. Dandelion stimulates bile flow and reduces bile duct inflammation, liver congestion, and gallstones. These improvements are relevant to the treatment of jaundice, mild hepatitis, and edema caused by liver toxicity. The leaves may be eaten as a salad green or steamed like spinach or a tea may be brewed from the roots. Dandelion can also be taken in capsule form.

Milk thistle (*Silybum marianum*) has over 2,000 years of medicinal use and is the subject of over one hundred clinical trials. It contains three powerful liver protective flavonoids known collectively as silymarin. Silymarin imparts potent therapeutic benefits as an antioxidant, by regenerating liver cells (hepatocytes) and by inhibiting inflammatory enzymes. Research has found that silymarin neutralizes the toxic effects of a wide variety of poisons including alcohol, excessive iron, industrial poisons, such as carbon tetrachloride, acetaminophen (Tylenol) overdose, and the deathcap mushroom, *Amanita phalloides*.

Silymarin prevents the depletion of the key liver antioxidant glutathione. In fact, silymarin has been shown to increase liver levels of glutathione by up to 35 percent. The higher the glutathione levels, the greater the liver's ability to detoxify. Studies indicate that Silymarin has benefits in treatment regimens for liver disease, cirrhosis, hepatitis, jaundice, fatty degeneration of the liver, and indigestion. I predict silymarin will one day likely become standard preventive treatment taken with any liver-toxic drug.

Mountain mahogany (Cercocarpus, various species) is an herb growing on the lower slopes of the Rocky Mountains. Indians of the region customarily chewed the tender leaves for stamina during long treks through the mountains. It is quite supportive for the liver and overall endocrine system.

Phyllanthus (*Phyllanthus amarus*) is an ancient Ayurvedic herb known for its liver-strengthening abilities. Phyllanthus is a mild, slow-acting herb ideal for individuals who need to detoxify in a gradual manner. In other words, phyllanthus does not aggressively and hastily flush toxins out of the system, but does so in a gentle process that does not overwhelm the body. It is helpful for many liver conditions, as it protects the liver cells against damage and disease. Phyllanthus is available in capsule form. This botanical has a long history as a liver-supportive herb. However, the jury is still out on its specific therapeutic applications.

Schizandra (*Schizandra chinensis*) is one of the most beneficial of the Chinese herbs for the liver, containing a dozen active compounds that are liver-protective. In Chinese medicine, schizandra has many uses, including its role as a tonic for both men and women and for viral hepatitis. It may be taken in capsule form or the dried berries can be found in herb shops. When taken for acute conditions, the herb is divided into several doses throughout the day.

Turmeric (*Curcuma longa*) is honored in Ayurvedic medicine as one of the foremost digestive tonics and overall remedies. It quiets indigestion and helps to reduce gas, bloating, and inflammation. Turmeric lowers cholesterol and is a general antimicrobial agent. This herb stimulates bile flow, helping digest oils and fats. These benefits make it relevant to the treatment of hemorrhoids. Animal studies show that it protects and detoxifies the liver. Curcumin, an active compound in turmeric, is reported to directly inhibit carcinogens.

Curcumin suppresses prostaglandin synthesis, which reduces pain in a manner similar to aspirin or ibuprofen, only milder. At high doses, Curcumin stimulates the adrenal glands to release cortisone—the body's natural anti-inflammatory and pain management agent. If you consume alcohol, smoke, or take frequent doses of prescription drugs or Tylenol (acetaminophen), you may want to include turmeric or milk thistle in your daily regime. However, individuals suffering from gallstones or bile duct blockage do best to avoid turmeric and also curry powder which is typically one-third turmeric. For sensitive types, turmeric may be best tolerated in combination with a product by NOW called Silymarin (with turmeric included in the ingredients).

HERBS FOR ULCERS

Fresh raw **cabbage** (*Brassica oleracea*) juice contains two compounds that are used as anti-ulcer agents, the amino acids glutamine and S-methyl-methionine. In a recent study, 92 percent of patients with ulcers showed a marked improvement within three weeks on a program of daily cabbage juice, compared with 32 percent drinking a look-alike placebo. Cabbage soup can also be helpful, especially with the addition of ginger, cloves, and just a hint of licorice. Typically two to four cups of the fresh cabbage juice are taken daily or eaten in soup form.

Ginger (*Zingiber officinale*) is reported to relieve inflammation and has the potential to protect the digestive system from ulcers. Ginger contains eleven different active constituents with proven anti-ulcer properties.

Licorice root (*Glycyrrhiza glabra*) is approved by German Commission E as an ulcer treatment. The preferred form is deglycyrrhizinated licorice root (DGL), which does not increase blood pressure rates. DGL promotes healing of the sensitive mucosal membranes of the GI tract. DGL is best taken in chewable tablets because the mixing of saliva with DGL activates the licorice's healing properties.

Meadowsweet (*Filipendula ulmaria*) is used extensively in Britain as an anti-ulcer agent. Meadowsweet contains tannins, which have been found to be antibacterial in research studies. Meadowsweet is a logical treatment for ulcers, since most are caused by a bacteria (*H. pylori.*).

Neem (*Azadiracta indica*) is a highly useful bitter herb that can improve digestion. In India, neem is used in cases of ulcers. It is also a respected immune stimulant and liver detoxifier, and helps diabetics lower their blood sugar levels.

Okra is a mucilaginous vegetable that is a potent gastrointestinal soother and healer. It is rich in chlorophyll and beta-carotene, and when eaten as a cooked vegetable assists in repairing the sensitive stomach and intestinal lining. The gelatinous quality of the vegetable tends to be quite healing.

Slippery elm (*Ulmus rubra*) also has an unusual gelatinous, mucilaginous content with traditional therapeutic use for ulcers, diverticulitis, ulcerative colitis, and Crohn's disease. It may be taken in capsules or prepared like oatmeal, adding hot water to the powdered bark to make a cereal.

Turmeric (*Curcuma longa*) is an excellent anti-inflammatory, anti-ulcer agent, and applied as a general healer for the GI tract in capsule or powder form.

BROAD SPECTRUM ANTI-MICROBIAL HERBS

All herbal roots and barks exert general antimicrobial properties. Otherwise, they would succumb to the widespread presence of microbes in the soil. Certain herbs exert an even stronger antimicrobial effect than others. The most potent of these herbs will now be discussed.

Black walnut (*Juglans nigra*) has traditional uses in Asia and America for its antiparasitic properties. Black walnut also possesses potent anti-yeast and mild antiviral properties. One study showed that fresh husks of the black walnut killed candida better than the commonly prescribed antifungal drug, without the side effects. In China it is used to kill tapeworms with good success. The black walnut's broad antimicrobial success is due to its high tannin content. The green hulls or the bark of the tree are used. Black walnut is usually effective in stopping diarrhea. It makes a good liver tonic and has been applied in cases of hemorrhoids and organ or tissue prolapse. Black walnut may be used in liquid extract form or in capsules.

Clove (*Syzygium aromaticum*) is the most stimulating and carminative of all aromatic spices (a carminative is an agent that dispels gas from the intestines). Clove possesses strong and proven general antimicrobial properties against fungus, bacteria, and parasites. Clove has a long tradition of use in China and in India, where cloves are used to stop diarrhea, gas, and bloating.

Clove acts as a restorative tonic to the digestive and circulatory systems. It is an excellent blood cleanser, relieves nausea and vomiting, and stimulates peristalsis. Often added to bitter herb-medicine preparations, clove tends to make them more palatable. Eating cloves is said to be an aphrodisiac. Caution: Do not use clove when pregnant or for children under 2 years of age. Clove is generally taken in capsule form.

Echinacea (Echinacea, various species) has a great range of activity against viruses, bacteria, fungi, and protozoa. It contains an antibiotic compound (echinacoside) with broad-spectrum activity, often compared to penicillin. Echinacea bolsters the immune defenses in various ways. (1) It strengthens the body's local defenses by use of a substance (echinacein) that deactivates germs' tissue-dissolving enzyme. This prevents germs from spreading and infecting other body tissues. (2) A study in *Infection and Immunology* showed that echinacea stimulated production of white blood cells and phagocytes and increased macrophage germ-killing activity. (3) A University of Munich study demonstrated that echinacea boosted production of infection-fighting T lymphocytes up to 30 percent more than standard immune-supportive drugs.

One study showed that echinacea has significant anti-yeast qualities. In Germany, echinacea is used to treat flu, colds, bronchitis, tonsillitis, ear infections and whooping cough, psoriasis, wounds, abscesses, and even meningitis and tuberculosis. The root of the plant offers the greatest healing potential. Root extracts of echinacea are believed to boost interferon levels, vital to the body's defenses. The German Commission E recommends echinacea to be used for short periods of time not to exceed eight successive weeks. It is best taken as liquid extract or in capsules.

Garlic (*Allium sativum*) is the botanical kingdom's best example of an herbal wonder drug for fighting infections. When the Russian army ran out of penicillin in World War II, garlic was their second choice, and they used it to treat typhus, dysentery, septic poisoning, and gangrene in battle wounds. Hence the nickname "Russian penicillin." Garlic contains several antimicrobial compounds, including allicin, one of nature's strongest broad-spectrum antibiotics. Research has found garlic to have antibacterial activity against bacillus, brucella, citrobacter, *E. coli,* hafnia, klebsiella, *Salmonella typhi,* shigella, *Vibrio cholerae,* and various forms of staph and strep.

At Bernares Hindu University in India, one of garlic's constituents, ajoene, was found to be almost as effective against mildew fungus as pharmaceutical antifungals. In test tube studies, garlic has demonstrated viricidal activity against many viruses, including rhino viruses and herpes simplex I and II. Garlic is often used in cases of food poisoning and GI tract infections. It exerts antiparasitic properties applied in treatment against pinworms, roundworms and certain protozoa, including *Entamoeba histolytica.*

Garlic is also used to help relieve gas pains and as an antispasmodic. It is most active in raw form as a food or a fresh-pressed juice. A few cloves may be juiced along with carrots to make the medicine go down easy. Or it can be taken in capsules, two to three per day as prevention, or two to three, three times daily, in acute situations. Note: To help counter the powerful smell, chew one or more of the following herbal breath fresheners: parsley, fenugreek, or fennel.

Ginger (*Zingiber officinale*) has been found to possess inhibitory action against various pathogenic microorganisms including the bacteria *E. coli*, salmonella, *Staphylococcus aureus,* and *Streptococcus viridans.* It also possesses anti-influenza, antiviral, antifungal and anti-yeast activity. Studies show ginger is quite effective against numerous parasites, including various protozoa. Remarkably this versatile herb also acts as a probiotic—promoting growth of friendly flora species like *Lactobacillus acidophilus.*

Grapefruit seed extract (GSE) is a general antimicrobial agent with specific antibacterial, antifungal, antiviral, and antiparasitic properties. This bitter herb is known for its excellent application against *Candida albicans.* In lab testing, GSE has shown effectiveness against a long list of other microorganisms as well, including *Staphylococcus aureus, Salmonella typhi, E. coli, Proteus vulgaris, Pseudomonas aeruginosa, Aspergillus parasiticus, Entamoeba histolytica, Giardia lamblia,* herpes simplex type 1, and influenza A virus. Applications also include controlling diarrhea. It's especially helpful for infections of unknown cause, because it is nontoxic and its activity is so broad.

GSE offers a safe, simple way to disinfect drinking water when camping or traveling. Available water should first be filtered (at the least, let suspended water particles settle). Retain the clear water and add 10 drops GSE for each gallon of water. Shake vigorously and let stand for a few minutes before drinking.

GSE may be used in liquid concentrate form or in capsules. GSE may be taken internally, in minute doses such as 2 to 4 drops twice daily diluted in at least 4 ounces carrot, orange, pineapple or grapefruit juice.

Licorice root (Glycyrrhiza glabra) helps prevent and remedy infections, fevers, and inflammation. It has broad antimicrobial activity against viruses, bacteria, yeast, and fungi. Licorice contains at least eight antiviral and twenty-five antifungal compounds. Licorice's active fungicidal constituents are greater than those of any other herb. Licorice also possesses antiviral compounds that promote interferon release, part of our body's antiviral arsenal. A Japanese study showed licorice to be effective against *Staphylococcus aureus* which was already resistant to penicillin and streptomycin. Furthermore, licorice remained just as effective against successive drug-resistant generations of the same staph.

In Chinese medicine, licorice is called the great unifier. It is used in small amounts in numerous herbal formulas for its exceptional harmonizing and synergistic qualities. Licorice heightens the beneficial effects of other herbs it is used with.

By itself, licorice is a dynamic herb which should only be used for short periods of time. Caution: Use only DGL (deglycyrrhizinated licorice) if you have high blood pressure. Avoid licorice altogether during pregnancy, or if you're diabetic or have glaucoma, water retention, heart disease, or a history of hypertension or stroke. Licorice has a naturally sweet taste and it may be taken as tea, liquid extract, or in capsules.

HONORABLE MENTION ANTI-MICROBIALS

Astragalus (Astragalus, various species) is a supremely versatile and potent immune strengthener. Astragalus builds up the body's vitality, prevents and hastens infection's exodus. Research in China shows **baikal skullcap** (*Scutellaria baicalensis*) has broad-spectrum antimicrobial activity so it is associated with the treatment of pneumonia, flu, and other respiratory infections. It suppresses viruses and pneumonia-causing fungi. **Cinchona bark** (Cinchona, various species) was the primary source for quinine until the drug was synthetically produced. Cinchona bark has over twenty active compounds; in addition to quinine it has antiviral, antimalarial, antiprotozoal, and antiyeast properties. Use in capsule form.

Dandelion (*Taraxacum officinale*) is used against respiratory infections. It may be taken as a tea, in capsules or the fresh greens as a salad. **Honeysuckle** (*Lonicera japonica*) is much used in China to treat bacterial and viral conditions. It is taken as a liquid from flower extracts or as a tea. **Olive leaf** (*Olea europaea*) has general antimicrobial properties, providing relief against bacteria, virus, fungi and certain protozoa. For GI conditions, its leaves contain a rich amount of FOS (fructo-oligo-saccharides), which nourish the growth of the good bacteria and promote their growth.

ANTI-BACTERIAL HERBS

A number of outstanding bactericidal botanicals have just been discussed in the section on antimicrobials. Of these, the most important include **echinacea, garlic, ginger,** and **grapefruit seed extract**. Also antibacterial but milder in their effects are clove, licorice, honeysuckle, and olive leaf. Additional outstanding antibacterial herbs follow.

Chaparral (*Larrea divaricata*) is a powerful antimicrobial herb. It can be effective against a broad spectrum of infectious agents, viruses, yeast, and bacteria. One compound in chaparral, nordihydroguarietic acid, is a viable antiseptic. Chaparral is one of nature's best blood cleansers and is quite immune-supportive in general. The tea works well, but tastes bad, so capsules are usually best.

Goldenseal (*Hydrastis canadensis*) is the antibacterial herb in greatest demand today. Due to this popularity, it is greatly overharvested and nearing extinction in the wild. Goldenseal stimulates macrophage activity, the microscopic Pac-Men of our immune system that engulf and devour bacteria. Goldenseal contains the active compounds berberine and hydrastine, which are anti-inflammatory and antihistamine and stimulate bile flow.

Berberine is strongly antibacterial, amoebicidal, and somewhat antifungal and antiviral. It helps stop diarrhea. Berberine appears to work by staining microbes (to be targets for the macrophages) and by preventing the microbes from attaching to cells. Note: Other berberine-containing herbs are oregon grape root, barberry, and Chinese goldthread. Goldenseal has broad applications for the GI tract and liver and is a potent blood cleanser.

Goldenseal is too bitter as a tea and the active ingredients may not translate into the liquid extract form. Thus capsules are preferred. Use goldenseal only for brief intervals of two to three weeks at a time. When used longer, goldenseal is reported to deplete the body of B vitamins, and to a lesser extent, vitamin C. Goldenseal can also be harsh on the kidneys and should be used judiciously. If the herb causes stomach discomfort, mouth irritation, or other symptoms, use less or stop using it altogether. Do not use it when pregnant.

Goldthread (*Coptis chinensis*) is from Asia and is sometimes called Chinese goldenseal. It offers an excellent substitute for American goldenseal, as its berberine content is twice as high. Caution: Do not confuse Chinese goldthread with American goldthread (*Coptis groenlandicum*).

ANTIVIRAL HERBS

In addition to the herbs listed here, a number of outstanding viricidal botanicals were discussed earlier. Of these, the most important are: **echinacea, garlic, licorice,** and **astragalus**. Also antiviral but milder in their effects are Baikal skullcap, cinchona bark, ginger, grapefruit seed extract, honeysuckle, and olive leaf. Other outstanding antiviral herbs include:

Black elderberry (*Sambuscus nigra L.*) has been used in cases of flu, coughs, colds, and upper respiratory infections for over 2,500 years. Recent studies demonstrate black elderberry's effectiveness against all strains of influenza virus. An enzyme present in black elderberry (neuraminidase) has been found to inhibit the virus from piercing the cell membrane and entering. Black elderberry is most effective in either a syrup form or in lozenges.

Black-eyed Susan root (Rudbeckia, various species) is about to be discovered for its virus-fighting capabilities. A recent report showed black-eyed Susan to be a more potent immune system stimulator than echinacea.

Forsythia (*Forsythia suspensa*) is a traditional Chinese herb used when there are colds, flu, and other viruses. It is often mixed with honeysuckle (*Lonicera japonica*) and sometimes lemon balm and/or ginger as a tea.

Isatidis (*Isatis tinctora*) is one of the best-known Chinese antiviral herbs. Isatidis is an excellent remedy for any virus. Because it helps reduce both swelling and liver inflammation, it has been used against hepatitis. Isatidis is mild and can be used for children or those who don't tolerate heat well (described as *pitta* types in the Ayurvedic system). Less well known, isatidis is also a good antibacterial agent.

Leptotaenia (*Lomatium dissecutim*). Research in 1948 demonstrated leptotaenia inhibited the growth of all sixty-two strains of bacteria and fungi tested with varying degrees of success. An oil extract of leptotaenia was shown in a 1949 in vitro test to completely inhibit growth of ten microbes, equivalent to penicillin at the same strength. Leptotaenia is available in both capsules or liquid extract. Because of these properties it is applied in the treatment of a number of viral conditions, such as pneumonia, flu, colds, and bronchitis, as well as all viruses including herpes simplex I and II and hepatitis C. Leptotaenia also possesses activity against many forms of viruses and yeast.

Schizandra (*Schizandra chinensis*) has uses in Chinese medicine as an antiviral herb, in cases of viral hepatitis. Schizandra may be taken in capsule form or the dried berries may be found in herb shops.

ANTI-YEAST HERBS

A number of outstanding bactericidal botanicals were discussed in the Anti-Microbial section. Of these, the most important anti-yeast herbs are

garlic, grapefruit seed extract, and **licorice.** Also anti-yeast but milder in their effects are Baikal skullcap, black walnut, cinchona bark, clove, echinacea, ginger, and olive leaf. Additional anti-yeast herbs include:

Celandine (*Chelidonium majus*) is a well-known herb with benefits to the liver which can help detoxify and eliminate the waste by-products from candida treatment. Celandine also possesses active anti-yeast properties in its own right. It is usually taken in capsule form.

Cranberry (*Vaccinium macrocarpon*) contains the compound arbutin, which has anti-yeast and anticandida properties, so it is used in fighting urinary tract infections. Use the unsweetened juice or capsule form.

Gentian (*Gentiana officinalis*) is a bitter herb that acts as a first line of defense against yeast overgrowth. Gentian stimulates gastric juice secretions. When our stomach acids are sufficient, microbes and yeasts are destroyed, "cooked" in the highly acid gastric medium. Gentian may be taken in capsules or liquid extract form.

Goldenrod (*Solidago virgaurea*) is approved by German Commission E for prevention and treatment of urogenital ailments including yeast infections. Goldenrod contains a number of potent antiyeast compounds. Can be taken as a tea or in capsules or in drop form.

Licorice (*Glycyrrhiza glabra*) contains the largest number of antifungal compounds of any single herb. For these properties, it may be taken in capsules, liquid extract, or as a tea, but not as the supplement DGL.

Oregano oil (*Origanum vulgare*) is a potent antiseptic. Research shows this tasty spice packs a whale of a wallop against a wide range of fungi, yeasts, and bacteria, with some antiviral and antiparasitic properties as well. Caution: The vast majority of oregano oil is mislabeled, usually derived from thyme or marjoram, and not nearly as effective. Add a few drops of oregano oil into juice. Emulsified oil of oregano is now available in caplet form.

Pau d'arco (Tabebuia, various species) is a highly revered South American herb that excels in controlling candida and yeast overgrowth. It contains three antiyeast compounds—lapachol, beta-lapachone, and xyloidine—active against *Candida albicans* and other common fungi. Lapachol's anti-yeast action alone has been found comparable to the drug Nizoral (ketaconazole). In Brazil, pau d'arco is commonly used for a host of conditions, including constipation, colitis, ulcers, diabetes, arthritis, respiratory problems, and infections of all kinds. Pau d'arco exhibits antiviral and antibacterial properties. The herb is effective in tea, liquid extract, and capsule form. Start slowly with whichever form you use, to avoid strong die-off reactions.

Pseudowintera colorata is a New Zealand herb containing a powerful antifungal agent called polygodial. It has been found effective against *Candida albicans* and other fungi. When combined with anethole, the active constituent of aniseed (*Pimpinella anisum*), polygodial's effectiveness against *Candida albicans* was found to increase thirty-two times, as confirmed by studies at the University of California.

The combination of pseudowintera colorata and aniseed work by damaging the cell membranes of *Candida albicans* and other yeasts. The yeast's cell division is thus significantly impeded. Note: Pseudowintera Colorata and aniseed are together found in a product manufactured by Forest Herbs called Kolorex, typically taken at the end of a meal.

Spicebush (*Lindera benzoin*) is an Appalachian herb quite effective against *Candida albicans*.

Honorable mention herbs include **Ivy** (*Hedera helix*), whose leaves inhibit candida and many bacteria as well. **Tea tree oil** (Melaleuca, various species) has a history of use against topical yeast problems so it's applied in treating athlete's foot. Use cautiously to determine suitability for your skin type. **Uva-ursi** (*Arctostaphylos uva-ursi*) possesses antiyeast properties, and therefore is taken for urogenital disorders. Taken as a tea or liquid extract, or in capsules.

ANTIPARASITE HERBS

A number of prominent antiparasitic botanicals were discussed in the section on antimicrobials. The most important were **black walnut, garlic**, and **grapefruit seed extract**. Also antiparasitic but milder in their effects are cinchona bark, clove, ginger, and olive leaf. Additional outstanding antiparasite herbs include:

Artemisia annua, derived from the Chinese herb Qing-Hao, is used in Chinese medicine in treating a variety of protozoan infections caused by amoebas (amebiasis), giardia (giardiasis), etc. Also known as sweet Annie, artemisia has also been found in research at the Walter Reed Army Research Institute in Washington, D.C., to be effective in fighting malaria. The organism that causes malaria is a species related to the amoeba. Artemisia is in the wormwood family of herbs, all of which are extremely bitter. They are used for indigestion, heartburn, flatulence, gastric pain, and jaundice, for general weakness, and in stimulating appetite. Wormwood also stimulates liver and bile flow, as well as general circulation.

Caution: One member of the wormwood family, *Artemisia absinthium,* has been declared unsafe by the U.S. Food and Drug Administration, and its use was outlawed in France in the nineteenth century because of its adverse effects to the nervous system.

Chaparro amargosa (*Castela emoryi* and *C. Texana*) is used against some of the nastiest protozoa on the planet, including *Entamoeba histolytica* and giardia. Known in Spanish as bitter bush, chaparro amargosa is also helpful in rebuilding the intestinal tract after antibiotic therapy or a bout of gastroenteritis. It is an excellent preventative when traveling to avoid diarrhea. Chaparro amargosa is usually taken in liquid tincture form, followed immediately with a more pleasant juice or tea to withstand the taste.

Kamala (*Mallotus philippinensis*) is used in India and elsewhere because of its anti-parasitic properties. It is most effective when used as a part of an herbal combination remedy, usually in capsule form.

Quassia (*Picraena excelsa*) is a bitter herb with strong antiparasitic qualities. A tea is made from quassia wood chips. Historically it is used to kill roundworms (ascaris). Taken internally as an enema, it is used against pinworm.

Wormseed (*Chenopodium ambrosioides*) is one of the most highly respected antiparasitic remedies, known for its ease of use, and low toxicity. Wormseed is believed to act as a direct poison to parasites. Traditionally, wormseed oil has been used against roundworms and hookworms, paralyzing them and causing them to lose their grip on the intestines. A strong laxative, administered shortly after wormseed, is said to drive the parasites from the body. Wormseed is often found by the Spanish name epazote. Mexicans prize epazote for dispelling gas associated with bean consumption. The fresh or dried herb is added to bean and lentil dishes when they are almost done.

Caution: Wormseed is quite potent. An overdose of the oil can cause poisoning or even death. A 1-year-old baby died after taking a dose of four drops three times a day for two days. Wormseed is not recommended for pregnant or lactating women or children under the age of six. Often a strong laxative is taken after the last dose of the oil. Wormseed is also available in capsule form. Consult your doctor for proper dosage, as each product is slightly different.

Special note: Eliminating parasites successfully can be tricky business. To minimize the challenge, we strongly recommend consulting with an experienced health practitioner whose training includes herbology *and* a track record of success in treating parasites.

COMBINATION HERBAL REMEDIES

Individual herbs may be all that you need. However, most herbalists will agree that combination herbal remedies are even more effective due to the combined synergy of benefits. The potency of a single herb can usually be significantly enhanced when correctly combined with other herbs. The overall results are greatly augmented. Traditional Chinese medicine and Ayurveda offer classic examples of herbs specifically combined for their distinct synergistic and therapeutic effects. Combination herbal remedies offer state of the art clinical results and serve as the foundation and core of modern herbalism. Refer to the Resources for a list of professional companies that offer high quality, effective combination herbal remedies.

TIMOTHY KUSS, PH.D., is founder and director of Infinity Health Systems, a private nutritional practice, consulting with both doctors and patients on the therapeutic use of nutrition. He holds a Ph.D. in nutrition and an N.D. in naturopathy, is a certified nutritional consultant, and studied with the respected biochemist and herbalist Stuart Wheelwright. He is cofounder of the Institute of Bio-Energetic Research, dedicated to nutritional research, and is nutrition director for Recovery Systems, a clinic that uses diet and nutrients to aid recovery from addictive lifestyles. Author of *A Guidebook to Clinical Nutrition for the Health Professional* and articles on a variety of health topics, he also formulates herbal and nutritional supplements. Timothy Kuss is available by phone for herbal and/or nutritional consultations at Infinity Health in the Denver area at 303-346-7212.

38

Treating Allergies with EPD Immunotherapy

W. A. SHRADER, JR., M.D.
INTERVIEWED BY NANCY FAASS

E PD (enzyme-potentiated desensitization) is a treatment developed to address allergies and digestive disorders. This method was established in England thirty years ago and has been used in the United States for the past several years under the auspices of a research study to evaluate its safety and effectiveness.

Disclaimer: At the time of this interview, EPD is considered by the Food and Drug Administration (FDA) to be an investigational therapy. Dr. Shrader is the principal researcher in a study to evaluate EPD therapy, in research that is monitored by the FDA and conducted under the auspices of an investigational review board. In addition, an application is in process to study EPD as an investigational new drug. These are standard steps in obtaining approval for the use of any new treatment or medication.

Until a therapy or drug is approved by the FDA, researchers are required to maintain scientific neutrality and cannot make claims regarding the efficacy of the treatment. Dr. Shrader has agreed to be interviewed, but the editors wish to make it clear that the content and wording are theirs and not his. Until the research is completed, no final conclusions can be drawn on the effectiveness of this therapy. Therefore, this chapter is intended to be informational only.

Specifics regarding EPD in this chapter reflect current statistics collected for more than 9,000 patients over a six-year period. Since the study is still in progress, this information should be viewed with the same neutrality one would employ for any treatment under evaluation.

EPD DEFINED

EPD therapy is an innovative method for treating allergies and digestive disorders, developed by the brilliant British allergist Dr. Leonard McEwen. The research to date shows that EPD may well have a higher rate of success for most conditions treatable by immunotherapy than that demonstrated by other available immunological therapies. Researchers believe that EPD works by desensitizing the body with extremely small doses of substances known to trigger allergies (allergens). An enzyme (beta-glucuronidase) is added to these allergens to activate the treatment. The body develops a certain degree of immunity to the allergens, and as a result, seems to be much less reactive when exposure occurs.

CONDITIONS TREATED WITH EPD

In the research to determine the level of effectiveness of EPD, success is measured by patient self-evaluation questionnaires, asking them to

---

The Possibilities of EPD Therapy

At 19, Sarah had a severe case of juvenile-onset rheumatoid arthritis, severe enough that she was unable to stand in our waiting room without help. We began her treatment using nutritional and dietary techniques in an attempt to reduce her symptoms. She improved somewhat using primarily dietary therapy.

Sarah's history also indicated bacteria as another possible causative agent. Specific research has found that 70 percent of people with rheumatoid arthritis test positive for antibodies to proteus bacteria. With juvenile arthritis such as Sarah had, the association with this particular bacteria is not necessarily present, but other factors or bacteria can be causal agents. In Sarah's case, another bacteria was implicated, so in preparation for EPD therapy, we first prepped her with the antibiotic vancomycin for ten days prior to the first scheduled treatment.

To our surprise, she was almost in total remission by the end of the course of vancomycin. As a result, it was decided we should take a wait-and-see attitude, and her EPD therapy was postponed. Her remission following the drug treatment lasted for about four months, at which time her symptoms returned. We repeated the antibiotic preparation and then began EPD immunotherapy.

Sarah received quite excellent relief with the EPD injections. By the end of a two-year period, she no longer required EPD. She has remained in remission for more than two years at this writing.

rate their condition before and after each EPD treatment. Self-assessment may range from "terrible" to "excellent." Responses of "good," "very good," and "excellent" are all considered indications of patient satisfaction with the treatment and a "successful outcome." Statements about success rate are based on data available at the current time. At the time of this interview, over sixty-five conditions have been identified that appear to be treatable with EPD therapy.

A number of digestive disorders seem to respond well to EPD therapy, including Crohn's disease, ulcerative colitis, irritable bowel syndrome (IBS), and chronic constipation. Food intolerance is the condition most frequently treated with EPD, and the data at this point in the study demonstrates that it works well for a majority of the patients with this condition. More importantly, the study data shows it also works for true food allergies (those triggered by IgE antibodies). These are typically difficult to treat; they are traditionally treated by complete avoidance. True food allergies can be life threatening or even fatal.

SUCCESS RATE

In the first 9,000 cases treated, EPD appears to have an overall average success rate of 70 percent to 76 percent in treating known allergies, intolerance, or adverse reactions. For those true life-threatening IgE-associated food allergies, EPD appears to be the only safe method of active immunotherapy available anywhere in the world. The same data demonstrates that this therapy can be extremely effective for numerous gastrointestinal conditions. Evaluations of long-term efficacy in Dr. McEwen's follow-up studies over the past twenty-five years suggest that EPD has much greater long-term success than any other current method of immunotherapy in use.

EPD Often Appears to Be a Successful Treatment For

- Chronic constipation
- Crohn's disease
- Ulcerative colitis
- Food allergies (IgE-associated)
- Food intolerance and sensitivities
- Irritable bowel syndrome (IBS)
- Gastrointestinal infection or overgrowth
- Yeasts like candida
- Autoimmune disease associated with certain bacteria such as proteus, klebsiella, and bacteroides

---

In addition, EPD appears to be an effective means of addressing many difficult-to-treat illnesses, such as attention deficit disorder, hyperactivity, Tourette's syndrome, and autism. EPD also appears to remediate a variety of autoimmune disorders. The study data available at this time also reflects success rates well above 70 percent for the treatment of hay fever, dust mite allergy, perennial rhinitis, urticaria (hives), eczema, dermatitis, asthma, and anaphylactic reactions (life-threatening swelling, often involving the airways). Generally, the study data indicates a success rate near 70 percent when treating individuals with chemical sensitivity, migraine, and other headaches. Spinal arthritis (ankylosing spondylitis) and systemic lupus also appear to respond well to EPD.

A TYPICAL TREATMENT WITH EPD

The EPD injection consists of minute doses of a mixture of the substances that have the potential to cause allergic reactions (called allergens). The contents can be tailored to the needs of the individual, based on test results and medical history. EPD mixtures may include extracts of foods, food additives, common chemicals (except pesticides and herbicides), formaldehyde, detergents (for skin sensitivity), inhaled pollens, danders, dust, and dust mites, as well as a wide range of bacteria, fungi, yeast, and molds. The physician can select from a variety of antigen mixtures that tend to act quite universally.

EPD therapy is administered by minute injections or absorption through the skin. Each injection is exceptionally small—$^1/_{20}$ of a cc—and extremely dilute. That is 20 times *smaller* than a typical 1 cc injection given at a doctor's office (in a flu shot, for example). Generally, one to five of these injections are given at any one time. Highly sensitive patients (those with the potential for anaphylactic shock) are treated through the skin, rather than by injection. EPD has an exceptional record of safety—at present, more than 300,000 doses of EPD have been given to patients worldwide without any deaths or life-threatening reactions.

The treatments are typically given once every two or three months for the first year, and then at longer intervals. Like many allergy treatments, EPD may need to be continued periodically over several years. Eventually treatments are only once a year or less often. Many adults average about sixteen to eighteen treatments before they discontinue EPD or extend their treatments to very long intervals (one to five years). Since treatment is so infrequent, patients usually feel that the regimen is not problematic.

Childhood allergies are also appropriate for treatment with EPD. The researchers have observed that for children in the study, allergies or health problems often tend to resolve more rapidly and completely than for adults. Many of the children complete their therapy with five to eight treatments at two- to five-month intervals.

EPD OFFERS A DIFFERENT APPROACH TO THE TREATMENT OF ALLERGY

In the past, classical allergists have acknowledged the effects of immediate food allergies (those that trigger IgE antibodies). The standard treatment for identifiable food allergies has been to avoid them. This is certainly a commonsense approach.

However, patients with life-threatening IgE-mediated allergies can experience anaphylaxis, which can be fatal, if they unknowingly consume an allergen. Avoidance is often difficult, because processed and restaurant foods may contain a complex mix of ingredients. In highly allergic individuals, common foods that may cause these fatal reactions include peanuts and shrimp, which are frequently found in dishes such as sauces, egg rolls, and stir-fries.

EPD has been used to treat many people with IgE allergies, and to date, only one of these patients has been recorded to experience a possible adverse effect. The data suggests generally that patients who accidentally or intentionally consume dangerous allergenic foods after the first year of therapy do not experience serious ill effects. The researchers feel that this is definitely one of the greatest potential values of EPD immunotherapy.

There are a number of other situations in which EPD appears to be of benefit:

◆ Some people have allergies that are difficult to identify, so classical immunotherapy (targeted at specific allergens) may not be feasible.

◆ Others have food intolerance rather than true allergies. Intolerances are believed to trigger a number of antibodies and stimulate other physiological mechanisms of response. Although the mechanism for many of these responses is unknown, patients must cope with the symptoms.

◆ Classical immunotherapy is typically not used to treat food allergy or intolerances.

These are important concerns to the many patients and doctors who must cope with the reality of food intolerance. EPD appears to offer a means of addressing both food intolerance and true, IgE-mediated food allergy.

HOW IT WORKS

British research strongly suggests that EPD inhibits overreaction by the immune system. Researchers have found that EPD treatments act on cells sometimes described as T suppressor cells. Their specific job is to shut off the T helper cells, which act as immune "defenders." T helpers can overrespond if there is no "off" switch, causing symptoms such as allergy, asthma, or autoimmune disorders.

The T helper (or T effector) cells may react inappropriately, mistakenly identify an otherwise nonallergenic substance as harmful and signal other T cells to mount an immune response. This may result in the production of certain cell mediators, such as various types of interleukins and histamine, which either produce the allergenic response directly or activate other immune mechanisms (such as mast cells that produce histamine).

An overly enthusiastic immune response can actually be harmful to the body. The natural defenses of the system may cause inflammation and swelling. If the response continues too long, tissue damage can occur; an example of this dynamic is the chronic synovial (joint) inflammation present in patients with rheumatoid arthritis.

The allergens used in EPD therapy are given in extremely small concentration. The dilution is comparable to low-potency homeopathic remedies (6× to 12×). Adding an enzyme, *beta-glucuronidase,* activates the material injected, which then serves as a cell-signaling agent, or *leukotriene.* The enzyme is the critical activating agent in EPD immunotherapy. Researchers believe that the enzyme transmits a signal to the developing T cells, faciliting a more appropriate immune response.

In this way, EPD can prevent damage from autoimmune reactivity. Autoimmune conditions can occur when the T cells misidentify an organ or tissue as foreign to the body. (This is called molecular mimicry.) The actual causative agent can be almost anything: bacteria, a parasite, a virus, even foods or other agents. T helper cells attack the tissue of the body instead of (or in addition to) the initial triggering agent. Research has established this curious phenomenon beyond question.

In the case of rheumatoid arthritis, the bacteria proteus has been associated with this condition in up to 70 percent of cases. The bacteria may be the stimulating agent, but T helper cells are fooled into attacking joint tissue (the synovial membrane). The preliminary EPD study data show that these conditions can usually be improved—often dramatically—using EPD therapy.

TREATMENT FOR COMPLEX GI PROBLEMS

This research suggests that a number of GI problems can be treatable with EPD immunotherapy, including those associated autoimmune disorders and chronic fatigue. For some of these conditions, EPD must be used in combination with other medications (antibiotics, antiparasitics, or antifungals).

In the early days of establishing treatment protocol, some patients did not respond as well as anticipated to EPD therapy. Doctors in the EPD study group realized over time that treatment failures were most often caused by inappropriate physiological or immune response to yeast, bacteria, or other organisms in the GI tract (dysbiosis). They found that many people with these symptoms didn't really improve until this dysbiosis was addressed.

In these cases, doctors first prescribe drug and/or herbal therapy to treat any significant dysbiosis, and then follow it immediately with EPD therapy. The data now indicates improved outcomes in treating patients with Crohn's disease, irritable bowel syndrome, ulcerative colitis, and other GI problems that in the past have not been as responsive to EPD immunotherapy. Using a combination of therapies appears to better address illnesses associated with yeasts, parasites, bacteria, or potentially harmful organisms.

So much of the answer lies in the complexity of the digestive system. We may have underestimated bacteria's general capacity to do harm. Although much attention has been focused on bacteria such as pathogenic *E. coli*, it seems we have not fully appreciated the capacity of other organisms such as klebsiella, proteus, and *H. pylori* to cause infection, damage, and autoimmune disease.

Most of the potentially harmful bacteria in the GI tract escape detection by lab testing. The vast majority of flora in the GI tract survives without oxygen (anaerobic) and is usually difficult to culture in lab tests. Certain highly specialized labs can now identify many of these organisms through special cultures, complex antibody testing, testing for metabolic by-products, and other methods. Only a very small fraction of the organisms in the GI tract can be identified by the lab testing most commonly available to physicians.

The medical literature has demonstrated that autoimmune disease is often associated with specific GI organisms. EPD therapy may contain antigens to specifically address the effects of bacteria that often evade detection, including proteus, klebsiella, and bacteroides. Preliminary data indicates that this approach can be beneficial in treating a variety of autoimmune conditions caused by organisms present in the GI tract.

FREQUENCY AND EFFECTIVENESS OF TREATMENT

Dr. McEwen, director of the EPD research studies in England, has found that EPD can be permanently discontinued for over half of his patients after about sixteen to eighteen treatments without recurrence of symptoms. Dr. McEwen has observed through his follow-up studies of twenty-five years that EPD has a greater long-term success than other current methods of immunotherapy in use.

TREATING GI PROBLEMS WITH EPD

The preliminary data collected on 900 patients diagnosed with food intolerance has shown that EPD therapy can be effective for the treatment of heartburn, gastritis, esophageal reflux, abdominal pain and cramping, gas, bloating, and chronic diarrhea or constipation *when due to food intolerance*.

Other digestive conditions under specific investigation that have also been shown to respond to EPD therapy are irritable bowel syndrome, gut fermentation syndrome, ulcerative colitis, and Crohn's disease.

W.A. SHRADER, JR., M.D. is board-certified in environmental medicine and a fellow of the American Academy of Environmental Medicine. He practices medicine in Santa Fe, New Mexico, specializing in nutritional medicine, clinical immunology, and EPD therapy. Dr. Shrader attended medical school at the University of Tennessee, followed by an internship and general surgery residency in Hawaii, where he maintained a practice in family medicine and allergy treatment from 1975 until 1986. He has taught immunology and nutrition for the American Academy of Environmental Medicine since 1992. Considered to be the American authority on EPD immunotherapy, he is principal investigator for the research project to evaluate EPD, a study in which more than 9,000 patients have participated to date.

The **American EPD Society** is a nonprofit organization whose purpose is to monitor patients receiving EPD immunotherapy and assist physicians who administer it. A list of physicians trained to provide this treatment can be obtained by sending a $10 tax-deductible donation and a self-addressed, stamped envelope to: American EPD Society, 141 Paseo de Peralta, Suite A, Santa Fe, NM 87501; 505-984-0004. Further information is also available on the society's website at www.epdallergy.com.

39

Medicine for the Future: Bioelectromagnetic Therapy

TRENT NICHOLS, M.D.

◈

THE USE OF MAGNETIC ENERGY IN MEDICINE

The use of magnetic and electromagnetic devices has many medical applications and has proven to be one of the safest, most effective means of diagnosing human diseases. The MRI (magnetic resonance imaging) provides an effective method of imaging that is replacing X-ray diagnosis because it doesn't involve radiation and yet is more accurate. As a result, MRI technology is frequently used instead of earlier technology—the CT or CAT scan (computer axial tomography). Similar technology is now challenging the EEG as the preferred technique for recording brain activity.

Other familiar applications of electromagnetics in diagnosis include the ECG (electrocardiography) to record the functioning of the heart, the EEG (electroencephalography) for the electrical activity of the brain, the EGG (electrogastrography) for the stomach, and the EMG (electromyography) to evaluate muscle function.

Electrogastrography (EGG) is not as well known as its cousins but is an excellent tool for diagnosing patients with nausea who have an abnormal gastric pacemaker—a natural function in the body—and have a slower (bradygastria) or faster (tachygastria) rhythm. In the future, more gastroenterologists will become acquainted with electrogastography and artificial external gastric pacemakers may become common.

GENERAL THERAPEUTIC APPLICATIONS

Therapeutic applications of magnetic devices include the relief of diabetic neuropathy and the reduction of pain and swelling for post-polio patients. These therapies were recently described in respected peer-reviewed medical literature in the United States.

In Japan and China there has been decades of experience with magnet therapy. One in eight Japanese uses magnetic therapy in his or her daily life, and either sleeps or walks on magnetic products. A controlled scientific study in Japan on magnetic sleep pads in 154 patients with low back pain found demonstration of efficacy in one to three weeks and was published in *The Journal of Orthopedic Surgery* in 1975. One company selling magnetic products worldwide has experienced billions of dollars in sales.

Here in the United States, Vanderbilt University School of Medicine has now a magnetic research laboratory and a professor of neurology there, Dr. Robert Holcromb, has patented a static magnetic product for the relief of pain. At present, there are four centers in North America that provide magnetic therapeutics as part of a large nationwide clinical trial, treating conditions ranging from brain injury to tissue regeneration.

MAJOR NEW APPLICATIONS

Eight major new applications of the use of electromagnetic fields in medicine include:

- ◆ Wound healing
- ◆ Tissue regeneration
- ◆ Immune system stimulation
- ◆ Neuroendrocrine modulations
- ◆ Treatment of osteoarthritis
- ◆ Bone repair
- ◆ Electro-acupuncture
- ◆ Nerve stimulation

A number of these applications are relevant to the healing of GI illness.

A device to restore bone tissue using pulsed electro-magnetic fields (PEMF) was approved for the treatment of fractures in 1979. Since that time, success rates have averaged 80 percent. The concept was developed by Dr. Andrew Bassett and the electro-chemist Arthur Pilla at Columbia-Presbyterian Medical Center in New York. A detailed account of this research and others is described in the book by Dr. Robert

Becker, *The Body Electric: Electromagnetism and the Foundation of Life*, which also tells of work in the restoration of nerve and bone tissue.

Electro-Acupuncture for Pain

TENS units are now prescribed by doctors for the control of pain in patient self-care. The TENS unit (which stands for transcutaneous electrical nerve stimulation) uses a small portable electrical generating device. A new application is a handheld TENS unit with a sensor enabling treatment of acupuncture meridians and points. In the Orient, safe, low-frequency units are widely available and are used by both doctors and patients. This device is been used by the author in his practice and found to be very effective in pain control. Patients are instructed in how to use the unit at home, which has led to the successful elimination of narcotics for patients with chronic pain.

Ann Ooyang, M.D., has published an abstract on the treatment of achalasia, a disease of the esophagus in which the lower esophageal sphincter does not relax, with a TENS at LI 4, which is an acupoint between the thumb and first finger. The author has also treated many patients with nausea using the acu-stim unit on specific acupuncture points (particularly the point known as P6—Neiguan).

Another style of commercial unit is designed to control symptoms of motion sickness. It is available as a wristband that electrically stimulates this same acupuncture point (P6) at the wrist. The unit was designed by Dr. Ken Koch at Penn State University. Such a unit to control nausea was used by Senator and astronaut John Glenn for his historic reentry into space.

Wound Healing and Immune Enhancement

Wound healing, tissue regeneration, and immune enhancement using the MME (magnetic molecular energizing) is a treatment method developed by Dr. Dean Bonlie for the Advanced Magnetic Research Institute, Calgary, Alberta. The MME device resembles MRI equipment. It consists of two strong electromagnets that create a therapeutic magnetic field that leads to enhanced electron transfer and accelerated chemical reactions in the body. This improves the body's oxygen capacity, the assimilation of nutrients, the removal of metabolic waste, the reduction of free radicals, the increased manufacture of enzymes, tissue regeneration, and healing. This technique is now being used in an FDA-approved clinical trial. Patients are receiving therapy for spinal cord injury, brain injury, stroke impairment, multiple sclerosis, muscular dystrophy, cerebral palsy, Alzheimer's and Parkinson's disease, and orthopedic conditions involving bone and joint repair. One patient treated for liver fibrosis has experienced complete clearing of symptoms and an absence of abnormal liver enzymes.

Microwave Resonance Therapy

Microwave resonance therapy is being studied for bone repair in trials under way in the United States. This research was begun in Russia using low-intensity radiation (continuous or pulsed-modulated) to treat ulcers, esophagitis, chronic pain, hypertension, arthritis, cerebral palsy, neurological disorders, and the side effects of cancer chemotherapy. Thousands of Russians have been treated by this therapy, which uses low-level microwaves applied at certain acupoints.

Dr. Bjorn Nordenstrom of a prestigious hospital in Sweden has published his work on the body's electrical circulatory system and cancer therapy using electrical currents. Dr. Sodi-Pallares, a master cardiologist in Mexico, has combined electromagnetic therapy with nutritional approaches and is achieving incredible results in patients with far-advanced metastatic malignancies. Patients awaiting heart transplants who opted for his therapy for end-stage cardiomyopathy have found they no longer need the transplants. In *Magnet Therapy, The Pain Cure Alternative*, Drs. Paul Rosch and Ronald Lawrence describe a number of other promising applications of magnetic therapy.

SOURCES OF MAGNETIC ENERGY

Magnetism is one of the fundamental forces of nature and has been studied and used since antiquity. A magnetic field is defined as a field of magnetic force extending out from a permanent magnet or produced by moving electrical currents. Biomagnetism exists in all living organisms and the earth is surrounded by magnetic fields. The core of the planet generates a magnetic field. Changes in the weather generate others. Solar storms also have powerful magnetic effects on the earth.

THE BODY ELECTRIC

The human body produces subtle electromagnetic fields that are generated by the chemical reactions within the body. This electromagnetic energy travels from the nerve cells of the brain (astrocytes) down the cells covering the nerves of the spinal cord (Schwann cells) out to organs and limbs. The energy is returned by the connective tissue. These routes of electromagnetic transmission in the body were first defined more than 2,000 years ago by Oriental practitioners as meridians.

PRACTICAL APPLICATIONS

Magnetic fields are also created by electrical devices: motors, television, office equipment, computers, microwave ovens, electrical wiring and lights, and the power lines that supplies them. Medical magnetic devices differ from these appliances and industrial applications by the use of low frequencies.

It has been long known that exposure to strongly ionized electromagnetic radiation can cause extreme damage in biological tissue. Only recently has it been discovered that pulsed electromagnetic fields (oscillating nonionizing fields) in the extremely low frequency range can have a vigorous beneficial effect on biological tissues and thus be therapeutic. Our system appears to require a certain amount of low electromagnetic current that the brain transmits every night in cycles to regenerate various organ tissues during sleep. (Researchers have actually measured this current and found it to be comparable to DC current of about 8 to 2 hertz.)

Dr. Andrew Bassett made this prophetic statement in a 1992 article:

> In the decade to come, it is safe to predict bioelectromagnetics will assume a therapeutic importance equal to, or greater than, that of pharmacology and surgery today. With proper interdisciplinary effort, significant inroads can be made in controlling the ravages of cancer, some forms of heart disease, arthritis, hormonal disorders, and neurological scourges such as Alzheimer's disease, spinal cord injury, and multiple sclerosis. This prediction is not pie in the sky. Pilot studies, and biological mechanisms already in primordial terms, form a rational basis for such a statement.

DR. NICHOLS is currently developing a center for magnetic molecular research and therapy. He can be reached for consultations by calling 717-632-0300.

40

Chinese Medicine and Digestion

EFREM KORNGOLD, O.M.D.

❖

THE VIEW OF CHINESE MEDICINE

Chinese medicine is a complete medical system that has been practiced continuously throughout Asia for more than twenty-three centuries. Not only has it successfully treated and prevented illness among Asian people, it has become part of the health care of millions of Westerners in Europe, North and South America for more than one hundred years. Chinese medicine alleviates sickness while enhancing immunity and recuperative power—in other words, it *promotes* health.

It is the ability of the body to resist illness and disease, as well as to repair and regenerate itself that enables it to remain adaptable and well. The capacity to recover *balance* or physiological homeostasis, and to restore the body to a healthy condition is entirely dependent upon the quantity and quality of Qi (pronounced "chee"), often translated as vital force or vital energy. Qi is the fundamental power that we are endowed with at birth and that we strive to maintain and increase by cultivating a healthy and satisfying lifestyle. All healing in Chinese medicine is directed toward conserving, protecting, restoring, and regulating Qi. And in the broadest sense, Qi refers to all the substances, resources, and capacities within our bodies that we use to remain alive and well.

HOW THE BODY IS ORGANIZED

Chinese medicine maintains that preserving the strength and integrity of the body as a whole is the most important defense against disease. This means that while acupuncture, herbal medicine, appropriate diet, and exercise are used to relieve symptoms and heal sickness, an equal or greater emphasis is placed upon replenishing the body's natural substances or body constituents (called Shen, Qi, Moisture, Blood, and Essence) and optimizing the function of the body's primary organ systems or *networks* (known as the Liver, Heart, Spleen, Lung, and Kidney Networks).

♦ Shen is our spirit or charisma, mirrored in our thoughts, feelings, sensations.

♦ Qi, our vital force, is observed in the body's warmth, movement, and metabolic activity.

♦ Moisture encompasses all of the fluids and internal secretions that lubricate the joints, and form tears, saliva, urine, and cerebrospinal fluid.

♦ Blood contains all of the nutritive elements from which the body's tissues are made and provides the structural components that form skin, muscles, vessels, nerves, bones, and visceral organs.

♦ Essence is the basic *stuff* that enables us to maintain primary vital functions such as growth, repair, reproduction, metabolism, sensation, and imagination.

These five body constituents are managed or *organized* by the five organ networks:

♦ The Heart network governs Shen, maintaining awareness and propelling the Blood through the vessels.

♦ The Lung network governs Qi, establishes the rhythm of breathing, and maintains the integrity of skin and mucous membranes.

♦ The Spleen governs Moisture, distributing fluids and nutrients and maintaining the integrity of muscle.

♦ The Liver governs Blood, regulating the smooth circulation of Qi and Blood.

♦ The Kidney network governs Essence, providing the basic foundation for life in all of its aspects, physical, mental, emotional, and spiritual.

DISHARMONY: THE ROOT OF DISEASE

The colloquial use of the term *stress* actually suggests a state of distress—a sometimes vague, sometimes distinct sense of disquiet, discomfort, and disequilibrium that is often a prelude to the overt outbreak of an illness. The notion of stress is parallel in meaning to the classical Chinese medical concept of disharmony or imbalance. By the time stress is experienced as an impediment, a variety of symptoms may occur, depending upon the tissues and organ systems that are already weak or vulnerable.

Health is a result of the harmonious interaction of the five body constituents and the five organ networks. In contrast, illness is the result of a depletion, obstruction, or abnormal alteration of the five body constituents and a disturbance of the coordinated activity of the organ networks. Chinese medicine considers all sickness to be a consequence of the body's inability to preserve its own equilibrium in response to constant and inevitable changes, internally and externally—in other words *stress*, the stress of living.

THE MISSION OF CHINESE MEDICINE: TO PRESERVE INTEGRITY, STABILITY, FLEXIBILITY, ADAPTABILITY

It is the central purpose of Chinese medicine to invigorate the individual's power to function in a natural and integrated way. This is facilitated through a number of methods:

- ◆ Acupuncture (the insertion of thin stainless-steel needles at specific locations along the meridians that traverse the surface of the body in order to regulate the body's vital energy or Qi)
- ◆ Herbal medicine (natural plant, animal, and mineral substances combined into specific formulas that are taken in the form of teas, powders, pills, and tablets to strengthen the body and antidote the disease process)
- ◆ Diet therapy (the use of special combinations of foods and herbs to nourish and strengthen the body)

The practitioner of Chinese medicine seeks to enable the body to restore itself to a condition of stability, flexibility, and adaptability. And while a condition of perfect health is not always completely attainable, these gentle and noninvasive methods of treatment will almost always restore or enhance immunity, vigor, and functionality. In addition, Chinese medicine can prevent or reverse many of the harmful effects of medical treatments that may be necessary to preserve and prolong life. In fact, using Chinese medicine in combination with Western medicine enables a person to better withstand the impact of aggressive medical interventions such as chemotherapy and surgery by building strength and accelerating the rate of recovery, maintaining the quality of life, and increasing the likelihood of long-term survival.

THE DIGESTIVE SYSTEM IS THE SOURCE OF QI

Each cell of our nervous and digestive systems must function appropriately every minute to assure coordinated muscular movements of the gut and the proper secretion of enzymes, hormones, and mucus. Digestion is therefore a crucial aspect of our intelligence.

According to Chinese medicine, Qi is the intelligent power of the body. So if Qi is adequately distributed throughout the body, then the

---

Chinese Medicine in Action: The Case of Elaine

◈

In 1991, Elaine was diagnosed with proctitis, and in 1993 she was diagnosed with ulcerative colitis. After four years of treatment with prednisone, steroid enemas, Rowasa suppositories, Asacol, and mercaptopurine, she was told that she needed to undergo surgical removal of her colon. At this point she decided to try something different—Chinese medicine.

When she began treatment with acupuncture and Chinese herbal medicine in 1997, Elaine was experiencing constant abdominal bloating and gas, intestinal pain and sensitivity, urgency and frequent bowel movements, very low energy and stamina, depression, and anxiety. Not only was she not responding well to her medications, she was having trouble figuring out what to eat that didn't aggravate her condition.

After ten acupuncture treatments over a period of eleven months, along with dietary modification (basically elimination of all grains, starchy vegetables, and milk products) and herbal formulas in the form of pills and liquid extracts, she has improved enormously. She rarely has gas, bloating, urgency, or diarrhea and she has no pain, intestinal bleeding, or mucus in her stool. She has reduced her medications considerably, but still relies on a daily dose of mercaptopurine, which has been reduced from 75 to 50 mg, and Asacol, which has been reduced to once every four days.

More important, her energy, stamina, and sense of hopefulness and optimism have returned, enabling her to go back to work, expand her spiritual life, and think about changing her career. All of this has occurred without major surgery and with a decreasing need for medication. The longer she continues with acupuncture, herbal medicine, and an appropriate diet, the more functional she becomes and the stronger she feels.

body will know what to do in each of its parts all the time. Each of us has an operating system, an organizing power (Qi) that has much in common with other beings but is unique to each individual. Every moment that we are alive, we're literally re-creating ourselves, and we do it a little differently every day—*we don't remain exactly the same*. Because our world is always changing, we must continually adapt, so one of the indications of disease is the loss of adaptability—when we're no longer able to adjust comfortably and naturally to the shifting circumstances of our lives. The health of the digestive system is crucial to maintaining our ability to adapt and to be well, for a lifetime.

It is the Spleen network that governs all digestive processes, including those of the mouth, esophagus, stomach, small intestine, large intestine, and pancreas. The Spleen network is subdivided into two organ systems: the Stomach, which regulates the digestion of food and fluids, and the Spleen, which regulates the absorption of nutrients and their distribution within the body. It is the job of the Spleen network to supply the body with the raw materials it needs on a daily basis to produce all the substances of the body, primarily Qi, Moisture, and Blood. So the digestive system is the source of all that we require for daily living, including the nutrients we need to grow and mature.

THE THREE PILLARS OF HEALTH

Because it supplies us with Qi, the digestive system is one of the three pillars of health—what are known as the Three Treasures—the other two being Shen and Essence. Shen is our spirit or charisma—what we experience as emotional warmth and presence of mind. Essence is the vital power and substance that we are endowed with at birth—what we "inherit" from our parents and from our mother while we're growing in her womb—and it enables us to have children, to be imaginative and creative, and to develop into mature and competent adults.

The signs of good digestion are:

◆ *Feeling good in the belly.* Your stomach and intestines, your upper and lower abdomen, feel comfortable, especially after eating or eliminating—so comfortable, in fact, they actually induce pleasurable sensations.

◆ *Experiencing regular and distinct feelings of hunger.* When you're hungry, you have a clear sense of what it is that you want and need to eat. When you eat and drink what is appropriate and nourishing *for you*, you feel satisfied, better after eating than you did before. You become revitalized and happy, ready to work and play.

♦ *Feeling good in the mouth.* You have a pleasant taste in your mouth, it feels comfortably moist, and your breath smells good.

Frequently when people feel unwell, if there is no clear evidence of illness or disease from a conventional Western medical perspective, their distress may be viewed as if it were merely a psychosomatic problem. It can be distressing to experience poor digestion and not recognize the cause. It is in situations like these, in which there is no clear understanding or diagnosis, that Chinese medicine can often be helpful. Vague complaints—the kind that mysteriously come and go or simply make us uncomfortable and discouraged—are taken to heart by the practitioner because they're seen as the vanguard of what could develop into a more serious condition. The goal is to treat problems before they become severe. One of the strengths of Chinese medicine is that it can offer interventions at the early stages of nonspecific illness, whereas conventional Western medicine is geared more to treat problems that are full-blown and therefore easier to identify with objective tests and diagnostic procedures.

TONGUE DIAGNOSIS: A SIMPLE WAY TO EVALUATE DIGESTIVE HEALTH

In Chinese medicine, the tongue is perceived as a window through which the signs of health or sickness can be directly seen. The condition of the tongue and its coating—the tongue fur—indicates quite clearly whether or not the digestive system is functioning well. By carefully noting the shape, color, and moisture of the tongue and its fur, we can tell if there is a disorder of the stomach or the intestines. If there is congestion in the stomach due to a lack of digestive secretions, inhibited peristalsis, toxins in the food, poor quality food, or food that is staying in the stomach or intestines too long and beginning to ferment or putrefy, it will appear as a change in the moisture, texture, thickness, and color of the fur.

A healthy tongue is a ruddy pink color, lays comfortably in the mouth (is neither too large or fat nor too small or thin), and has an even shape, a smooth texture, and a thin, moist, light white fur that covers its surface evenly from the back to the front. The appearance of coarse, thickened, wet, dry, absent, or discolored fur (translucent white changing to opaque white, gray, yellow, or brown) is an early sign of congestion in the stomach and of poor digestion. By examining the tongue fur each morning and evening, you will know whether your digestive health is improving or worsening. Usually, if the tongue fur is becoming thicker and/or more yellow, it indicates either a disturbance of digestion and elimination, the development of an acute illness like stomach or intestinal flu or both. If the fur is becoming progressively thinner, whiter, and clearer it represents a general improvement in the entire condition of the body as well as the digestive system. On the other hand, if the fur becomes very thin, patchy, or entirely absent, it represents a worsening of health in general, and a weakening of the Qi of the whole body.

Very often visible signs on the tongue are associated with a subjective experience of distress, generally as well as locally in the digestive organs. A sensation of bloating in the stomach or belly, belching or flatulence, irregular bowel movements, strong food aversions or cravings, irritability, and pain are symptoms of congestion, whereas feelings of fatigue and weakness, chilliness, melancholy and dull thinking, vague discomforts that can't be easily localized, slow or infrequent bowel movements, loose stools, and cravings that are difficult to describe or satisfy are symptoms of depletion. Another early warning of poor digestion is a sense of dissatisfaction, irritability, or malaise after eating—lingering hunger, queasiness, or feeling as if you ate something spoiled or improperly cooked.

HOW DIGESTIVE PROBLEMS BEGIN

From the point of view of Chinese medicine, disorders such as esophagitis, gastritis, ileitis, and colitis are all variations on a theme—the disordered function of the stomach and intestines (the Spleen network). These organs can become disturbed for a multiplicity of reasons: poor diet; irregular eating habits; physical and mental strain; a viral, bacterial, fungal, or parasitic infection; allergies; toxicity; and harsh medications like antibiotics (tetracycline, metronidazole, Biaxin), anti-inflammatory drugs (aspirin, Motrin, Indocin, Asacol), steroids (prednisone, cortisone), chemotherapy drugs (methotrexate, cisplatin, 5-FU, Adriamycin). These influences can undermine the health of the digestive system in the short term—as in diarrhea and nausea caused by antibiotics or chemotherapy—and if present over a

The Tongue and Its Fur

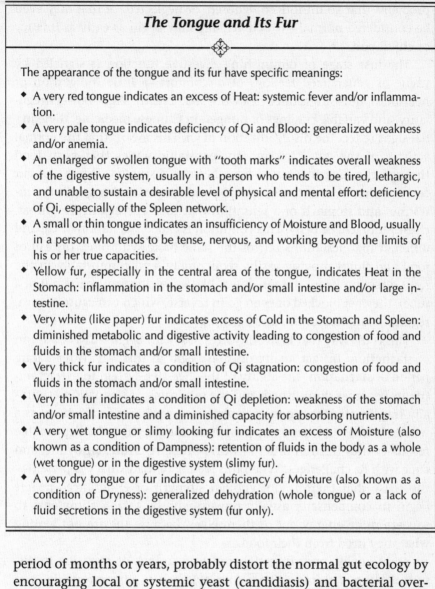

The appearance of the tongue and its fur have specific meanings:

- A very red tongue indicates an excess of Heat: systemic fever and/or inflammation.
- A very pale tongue indicates deficiency of Qi and Blood: generalized weakness and/or anemia.
- An enlarged or swollen tongue with "tooth marks" indicates overall weakness of the digestive system, usually in a person who tends to be tired, lethargic, and unable to sustain a desirable level of physical and mental effort: deficiency of Qi, especially of the Spleen network.
- A small or thin tongue indicates an insufficiency of Moisture and Blood, usually in a person who tends to be tense, nervous, and working beyond the limits of his or her true capacities.
- Yellow fur, especially in the central area of the tongue, indicates Heat in the Stomach: inflammation in the stomach and/or small intestine and/or large intestine.
- Very white (like paper) fur indicates excess of Cold in the Stomach and Spleen: diminished metabolic and digestive activity leading to congestion of food and fluids in the stomach and/or small intestine.
- Very thick fur indicates a condition of Qi stagnation: congestion of food and fluids in the stomach and/or small intestine.
- Very thin fur indicates a condition of Qi depletion: weakness of the stomach and/or small intestine and a diminished capacity for absorbing nutrients.
- A very wet tongue or slimy looking fur indicates an excess of Moisture (also known as a condition of Dampness): retention of fluids in the body as a whole (wet tongue) or in the digestive system (slimy fur).
- A very dry tongue or fur indicates a deficiency of Moisture (also known as a condition of Dryness): generalized dehydration (whole tongue) or a lack of fluid secretions in the digestive system (fur only).

period of months or years, probably distort the normal gut ecology by encouraging local or systemic yeast (candidiasis) and bacterial overgrowth in the stomach and intestines, decreasing enzymatic functions (inhibiting fat, protein, and carbohydrate digesting enzymes), and compromising gut immunity (decreasing immunoglobulins and increasing antibodies that cause allergic reactions to food and other substances). It's unusual for chronic problems to arise out of a single acute incident, although they may appear that way to the individual. Invariably there is a history of symptoms—minor, but persistent or recurring problems that go unnoticed, ignored, or neglected, or that may even be considered normal—which actually may begin as early as infancy or childhood.

The first stage of diminishing digestive function is signaled by vague or generalized feelings of discomfort—a little indigestion or heartburn, queasiness once in a while, bad breath, slight bowel irregularity, and variable cravings or hunger. In Chinese medicine, these initial signs reflect the disorganization of Qi. This means that the normal activity of the gut—the smooth, peristaltic waves that push food through the digestive tract—have become disrupted. When the gut ceases to function naturally, people begin experiencing gas in the intestines and stomach or a sensation that food is stuck in the throat, chest, stomach, or belly. This condition is called stagnation of Qi, and different manifestations mirror the same basic syndrome. Instead of food and fluids moving easily, sequentially, and comfortably in the right direction (from the top down, like squeezing toothpaste out of a tube), they get blocked or even go in reverse, which can cause nausea, regurgitation, heartburn, and belching.

This is the way that many digestive problems begin—as a condition of stagnation. In fact, many diseases begin in this way. After a long period of stagnation, the ability of the digestive system to extract nutrients becomes diminished, and the syndrome of stagnation eventually transforms into a one of depletion, a weakness of the body as a whole. When that happens, people no longer have the dependable resources they need in order to work, think, re-create, enjoy life, and cope with its challenges. When this feeling of inadequacy is present— the sense that there is not enough strength or endurance—people begin to compensate, usually unwittingly, by taking stimulants to squeeze more energy out of themselves, because they're not getting what they need from their food.

Additionally, poor digestion can lead to lack of rest, due to disturbed sleep patterns. When your stomach is uncomfortable, you don't sleep as well. Because of work schedules or long commutes, many people eat too late and too much before they go to bed, allowing excess food to remain in the stomach and intestines while sleeping. Ordinarily, digestion is facilitated by getting up and moving around after eating, whereas eating just before going to sleep can interfere with this process.

WHEN AND HOW TO EAT

The Chinese medical model describes an optimum time for each organ system during the 24-hour cycle of day and night. Ideally, soon after you awaken in the morning, you have a bowel movement. That way the gut is emptied and prepared to receive the first food of the new day. Between seven and nine A.M. is the optimum time to empty the bowels. The optimum time for eating and digesting is from mid-morning to early afternoon, nine A.M. to three P.M. This is the time of peak activity for the stomach and the small intestine. So from the point of view of the digestive organs, breakfast and lunch are the most important meals. The midday meal should be the largest, breakfast should be moderate, and dinner should be the lightest and easiest to digest.

Most of us eat breakfast fairly early, somewhere between seven and nine o'clock in the morning when we're not yet ready physiologically for a large meal. We need to eat something nourishing and filling in the morning because we're empty and somewhat weak after sleeping for eight hours, but we should eat just enough to get the juices flowing. As a general principle, you should eat a small meal for breakfast. On the other hand, it's important not to go without breakfast, because you'll be too hungry for lunch and end up overeating. The better you keep to a regular schedule of meals, the better you'll feel.

Another issue is how quickly we eat. Many people eat too fast—they're always in a hurry. The only time they're not rushing is late in the evening, when they're physically and mentally worn out from the day. Not only do you feel weary in the evening, your digestive system is at a low ebb because its prime time is long past. Yet when the evening meal is delayed, you'll be even hungrier and tempted to overeat. If you overload yourself with food at that time, your body will perceive it as a burden, not as a pleasure.

CARING FOR THE STOMACH

Another habit that Americans indulge in that can have damaging effects on digestion is eating too much cold and raw food, especially in the beginning of the day—like reaching for the orange juice right out of the refrigerator first thing in the morning, or having cold yogurt or a piece of chilled fruit or all three. Sometimes the cold and raw food is chased with a hot cup of coffee. And even though a cup of hot coffee warms things up, it's often so intensely hot that it is an insult to the stomach. Drinking something extremely hot right after eating something very cold is a little like running cold water over a very hot cast-iron frying pan, which can sometimes crack under the strain. Such a sudden and extreme change can damage the stomach Qi and lead to Qi stagnation syndrome, causing chronic indigestion over the long term.

Raw foods, like refrigerated and frozen food, are also considered to have a cooling influence on the body. A diet that consists primarily of raw and cold foods will often lead to persistent diarrhea with abdominal gas and bloating. Cooling or cold food may be appropriate when the body is overheated in hot weather or during an acute illness with a high fever. For example, eating watermelon on a hot day helps to cool us down, and watermelon juice can actually bring down a fever that comes as a result of being too long in the sun.

The inherent coldness of raw and refrigerated foods chills the stomach, and instead of helping to increase its blood supply for effective digestion and activate its digestive secretions, it causes the stomach to contract, to reduce its blood supply and inhibit its secretions. The mixing of hot and cold foods in quick succession can easily lead to Qi stagnation syndrome and may ultimately result in chronic indigestion.

A more healthful morning ritual would be to first drink something warm, even plain hot water. What this does is to prepare the stomach—it "wakes it up," just as a hot shower invigorates you and gets your blood moving. The hot shower invigorates you from the outside and drinking something hot invigorates you on the inside. After drinking something hot, eat something else that's warm, like cooked cereal or steamed vegetables or even stewed fruit—something that you can digest easily and that provides more nutrients than a piece of toast or a muffin with a cup of coffee. Cooked foods have a warming influence that helps the stomach and intestines function more effectively. Then, if you want to finish your morning meal with something fresh, like a piece of fruit or some yogurt, as long as it's at least room temperature, that's fine, because the digestive organs are already "warmed up." If you must eat something cold—because you're in a hurry or feeling hot or thirsty—always eat or drink something hot first.

Throughout Asia, hot water is considered to be the universal remedy for any illness, as well as being a simple health tonic. Just sipping hot water (or hot lemon water, vegetable broth, diluted fruit juice, or even weak green tea) throughout the day is very good therapy for your digestion. The reason that the frequent ingestion of warm or hot (but not scalding) liquids is so beneficial is that it restores and maintains natural condition of the digestive organs. For example, recall how you feel when you go into a cold environment and you're not dressed warmly enough: You become rapidly chilled and begin to feel lethargic or even sleepy, like you want to curl up in a ball in order to get warm and conserve your body heat. Exactly the same thing happens to the internal organs when they're subjected to cold influences.

When I was a child, I loved ice cream, and I would always ask to have ice cream for dessert. I was a rather thin child, so when we would go to a restaurant, my father would always say, "Now if you get ice cream, you're going to feel really cold when you go outside." I would never believe him. And every time I'd walk outside and get really cold. The point is that eating cold things makes us cold. And, naturally, our body responds defensively: It contracts, the pulse slows down, and metabolic activity becomes depressed. The more the body slows down, the harder it is to eat, digest, assimilate, and transform the food nutrients into energy, blood, and tissue.

THE MAIN FACTORS IN GOOD DIGESTION

The primary factors that promote good digestion include:

- ◆ Timing—when you eat
- ◆ Manner—how you eat
- ◆ Quantity—how much
- ◆ Condition of the food—whether it's raw, cooked, warm, or cold
- ◆ Quality—whether the food is fresh, clean, and pure
- ◆ Appropriateness—whether the food is compatible with your digestive capacity and relevant to your nutritional requirements

The quality, quantity, condition, and appropriateness of your food are all important from the Chinese medicine point of view. But even more crucial are the conditions of eating—the manner in which you eat, how quickly you eat, whether you're standing or sitting or moving about, whether you're paying attention to your food or continuing to work. If you continue to work while you eat—to engage in intense problem-solving or read something that makes you tense—you are depriving the digestive system of the energy it needs to perform its function. If reading or conversing while you eat relaxes you, then it's good; if not, then it's an unnecessary stress and potentially harmful.

If you're trying to work while you eat, you're forcing the body to divide its resources between action or thinking and the work of digestion. This uses up the Qi instead of restoring it, so that you wind up competing with yourself. People who eat and run or who eat on the run will progressively begin to lose energy and digestive power. This is also true of those who eat without stopping or who eat and then immediately get up and go back to work, without allowing time for digestion. The consequence of this is an increased risk of diminished physical capacities and deteriorating health. Chronic health problems generally originate very early in life because that's when our habits around food and eating are established, like not chewing well and eating too fast.

In my family, my father ate so fast that he was always finished before everybody else and couldn't tolerate leaving the food and dishes on the table. He immediately began to wash the dishes and put the leftovers away. So if I didn't finish quickly, I wouldn't get to eat all of my food, and I was a dreamy child who ate particularly slowly. Eventually I learned to eat very quickly; and as a result, I've had to learn to undo that conditioning in my adult life. Being tense and gulping your food leads to a lot of discomfort, especially for children, who often get stomachaches after eating too much and too quickly—often in response to messages like "You can't leave the table until you eat everything on your plate."

WHEN THERE'S NO TIME TO EAT

If you're in a hurry, if you really don't have time to sit down, it is better to drink your food rather than eat it. Drink something warm, like soup or even plain broth. If you have to eat in a hurry, it's a lot easier to digest cooked vegetables than raw salads. Later, when you have time to sit, to calm down, and to chew thoroughly, then you can eat more dense, solid food—and you'll be able to digest it.

Even before you put something in your mouth, you should feel good in your belly. This good feeling comes as a sign that the body is getting ready for the food. When you begin to put the food in your mouth, chew, and swallow, you'll start to feel even better: as the food slides smoothly down the esophagus and into the stomach, it should induce pleasurable sensations all along the way. Then as you eat more, it gets pushed along and pushed along, and eventually you say to yourself, "That's it, I'm finished. I'm not hungry anymore."

RESTORING VITALITY, RESTORING QI

People with digestive disorders often miss the pleasurable experience of eating, but they certainly want to regain it. The purpose of acupuncture, herbal medicine, and dietary modification is to restore the normal activity of the Qi, to relieve stagnation—to promote the normal secretions and peristalsis of the digestive tract. This is essential to good health.

To restore the Qi means to restore the normal pattern of movement: the movement of blood and fluids and the activity of the organs themselves. One of the early signs of poor digestion is *reflux*, which means that food, air, and fluid are reversing their normal direction, going up instead of down. This is what causes problems such as esophageal irritation and spasm. On the other hand, when the gut is hyperactive, food and liquid is passing through too quickly to be properly transformed and absorbed. This is also *abnormal* movement. Gut hyperactivity can be a manifestation of irritability and anxiety; and, under these conditions, food is experienced as an irritant and the body tries to get rid of it as quickly as possible, resulting in urgency and diarrhea.

THE IMPORTANCE OF IMMUNITY

The gut is not only a digestive organ, it is also an essential component of the immune system. It functions as a boundary, a permeable membrane, just like the skin, except it's on the inside of the body instead of the outside. In fact, the lining of the gut—its surface area—is much greater than that of the skin. If you were to lay out the entire gut, it would fill up the area of a tennis court. In comparison, the skin would only cover a desktop. So even though the gut is considered to be an internal organ, it is exposed to the external environment by direct contact with the gases, liquids, and solids that enter the digestive tract. Thus, the gut is the body's first line of defense against multitudes of invading pathogenic organisms including viruses, bacteria, fungi, and parasites. And since the gut functions as an immunological boundary, it's normal for there to be bacteria in the mouth, the throat, the stomach, and the intestines. But these organisms should remain on the surface, outside the digestive barrier, not inside of it. And if the lining of the gut is in some way compromised, our resistance is diminished and we become subject to infection and the toxic metabolic by-products of those same microorganisms.

There are many factors that can lower our resistance or diminish the integrity of our boundaries—illness, improper diet, stress, exposure to damaging toxins (poisons in the food or bad medicine), or a combination of these things. Take, for example, a sunburn. Once the skin becomes damaged by exposure, some people become more prone to herpes or vulnerable to other kinds of problems like warts, fungi, or bacterial infection. Similarly, damage to the lining of the digestive tract can make us more vulnerable to other conditions.

Because everything in the body is interconnected, what happens to the body that's good benefits the whole body, and what happens to the body that's bad ultimately harms the whole body. When one aspect of function is impaired, the others are also diminished. You can't separate them: Poor digestion also weakens immunity. Compromise of the immune function of the membrane of the gut eventually leads to disturbed digestion and absorption. From the Chinese medicine point of view, resistance—the ability to defend oneself against what is "not me"—is completely dependent on the quality of Qi; and the quality of Qi is completely dependent on digestion, which is its source.

MANAGING STRESS

It's not just what you do specifically to improve your health that's important, it's everything you do. You're not healthy just because you're taking digestive enzymes or beneficial intestinal bacteria or herbs to improve digestion and elimination. These may all be very good for you, but they're just parts of the picture, not the whole view. That is the typical approach of Western medicine and even some forms of alternative medicine—a tendency to be simplistic or reductionistic, being more concerned with the parts rather than the whole.

How you take care of yourself, how you manage yourself physically from day to day, is as important to your health as any medicine or therapy. For example, some people with Crohn's and colitis know that their condition is aggravated by mental, emotional, and physical stress. Yet a lot of people with these problems lead very strenuous lives. In spite of their illness, they continue to push themselves, to overextend themselves, and to put themselves in situations which make them feel inadequate.

It may be that the vast majority of people have these same habits, but not everybody has inflammatory bowel disease. Other people get problems that may be just as serious, but they arise elsewhere in the body. And so the issues of stress and lifestyle are ever-present factors that are always influencing our health.

Wherever your weakness lies, that's where the greatest distress is going to appear. This means that conducting your life so that you are not overextending and weakening yourself is fundamental to managing these kinds of illnesses successfully. Success doesn't mean achieving a complete cure, but it does mean enabling people to be functional. The goal is to become competent to the degree that the illness is no longer a disability. After all, nobody's perfect and very few of us are going to get through life without some kind of injury or insult.

Part of the problem in our culture is that we're always looking for a total cure—it's all or nothing. Yet a complete cure may be an unrealistic expectation for many people with chronic illness. People need to learn how to cope with their impairments realistically and not feel defeated by them. The goal is to increase our capacity to the point where our limitations will not prevent us from fulfilling our purposes in life.

THE BODY'S COMMUNICATION SYSTEM

In Chinese medicine, the body is conceived of as a microcosm of society in which the organ systems interact like the members of a family. In order for the family to work together harmoniously, there must be cooperation, coordination, and accommodation. The basis of this is communication.

Adequate circulation plays an essential role in healing, because circulation is an important form of inter-body communication. Candace Pert, a respected NIH researcher, discovered that there are chemical messengers called peptides that circulate in the blood. Every tissue makes these same chemical messengers. So the blood is not only a vehicle for transporting nutrients, it's also a medium for delivering information. Every cell is constantly sending messages to every other part of the organism.

If circulation to a certain part of the body is reduced, then there will be a breakdown in the information network. As a consequence, a process of isolation due to a loss of contact begins to occur that can eventually develop into a condition of confusion and conflict within the body. Disease is a breakdown in the process of coordination that binds the organism together. The body should function as if it were a unified entity, and when it begins to function as if it weren't, the process of disease begins.

IMPROVING COMMUNICATION WITHIN THE BODY

Qi is the vital force that heals us and Qi is also a kind of intelligence. It is the mind or consciousness. It's the body being aware of itself. You're able to be self-aware because all the parts of you are linked together by Qi, the dynamic intelligence of the organism. Qi is everywhere, all the time, as it flows with the blood through a special system of channels or meridians.

Immunity is an important aspect of that intelligence which is able to distinguish between what is you and what is not you, what is of benefit to you and what harms you. Acupuncture restores the circulation of Qi, which in turn renews the integrity of mind, self, and body, invigorates immunity and enables healing to occur.

Illness is a consequence of the disorganization of Qi—a kind of disintegration. Acupuncture can often reorganize the Qi and reestablish bodily unity. The more consistently a person receives acupuncture, the more long lasting the effects. The experience of well-being that follows an acupuncture treatment is the renewed feeling of being integrated, as if your body has been reunited, rather than continuing to be an assemblage of conflicting and competing parts.

When a part of our body is in pain or inflamed—like a shoulder with bursitis or an irritable colon—then it becomes our whole world, taking over a large portion of our waking life. A process of self-alienation begins in which there is a desire to disassociate from the offending bodily part; it becomes like an adversary that we begin to resent for the discomfort it creates. In fact, the shoulder and the stomach are still part of us, but there's been a breakdown in the sense of unity between the self and the body.

What acupuncture works to restore is coordination and communication within the body, brain, and mind. Once that begins to happen, the natural mechanisms for repair, recovery, and regeneration are permitted to function again. The shoulder that aches and the colon that cramps are brought back into contact with the rest of the body, which greets them lovingly as if to say, "Now I remember. You're really part of us. We're going to help you. We can't live without you. You can't live without us. So we'll make you well."

EFREM KORNGOLD, O.M.D., has been practicing Chinese traditional medicine since 1973 at his clinic, Chinese Medicine Works, in San Francisco. He received his early training in the United Kingdom and has twice traveled to China for advanced studies. A diplomate in acupuncture and a doctor of Oriental medicine, he has contributed his expertise as an examination consultant to the National Commission for Certification in Acupuncture and Oriental Medicine. He is co-author with Harriet Beinfield, L.Ac., of the book *Between Heaven and Earth: A Guide to Chinese Medicine* (Ballantine, 1991), and the herbal guide *Chinese Modular Solutions Handbook for Health Professionals* (available through K'AN Herb Company). Dr. Korngold is currently on the faculty of the American College of Traditional Chinese Medicine in San Francisco and a peer reviewer for the journal *Integrative Medicine*, edited by Dr. Andrew Weil.

41

Homeopathic Remedies*

MAESIMUND PANOS, M.D., AND
JANE HEIMLICH, M.S.

❖

Homeopathy is reemerging as a vigorous field within medicine. France has nearly 800 homeopathic physicians, and the movement is also active in Germany, Austria, and Switzerland. In England, members of the royal family have been cared for by homeopathic physicians since the reign of Queen Victoria. There are about 200 homeopathic physicians in Britain; the principal hospitals offering homeopathic treatment are in London and Glasgow.

India is a stronghold of homeopathy. In 1980, there were 124 homeopathic medical schools there. Central and Latin America are also important centers. In Mexico, there are three homeopathic medical colleges, two of which are state supported. There is a similar school of medicine in Brazil. Around 450 Argentine physicians are homeopaths. Homeopathy is on the rise all over the world in response to the need for new safe and effective approaches to healing.

HOW HOMEOPATHY WORKS

The Office Visit

If you're continually experiencing one upset after another, you could be wise to seek homeopathic care. The constitutional remedy, being suited to the individual's entire being, often resolves recurring com-

*From *Homeopathic Medicine at Home* by Maesimund Panos & Jane Heimlich. Copyright © 1980 by Maesimund Panos & Jane Heimlich. Used by permission of Putnam Berkley, a division of Penguin Putnam Inc. Homeopathy is based on timeless scientific principles, so we found that none of the information in the original text had become dated. The need for this information is greater than ever.

plaints and promotes increased vitality and well-being. On your first office visit, you'll probably notice that the homeopathic physician is an excellent listener. Your symptoms are considered thoughtfully and recorded carefully. However, the purpose of this symptom-taking is somewhat different than in other medical practice. In homeopathic prescribing, the ultimate healer is your own vital force, your energy. Symptoms are the basis for selecting a remedy that will activate your own immune system.

Homeopathic Remedies

Homeopathic remedies have been respected for more than a century because they are safe as well as effective. In contrast to pharmaceuticals, the remedies contain exceptionally minute doses that are said to influence the body on an energetic level.

The remedy is selected because of the symptoms it causes *in someone who is well*. In a person who is ill, a remedy is given that exactly matches their symptoms, making them slightly sicker, on a subtle physical level. The sudden subtle worsening of the illness is said to awaken the immune system. If a healing response isn't observed, the exceptionally small dose is given again periodically (for example, every four hours or twice a day) until the immune system is activated and the person begins to improve. Once there is clear improvement, the remedy is stopped, since the body's own defenses have been set in motion.

The Mechanism of the Remedies

Homeopathy was discovered by Samuel Hahnemann, a German physician in the early 1800s who practiced medicine in a time when the primary treatment for illness was to rid the body of "ill humors" or fluids by cauterizing, blistering, purging, and bleeding. When he found himself without a logical rationale to treat illness in his own children, he became so disillusioned that he gave up the practice of medicine and turned to medical translating for a livelihood.

Translating a text that described quinine, he realized that quinine, when *given to a well person,* duplicates the symptoms of malaria. Taking the remedy himself, he experienced fatigue, palpitations, anxiety, trembling, redness of the cheeks, prostration—all the characteristics of intermittent fever. Hahnemann reasoned that malaria was cured by quinine, not because of its bitter properties, but because it produces the *symptoms* of malaria. He devised a method of more safely using substances such as quinine by diluting them to almost infinitesimally small doses. By using minute doses to exaggerate the illness, the immune system is engaged more rapidly and the body's own healing mechanism can then address the condition.

If improvement occurs and then stops, the remedy is given again until the immune system is reactivated and progress is observed. If the symptoms change but still require healing (often following some observed improvement), a different remedy is given in response to the new symptom pattern.

The Minimum Dose

The substances selected as remedies are prepared in extremely diluted form, so that only traces remain. Consequently, the remedies are exceptionally safe. All the remedies have been tested repeatedly and systematically over the past 150 years in people who are well, in a process called proving—short for proving a remedy.

The remedy is given to the patient at consistent intervals. For example, a low-dose home remedy of 6x, 6c, 12c, or 30x strength may be given once every four hours until healing or a change in symptoms occurs. During the first fifteen minutes following the remedy, the symptoms may intensify slightly. Patients are encouraged to lie down and rest during this period. It has been suggested that this brief intensification of the symptoms is part of the process that calls the illness to the attention of the immune system more quickly and sets in motion its healing activities. Homeopathy is a noninvasive way to speed up our natural mechanisms.

Homeopathy and Self-Healing

Note that it is also important to complement the action of the remedies with self-care. It is essential to support the body and the immune function through good nutrition, sufficient rest and fluids, fresh air, and other resources that provide the raw materials for healing.

TREATING DIGESTIVE COMPLAINTS WITH HOMEOPATHY

Indigestion

"A meal a minute . . . fast take-out . . . the minute chef . . ." A stranger to our culture observing our commercial eating places might conclude that eating requires a stopwatch. Many of us follow the same pattern at home. The evening meal may be interrupted by phone calls or the pressure of PTA meetings. Singles frequently gulp a meal en route to an evening engagement.

If your frantic schedule is giving you indigestion, resolve to cut out the nonessentials. If you're still troubled by stomach distress, consider the following remedies, and choose one that fits you and your symptoms:

♦ *Bryonia.* Your stomach feels heavy after eating and is sensitive to touch. You have bitter risings and may vomit bile and water. You are thirsty for long drinks of cold water, but may vomit from warm drinks. The least movement makes your stomach feel worse.

♦ *Carbo vegetalis.* The plainest food disagrees with you and causes gas and belching about half an hour after eating. Any indulgence causes a headache. You have an aversion to meat, milk, and fatty foods and a craving for fresh air, and need to loosen your belt after eating.

♦ *Chamomilla.* An attack of indigestion follows a fit of anger and irritability. Your stomach is distended with gas and cramping in the abdomen; your mouth has a bitter taste. You have flushed cheeks and an aversion to warm drinks.

♦ *Ignatia.* You are tense, nervous, excitable, sensitive, and crave food that doesn't agree with you. Indigestion is caused by eating after receiving bad news or shock. Symptoms are rumbling in the bowels, sour belching. You have a tendency to take deep breaths or sigh frequently.

♦ *Nux vomica.* You're the hard-driving type who overindulges in food, coffee, liquor, or tobacco. Symptoms are heartburn, belching,

---

Everyday Healing—A Note from the Homeopathic Physician

I have seen homeopathic prescribing work dramatically. For example, take the case of a young woman named Ellen, going through the trauma of divorce. Ellen called me one day. "I have to appear in court this morning," she said weakly, "and I'm having diarrhea and throwing up at the same time." She was also in a cold sweat, she said, and felt as if she were going to collapse at any moment. I suggested she take the remedy Veratrum alb. and call me in a half hour. At that time, she reported that the vomiting and diarrhea had stopped, and she felt strong enough to face the ordeal ahead.

bloating of abdomen a few hours after eating. You may also be constipated.

◆ *Pulsatilla.* You are peevish and wake up in the morning feeling
as if you have a stone in your stomach; your mouth is dry with a bad
taste but you're not thirsty. You have some of the same symptoms as
Carbo vegetalis—pain in the stomach half an hour after eating, an aversion to fatty foods, and too snug clothing around the abdomen.

BEYOND FIRST AID. Abdominal pain may be a warning of appendicitis or other more serious problems. Therefore, when such pain persists
and especially when it is accompanied by slight fever, nausea, vomiting, or even loss of appetite, seek professional help.

Nausea and Vomiting

Eating and drinking too much or eating contaminated food are some
common causes of vomiting. The following remedies will help relieve
this condition.

◆ *Antimony.* Vomiting caused by eating to excess or eating an indi-
gestible substance. Patient vomits right after eating or drinking and
has a white-coated tongue.

◆ *Arsenicum.* Nausea, vomiting, and diarrhea caused by spoiled
food, especially bad meat or watery fruit. Burning pains in the stomach after eating are relieved by warm drinks.

◆ *Colcoynthis* (bitter cucumber). Agonizing pain in the abdomen
causes the patient to double up. Pressure and warmth applied to the
stomach ameliorate the situation.

◆ *Ipecac.* Nausea, griping pains in the intestines, with or without
vomiting. Nausea from looking at moving objects, or reading in a
moving vehicle. Tongue is clean, even though stomach is disordered.

◆ *Nux vomica.* "Wants to and can't." This is a keynote of Nux,
whether the condition involves vomiting, moving bowels, or urinat-
ing. The patient is wakeful after three A.M., falls asleep in the morning,
and awakens feeling wretched.

◆ *Phosphorus.* Great thirst for cold water, which is vomited as soon
as it becomes warm in the stomach. This remedy is also helpful in
serious cases involving vomiting of blood.

◆ *Veratrum album.* Patient alternates between vomiting and diarrhea. Cold sweat breaks out on the forehead, perhaps all over the body.

Collapse is possible. Other symptoms are cramps in extremities and continued retching.

GAS

If you are not digesting your food properly, air or gas forms in the stomach and intestines. This can cause abdominal pain, bloating, rumbling, belching, and passing gas—and a good deal of embarrassment.

Like indigestion, gas can be the result of eating too fast, eating while emotionally upset, or swallowing air while eating or talking. Dysbiosis can also be a major cause of gas and bloating. The wrong balance of GI flora can occur after a round of antibiotics—especially an extended course or intravenous antibiotics. Gas can also result from an overgrowth of normal bacteria or yeast or from an infection due to invading bacteria or parasites.

The digestive system is a marvelously synchronized effort, and each of its parts plays a distinct role in the process. If we don't chew our food thoroughly, the stomach, having no teeth, cannot break the food into small enough pieces to allow digestive juices to penetrate thoroughly, and thus the food passes into the intestines with its central portions undigested. Some of this undigested food will ferment and putrefy, causing unpleasant-smelling intestinal gas and discomfort. The following homeopathic remedies will help relieve this condition:

♦ *Carbo veg.* The stomach fills up with gas no matter what you eat, resulting in repeated belching.

♦ *China.* The stomach feels full of gas that won't come up or go down. The person's midsection feels distended.

♦ *Lycopodium.* There is a feeling of fullness even before you finish eating or after a light meal. Belt feels too tight and there is rumbling gas and discharge.

COMMONSENSE MEASURES. Some of the foods that are commonly believed to cause gas are onions, cooked cabbage, raw apples, baked beans, and cucumbers, as well as sulfur-containing vegetables such as broccoli and Brussels sprouts. If any of these foods or others affect you this way, eliminate them from your diet.

No remedy, homeopathic or otherwise, should be taken regularly. If you are frequently troubled with stomach disorders, resolve to change your eating habits. Chew your food thoroughly. If you must eat on the run, choose easily digested foods such as cottage cheese or yogurt.

Sip cold drinks—don't gulp. The lining of the stomach is well supplied with blood vessels; a large swallow of cold liquid can chill the stomach and cause it to go into spasm. Another commonsense rule: Don't eat when you're not hungry or when angry or overtired. You may have noticed that a dog will refuse food when frightened or exhausted from a chase. When you're tired, your stomach shares your fatigue; relax for at least a quarter hour before eating. If your condition persists, it may be a sign of intestinal infection by microscopic parasites or an overgrowth of yeast or bacteria.

Antacids Can Be Anti-Health

If, now and then, you get off your feed, don't just automatically take an antacid. Antacids do neutralize stomach acid. But in moderate amounts, stomach acid is not a villain; it is necessary for digestion. During digestion, the complex structure of our foods is broken down into simpler substances that can be absorbed and used by the body. Stomach acid also kills or inactivates many germs that are in our food, so it is desirable to have *some* acid in the stomach.

Neutralizing acid also has an undesirable side effect: acid rebound, which means increased secretions of stomach acid that may persist long after the antacid action has ended. Consequently, the stomach's acid-producing cells must work harder to keep up the acid supply, and the result is excess acid in the stomach.

Use of antacids has been linked to brucellosis infection, also called undulant fever. The disease can be contracted from drinking unpasteurized infected milk. In a medical journal, Dr. Robert Steffen at the University of California warns travelers who may be eating unpasteurized dairy products against heavy use of antacids. Stomach acid is our natural defense against bacteria; low levels of stomach acid have been linked with traveler's diarrhea, as well as more serious conditions.

Like many other drugs, antacids can be potentially harmful. These products taken over a prolonged period can cause either constipation or diarrhea, accompanied by nausea. Sodium bicarbonate (baking soda), a major ingredient in antacids, may lead to stone formation in the urinary tract and may also contribute to recurrent bladder infections. Magnesium-containing antacids can produce severe reactions, including lethargy, coma, circulatory collapse, and respiratory paralysis. All antacids are dangerous for persons with high blood pressure, kidney disease, a history of urinary stones, or gastrointestinal bleeding.

CONSTIPATION

The body's way of disposing of waste material, like all its functions, is a marvel of design. After food has been digested, the colon muscles contract in a wavelike action called peristalsis, which carries its contents toward the rectum. On the way, the colon absorbs excess liquid from the mass of substance that comes from the small intestine. If you have not drunk enough fluids, the stool becomes dry and difficult to evacuate.

Constipation isn't a modern problem. The ancient Egyptians used the aloe vera plant as a purgative. North American Indians, when in need of a cathartic, brewed the leaves of the senna plant. Judging by the TV commercials, we are still making a cripple of our poor colon by taking laxatives. As stated in a British medical journal: "The long-term use of laxatives ultimately leads to increasing constipation and the resort to even stronger purges." Severe chronic constipation can cause the colon to distend and lose more and more of its ability to contract.

Constipation can arise from organic causes, such as the narrowing of the intestine and obstruction from growths, but the vast majority of cases of constipation stems from easily modified causes. These are a diet lacking in fiber or fluids; a lack of exercise; negative emotional states; ignoring the body's signals; and low levels of beneficial flora or high levels of harmful flora. In addition, many people who are regular at home become constipated on a trip, perhaps due to the extended inactivity, the change in food, or exposure to unfamiliar microbes. Don't forget to try hot lemon water half an hour before breakfast.

◆ *Nux vomica.* You may be able to overcome constipation by changing your habits, but if you need immediate relief from constipation, choose a homeopathic remedy that stimulates a return to normalcy. If you're hooked on laxatives, Nux vomica will help break the habit. Take a dose on retiring, or better still, a few hours before bedtime; Nux acts better when mind and body are at rest. A daily dose may be needed for several days, but do not substitute a Nux vomica habit for your former laxative habit. If you require repeated doses over

a long period of time, you are not curing constipation, merely relieving it, and you need constitutional treatment.

◆ *Sulfur*. If it's painful to pass stool owing to a rectal fissure (a crack
in the lining of the rectum), sulfur will help restore the rectum to normal condition. People whose symptoms fit this remedy may find they
have an ineffective urging to stool, with burning at the anus, alternating with diarrhea. Feces are hard, dark, and dry, and there is a tendency to hemorrhoids.

◆ *Alumina*. If you have difficulty passing stool, although your stool
is so soft and sticky that a bowel movement requires quantities of toi-
let paper, consider Alumina. Repeated ingestion of small amounts of
aluminum can cause this symptom, so if you're using aluminum cook
ware, this may be the cause of your GI problem.

◆ *Bryonia*. A large, hard, and dry stool, dark as if burnt, may indicate a need for bryonia. Stools are passed with great difficulty owing
to diminished intestinal secretions and poor muscle tone. The person
is irritable and ill tempered. Children who are constipated often need
bryonia.

◆ *Natrum mur*. A keynote of Natrum mur is a hard, crumbly stool
that causes rectal bleeding, smarting, and soreness. There is contraction of the anus, bleeding, and pain.

◆ *Graphites* (from the mineral graphite). When there is no urge to
defecate, consider graphites. You may go for days without a bowel
movement, and when it finally comes, it takes the form of round balls
stuck together with mucus and painful to pass. Other symptoms are
fissures, or cracks, in the rectal mucosa, and hemorrhoids that burn
and itch. The anus aches after passage of stool and becomes sore from
wiping. The person who needs graphites is often gloomy and obese.

◆ *Silica*. An indication for silica is a "bashful stool" that starts out
and goes back. This difficulty is due to an insufficient expulsive power
of the rectum and spasmodic condition of the sphincter muscle that
surrounds and contracts the anus. There is soreness about the anus
and often oozing of mucus.

Laxatives Make Your Body "Lax"

Above all, avoid the chronic use of laxatives. The two main types produce an artificial action to stimulate peristalsis. One type, the irritant,
does so by irritating nerve endings in the wall of the colon. The other,
the saline cathartic, withdraws moisture from the intestinal lining,

and the large volume of fluid then stimulates peristalsis. Mineral oil, which lubricates the stool, thus facilitating evacuation, has the disadvantage of causing embarrassing leakage; continued use also cuts down on the absorption of vitamins.

All laxatives, no matter how they work, are taking over a job that the body should be doing. Don't delude yourself that you're doing something natural by taking an herbal laxative. All laxatives, whether herbal or synthetic, cause a lazy bowel and are habit forming. If constipation has continued a month or more, see your physician.

DIARRHEA

Diarrhea, the frequent and excessive discharge of watery stools, is most often an acute condition caused by eating something unfamiliar to the body, perhaps food that is highly seasoned or spoiled. The experience is unpleasant, but the next time it occurs, consider what an efficient way this is for your body to get rid of an undesirable substance. The following homeopathic remedies will help relieve the miseries of diarrhea without interfering with its cleansing action.

♦ *Arsenicum.* The stomach feels heavy; patient experiences nausea and vomiting; there is a feeling of weakness. This comes from eating spoiled food or excessive amounts of any fruit, particularly melons. Arsenicum will not interfere with the discharge of toxic substances but will bring about order in the irritated intestinal tract so that diarrhea is no longer needed.

♦ *Cuprum arsenicosum* (arsenate of copper). Symptoms are burning, cramping, colicky pains in the lower bowels, accompanied by vomiting and diarrhea, with cramps and sensation of collapse.

This remedy proved helpful recently for a young man who rushed into the office without an appointment and begged to see me. "I'm running late," I explained, but after hearing his plight, I relented. He had eaten a Mexican dinner the night before and, since early morning, had suffered diarrhea and weakness. He had taken Arsenicum, which had not helped. In the last hours, he had developed severe cramping, which indicated Cuprum ars. After taking the remedy, he lay down on the examining table, and within fifteen minutes the cramping had subsided. At my suggestion, he rested another half an hour and then left, feeling recovered.

♦ *Gelsemium.* Diarrhea from anticipation of even an enjoyable social engagement, or from fear of an ordeal. Loose movements may also follow a fright.

◆ *Podophyllum* (May apple). Diarrhea—yellow watery stools that are squirted out—occurs in the early morning or after eating. The patient may have cramps that are relieved by warmth and bending double. After having a bowel movement, the patient experiences a weak feeling in the abdomen and feels "all in."

◆ *Sulfur*. Stools are changeable; sometimes they are yellow and watery, other times slimy, with undigested food. Urgent need to defecate drives the patient out of bed first thing in the morning.

◆ *Veratrum album*. Symptoms are similar to Arsenicum, but in addition, the patient experiences a cold sweat and feels on the verge of collapse.

COMMONSENSE MEASURES. Restore fluid balance in the body by taking plenty of liquids such as water, herb tea, and clear soups. Avoid milk. When diarrhea eases off, add tea and toast, and follow with a bland diet.

BEYOND FIRST AID. The chief danger in diarrhea is that the person may become dehydrated, or if the condition becomes chronic, that it can lead to anemia and malnutrition. Should diarrhea persist more than a few days, consult your doctor.

If your diarrhea is severe and you do not have the necessary homeopathic remedy, a kaolin-pectin mixture is a helpful temporary measure. This combination prevents absorption of bacterial toxins by forming a film on the intestinal wall and itself absorbing some of these toxins.

Paregoric, a form of opium, paralyzes the action of the intestinal waves (peristalsis) and thus opposes the body's efforts to expel the toxic matter. *Do not use.*

HEMORRHOIDS

A hemorrhoid is an enlarged or varicose vein in the region of the rectum, an extremely sensitive area. These veins can become so distended that they protrude, rupture, and bleed. According to some estimates, half of all adult Americans suffer from hemorrhoids.

Fortunately, homeopathy can help this common affliction and has been doing so for over 150 years. To relieve painful hemorrhoids, take a sitz bath—a warm tub bath—for ten to fifteen minutes, at least twice a day. Then apply Aesculus and Hamamelis ointment. Aesculus is homeopathically prepared from the horse chestnut (*Aesculus hippocastanum*) and Hamamelis virginic is made from the witch hazel scrub. This preparation relieves itching, pain, and inflammation, and aids healing.

♦ *Aesculus.* Internal homeopathic remedies (tablets or powders) when indicated will also relieve discomfort and promote healing. The person needing Aesculus experiences a burning sensation in the rectum, a dull ache in the lower back, and sharp shooting pains upward. The lining of the rectum seems swollen and obstructs the passageway. The hemorrhoids look like a bunch of purple grapes.

British homeopath Dr. A. C. Gordon Ross, in his book *Homeopathic Green Medicine*, writes: "This is one of the best homeopathic remedies for piles, and I have gained whole families as lifelong patients just because a few powders of Aesculus hippocastanum cured grandfather's piles in a week."

♦ *Arnica*, which heals damaged tissue, is used for hemorrhoids that develop after childbirth. During childbirth, the pressure of the baby's head may cause trauma to tissues. I've seen tremendously swollen, angry-looking hemorrhoids in a new mother respond to Arnica.

♦ *Collinsonia* (a stone root) is indicated when the symptoms have the sensation of sticks in the rectum; the patient is usually constipated.

♦ *Nitric acid* is indicated when hemorrhoids feel like needles or splinters in the rectum.

♦ *Nux vomica* is characterized by itching; the hemorrhoids are better from cool bathing.

♦ *Sulfur* is the remedy for itching and burning around the anus made worse by bathing, an unusual symptom for hemorrhoids. The condition is also worse from rubbing and standing, and worse at night.

COMMONSENSE MEASURES. Hemorrhoids are generally caused by straining during bowel movements, which pushes out the veins. If your hemorrhoids are due to constipation, see the list of causes mentioned in the section on constipation and work on correcting those aspects of your condition. If the constipation has lasted more than a month, see the help of your health care practitioner.

BEYOND FIRST AID. Severe pain may mean that you have a thrombosed hemorrhoid (blood clot). You will obtain instant relief from a minor surgical procedure in which the surgeon nicks the skin of the vein, releasing the clot. If there is rectal bleeding, check with your physician to make sure there is nothing more serious than hemorrhoids.

Homeopathy as practice by a physician is both a science and an art that demand a lifetime of study. But self-help homeopathy is an approach that can be mastered by most anyone concerned with better health. It requires learning the basic principles of homeopathy and familiarizing yourself with the remedies most often indicated for minor ailments and emergencies, such as those listed here. In most cases, it is a simple matter to limit the degree of discomfort and prevent future trouble.

JANE HEIMLICH is a respected medical journalist. She is also co-author of *Milk, the Deadly Poison* (Argus Publishing, 1998), *What Your Doctor Won't Tell You* (HarperCollins, 1990), and *Oxycal vs. Arthritis* (Ralph Tanner Associates, 1984).

MAESIMUND B. PANOS, M.D., until her retirement, was a practicing homeopathic physician in Washington, D.C., and later in Cincinnati, Ohio. She trained in medicine at the Ohio State College of Medicine, and was the also the wife a homeopathic physician and the daughter of a homeopath. Dr. Panos was a superb practitioner and many can attest to her compassionate and insightful prescribing.

42

Ayurvedic Medicine*

VASANT LAD, M.D.

❖

Ayurveda is considered by many scholars to be the oldest of the healing sciences. In Sanskrit, Ayurveda means the science of life. Ayurvedic knowledge originated in India more than 5,000 years ago. It stems from the ancient Vedic culture and was taught for thousands of years in an oral tradition from accomplished masters to their disciples. Some of this knowledge was set in print a few thousand years ago. The principles of many of the natural healing systems now familiar in the West have their roots in Ayurveda, including homeopathy and polarity therapy.

Ayurveda places great emphasis on prevention and encourages the maintenance of health through close attention to balance in one's life, right thinking, diet, lifestyle, and the use of herbs. Knowledge of Ayurveda enables one to understand how to create this balance of body, mind, and consciousness according to one's own individual constitution and how to make lifestyle changes to bring about and maintain this balance.

Just as everyone has unique fingerprints, according to Ayurveda, each person has a particular pattern of energy—an individual combination of physical, mental, and emotional characteristics—which comprises his or her own constitution. This constitution is determined at conception by a number of factors and remains the same throughout one's life.

LEARNING TO MAINTAIN INNER BALANCE

Many factors, both internal and external, act upon us to disturb our inner balance and are reflected as a change in one's constitution from

*From *A Brief Introduction to Ayurveda* by Dr. Vasant Lad (Albuquerque, NM: The Ayurvedic Press, 1996). Copyright © 1996 by Dr. Vasant Lad. Used by permission of the author.

the balanced state. Examples of these emotional and physical stresses include one's emotional state, diet and choices of foods, seasons and weather, physical trauma, work, and family relationships. Once these factors are understood, one can take appropriate actions to nullify or minimize their effects or eliminate the causes of imbalance and re-establish one's original constitution. Balance is the natural order; imbalance is disorder. Health is order; disease is disorder. Within the body there is a constant interaction between order and disorder. Once one understands the nature and structure of disorder, one can reestablish order.

THE THREE FUNDAMENTAL ENERGIES OF THE BODY

Ayurveda identifies three basic types of energy or functional principles that are present in everyone and everything. Since there are no single words in English that convey these concepts, we use the original Sanskrit words *vata, pitta,* and *kapha.* These principles can be related to the basic biology of the body.

Energy is required to create movement so that fluids and nutrients get to the cells, enabling the body to function. Energy is also required to metabolize the nutrients in the cells, and is called for to lubricate and maintain the structure of the cell. *Vata* is the energy of movement, *pitta* is the energy of digestion or metabolism, and *kapha,* the energy of lubrication and structure. All people have the qualities of *vata, pitta,* and *kapha,* but one energy is usually primary, one secondary, the third is usually the least prominent. The cause of disease in Ayurveda is viewed as the lack of proper cellular function because of an excess or deficiency of *vata, pitta,* or *kapha.* In addition, disease can be caused by the presence of toxins.

BALANCING ENERGY

In Ayurveda, body, mind, and consciousness work together in maintaining balance. They are simply viewed as different facets of one's being. To learn how to balance the body, mind, and consciousness requires an understanding of how *vata, pitta,* and *kapha* work together. According to Ayurvedic philosophy, the entire cosmos is an interplay of the energies of the five great elements—Space, Air, Fire, Water, and Earth. *Vata, pitta*, and *kapha* are combinations and permutations of these five elements that manifest as patterns present in all creation. In the physical body, *vata* is the subtle energy of movement, *pitta* the energy of digestion and metabolism, and *kapha* the energy that forms the body's structure.

♦ *Vata is the energy associated with movement,* composed of Space and Air. It governs breathing, blinking, muscle and tissue movement, pulsation of the heart, and all movements in the cytoplasm and cell membranes. In balance, vata promotes creativity and flexibility. Out of balance, vata produces fear and anxiety.

♦ *Pitta expresses as the body's metabolic system,* made up of Fire and Water. It governs digestion, absorption, assimilation, nutrition, metabolism, and body temperature. In balance, *pitta* promotes understanding and intelligence. Out of balance, *pitta* arouses anger, hatred, and jealousy.

♦ *Kapha is the energy that forms the body's structure*—bones, muscles, tendons—and provides the "glue" that holds the cells together, metaphorically formed from Earth and Water. Kapha supplies the water for all bodily parts and systems. It lubricates joints, moisturizes the skin, and maintains immunity. In balance, kapha is expressed as love, calmness, and forgiveness. Out of balance, it leads to attachment, greed, and envy.

OUR AREAS OF INFLUENCE: LIFESTYLE AND DIET

Life presents us with many challenges and opportunities. Although there is much over which we have little control, we do have the power to decide about some things, such as diet and lifestyle. To maintain balance and health, it is important to pay attention to these decisions. Diet and lifestyle appropriate to one's individual constitution strengthen the body, mind, and consciousness.

AYURVEDA AS PREVENTIVE MEDICINE

The basic difference between Ayurveda and Western allopathic medicine is important to understand. Western allopathic medicine currently tends to focus on symptomatology and disease, and primarily uses drugs and surgery to rid the body of pathogens or diseased tissue. Many lives have been saved by this approach. In fact, surgery is also encompassed by Ayurveda. However, drugs, because of their toxicity, often weaken the body. Ayurveda does not focus on disease. Rather, Ayurveda maintains that all life must be supported by energy in balance. When there is minimal stress and the flow of energy within a person is balanced, the body's natural defense systems will be strong and can more easily defend against disease.

AYURVEDA AS A COMPLEMENTARY SYSTEM OF HEALING

It must be emphasized that Ayurveda is not a substitute for Western allopathic medicine. There are many instances when the disease process and acute conditions can best be treated with drugs or surgery. Ayurveda can be used in conjunction with Western medicine to make a person stronger and less likely to be afflicted with disease or to rebuild the body after being treated with drugs or surgery.

We all have times when we don't feel well and recognize that we're out of balance. Sometimes we go to the doctor only to be told there is nothing wrong. What is actually occurring is that this imbalance has not yet become recognizable as a disease. Yet it is serious enough to make us notice our discomfort. We may start to wonder if it is not just our imagination. We may also begin to consider alternative measures and actively seek to create balance in our body, mind, and consciousness.

BASIC PRACTICES OF AYURVEDIC MEDICINE

Ayurveda encompasses various techniques for assessing health. The practitioner carefully evaluates key signs and symptoms of illness, especially in relation to the origin and cause of an imbalance. He or she also considers the patient's suitability for various treatments. The practitioner arrives at diagnosis through both direct questioning, observation, and a physical exam, as well as inference. Basic techniques employed during an assessment include taking the pulse; observing the tongue, eyes, and physical form; and listening to the tone of the voice.

AYURVEDIC TREATMENT

Palliative and cleansing measures, if appropriate, can be used to help eliminate an imbalance along with suggestions for eliminating or managing the causes of the imbalance. Recommendations may include the implementation of lifestyle changes; starting and maintaining a suggested diet; and the use of herbs. In some cases, participating in a cleansing program, called panchakarma, is suggested to help rid the body of accumulated toxins to gain more benefit from other aspects of the treatment.

In summary, Ayurveda addresses all aspects of life—the body, mind, and spirit. It recognizes that each of us is unique, each responds differently to the many aspects of life, each possesses different strengths and weakness. Through insight, understanding, and experience, Ayurveda presents a vast wealth of information on the relationships between causes and their effects, both immediate and subtle, for each unique individual.

BASIC PRINCIPLES OF AYURVEDA

♦ *Everything in your life has an impact on your well-being.* From that point of view, problems with digestion are not simply a matter of digestion; other areas in your life are reflected in the thoroughness of digestion. Digestion is also influenced by the basic energy that is dominant in your particular personality (the doshas).

♦ *The choice of foods and food combinations is important.* Diet is an important area in the Ayurvedic system because it is relatively easy to change. There are simple things that people can do to enhance their digestion, such as changing their diet and practicing proper food combining. This change alone can make remarkable differences. Most of us never think about food combining, its impact on digestion, or even the impact of indigestion on the whole system. If the food you eat causes more toxins than your body can eliminate, then naturally you'll have problems.

Proper food combining and the resulting digestion influence the quality of your blood. The quality of the blood can have a big impact on your physical and emotional balance. Eating foods that your body can thoroughly digest and find calming and that are nourishing to your individual constitution will help you to be better able to cope in your day-to-day environment. The ultimate goal of better digestion is to avoid the buildup of toxins in the body.

♦ *Hatha yoga is viewed as a way to strengthen your body*, make it more flexible, and release tensions, so you can more fully enjoy your life. A lot of problems can be related to a lack of flexibility in the body. If we have strength and flexibility, then we can live better. Within hatha yoga, the system of the three energies can also be related to the yoga postures, using the postures to calm or stimulate. In this way, the postures become a means of restoring balance to the body.

◆ *Cleansing the body can release toxins and improve circulation.* One of the goals of the Ayurvedic physician is to determine where you're out of balance. For many, a five-day cleansing cycle is quite beneficial, including daily massage to move the energies and toxins out of areas of stagnation in the body, back into the gastrointestinal tract where they can be eliminated. Cleansing the GI tract is encouraged during this process through a number of specific techniques. In Ayurveda, cleansing is a discipline unto itself, the classic practice of Panchakarma. We have seen that it can produce remarkable results.

However, there are cases in which a person may not be strong enough for this cleansing or situations in which the detoxification process may actually worsen their condition. These conditions include pregnancy, menses, lactation, hypertension, lymphosarcoma, cancer of the lungs or testicles, melanoma, congestive heart failure, angina pectoris, HIV or AIDS, dehydration, obesity, or any active infectious disease. Check with your practitioner before embarking upon any cleansing program.

◆ *Cleansing the mind is an essential element in maintaining balance.* Many of the basic tenets of alternative health grow out of Ayurvedic philosophies, including respect for the importance of meditation and contemplation. For example, there is value in the practice of reviewing your day. All these habits help us mentally and emotionally process the things we haven't digested.

Mental and emotional digestion is as important as physical digestion. It also has an impact on the body because it is possible to accumulate psychological toxins. For example, the remnants of childhood psychological trauma can act as a form of mental toxin. Therefore, it is important to have a process built into our life for reflectiveness. It is essential to have a mechanism for processing and clearing stressful or traumatic experiences. This is a coping skill that can be extremely valuable in the midst of our busy lives.

◆ *Meditation and visualizations also have beneficial effects on the body.* They can be used to help people uncover areas that are unexamined and process them.

By clearing the mind and body, with new coping skills and new self-knowledge, you are provided with the tools to digest new experiences as they come along, as they occur, rather than later. Ayurveda provides the foundation for maintaining physical, mental, and spiritual balance.

DR. VASANT LAD, a native of India, has been a practitioner and professor of Ayurvedic medicine for more than twenty-five years. He attended Tilak Ayurvedic Medical College in Pune, India, where he later taught and was the residential medical officer at the college hospital. For the past eighteen years, he has served as director of a full-time program of study at the Ayurvedic Institute in Albuquerque, New Mexico. Dr. Lad has lectured extensively throughout the U.S. and has written numerous books and articles on Ayurveda. Dr. Lad's classic books are *Ayurveda: The Science of Self-Healing* (1984) and *The Yoga of Herbs* (1986). He is also the author of *Ayurvedic Cooking for Self-Healing* (2nd ed., 1997) and *Secrets of the Pulse* (1997). His most recent book is *The Complete Book of Ayurvedic Home Remedies*, published by Harmony Books (1998).

The Ayurvedic Institute in Albuquerque was founded by Dr. Lad in 1984 to promote the traditional knowledge of Ayurveda and offers an eight-month studies program, additional advanced study, weekend seminars and intensives, yoga courses, a correspondence course, the traditional cleansing program, and sales of Ayurvedic products and herbs. The Institute can be reached at PO Box 23445, Albuquerque, NM 87192, by phone at 505-291-9698, and on the Web at www.ayurveda.com.

43

Gentle Exercise

ROGER JAHNKE, O.M.D.

❖

One of the most profound pathways to healing or improved health is appropriate exercise. In the ancient cultures, exercise methods such as yoga, Qigong, and tai chi were developed to mobilize healing resources. Qigong from China has long been respected as one of the premier approaches to healing in the world. Yoga from India has also been used as a vehicle for healing for thousands of years. Although we typically think of exercise as vigorous, for building strength, for toning, or for losing weight, for healing, exercise must be modified so that it is more gentle, less intense. Done correctly, gentle exercise produces and circulates powerful physiological resources for healing.

The lessons that we have learned from ancient Oriental fitness traditions suggest that by slowing and deepening the breath, purposefully and gently moving the body, and focusing the mind, a tremendous health benefit can be gained. Mild fitness practices are at least as valuable as vigorous fitness practices, according to *The Surgeon General's Report on Exercise and Fitness* in 1996. In fact, they may be even better because there's lesser risk of injury and less need for special equipment. Vigorous exertion spends much of the healing energy that is created by the exercise. Gentle practices such as yoga and Qigong conserve energy. Whenever healing is the goal, energy conservation becomes a major focus.

Research shows that when you're unwell, it's important *not* to exercise vigorously. Free radicals can be produced as a natural by-product of exercise; they're also produced through digestion and many other basic processes. When we're well, we have the necessary "cushioning" in the cells to withstand potential damage from free radicals. However, in someone who is less well, the body may not be able to clear the free radicals as quickly as necessary, putting them at risk for oxidative stress, which can initiate damage to cells and tissues and even cause disease.

Yoga, Qigong, and strength training can be done anytime, anywhere. And each of these practices can be introduced very gradually, paced to your situation. Yoga and Qigong require no equipment of any kind. Strength training can be done with the use of inexpensive handheld free weights.

We include exercising with weights in this approach because of the spectacular results seen in 80- and 90-year-old people with chronic illness, working with researchers from Tufts University. We felt that if they can do it, you and your doctor might take a serious look at this breakthrough practice.

BEFORE YOU GET STARTED, CHECK WITH YOUR DOCTOR

If you have chronic illness or if you're over 40, be sure to get a checkup and clearance from a doctor who understands the benefits of exercise, before you begin a gentle exercise program. Even then, the truth is that nobody is ever going to know as much about your strengths and limitations as you do. So when you exercise, be mindful and monitor yourself carefully. Any form of pain is an important message from your body that something may not be right, like the red warning light on your dashboard. With all forms of gentle exercise, you must pay attention to the messages from your body and not push yourself. Stay in the zone of comfort. In addition, use the messages you get from your body to continually analyze your health and to help you create a personal strategy to solve your health challenges.

ALMOST ANY EXERCISE CAN BE GENTLE EXERCISE

The whole process that we're describing here typically involves understanding a more gentle approach to exercise. Almost any form of exercise can be modified to become gentle exercise. Vigorous aerobics become mindful low-impact aerobics. Running becomes purposeful walking.

Techniques such as yoga, Qigong, and tai chi are very gentle practices, yet highly effective. They typically involve three areas of focus:

♦ *Moving the body gently,* honoring the limits of a person's vital energy, structure, and physical capacity, and monitoring these limits very carefully.

♦ *Enhancing the breath* and focusing on it, so that it becomes deep and full, slow and relaxed, compared to the less relaxed, more urgent breathing of more aggressive exercise.

♦ *Encouraging the mind* and thought patterns toward a state of deep relaxation or meditation as you perform the movements.

With this approach, even modified aerobics, swimming, and walking can become a kind of yoga or Qigong. At that point, Western exercise and ancient practice merge.

Some people approach exercise as simply a function of the body and don't really factor in the role of the mind. Often we see people exercising on the Stairmaster while reading the paper or riding an Exercyle while watching television. We encourage a different approach. Mindfulness can add a meaningful dimension to exercise. With relaxation and mindfulness, exercise accelerates the mind/body interactions. Any increase in your awareness of your body and your health state can be brought to bear on the healing process in different ways—in reporting to your doctor or changing to more healthful behaviors. Mindfulness is an essential component of both yoga and Qigong. The importance of mindfulness is now acknowledged throughout the world of sports, from major-league football and basketball teams who use meditation to tennis and golf professionals who practice the Zen of the game and Olympic athletes who use visualization.

It is not unusual for people to believe that more aggressive exercise equals more gain—"no pain, no gain." And yet many are unable to do vigorous exercise due to health limitations. The primary reason for modifying aggressive exercise to gentle exercise is this: when you exercise, the body produces a powerful fuel, a healing resource. When you do vigorous exercise, you produce that fuel, that vital resource, but because of the vigorous nature of the exercise, most of that fuel is burned and expended by the muscles. When gentle exercise practices are done, you still produce that fuel, but instead of spending it on the exertion of exercise itself, your body uses this fuel as a healing resource, literally an inner medicine.

So, no matter what kind of exercise you have typically been doing or that you feel you should be doing, consider lightening the exertion a little and slowing the process down. Next, engage the breath in a meaningful sort of way, in a kind of rhythmic, deep, slow, relaxed fashion. Finally, adjust the mind toward a deep state of relaxation. By clearing the mind and refusing to engage in list-making and worry, you curtail the adrenaline-based aspect of your nervous system activity. This activates a whole array of inner healing factors.

THE BENEFITS OF GENTLE EXERCISE

When you do a gentle sort of exercise, natural physiological mechanisms are triggered. If someone loses their health, some of these mechanisms may become deficient, causing pain and other symptoms. The body's inherent system of self-healing, self-regulation, and self-repair can be stimulated and maximized, using simple and gentle exercise practices.

Oxygen

Perhaps the most important of the body's natural mechanisms of self-repair is the delivery of oxygen. Oxygen is one of the most vital internal healing resources there is. Many people who are suffering from chronic diseases are actually suffering from a kind of oxygen deficiency. There are several reasons why these oxygen deficiencies occur. The lack of activity decreases the circulation of oxygen-bearing blood cells. Or in other cases oxygen deficiency has metabolic causes, due to malfunction of the organs. But when you move gently, deepening the breath and relaxing the mind, oxygen is more effectively delivered to your entire system.

Vigorous and aggressive exercise is typically associated with the delivery of oxygen throughout the body—hence the term *aerobics,* meaning "with oxygen." But it is true that when the person does gentle exercise, it can also be aerobic. We are used to thinking that if we're not vigorously jumping around or using maximal exertion, we're not getting oxygen. That, frankly, is not true. When you go into this deep state of relaxation, along with the movement, the body turns on the mechanisms that deliver oxygen into the tissues. Instead of using all the oxygen to operate vigorously active muscles, that oxygen remains within the system to circulate as a healing resource. In addition, when you are relaxed, the blood vessels expand, carrying more oxygen deeper into the organs and glands.

Cleansing the Cells and Tissues

The second healing benefit of gentle exercise is its positive effect on the lymph system. When you do the deep-breathing practice in combination with gentle motion, it very effectively pumps the lymph. The lymph has two big jobs in the human body. First, it delivers the immune cells to their sites of activity. Second, it eliminates toxins from our system—minimizing pathogens, by-products of metabolism, and any kind of pollution that's gotten into the interior of the system. So when you take that deep breath and when you move the body around gently, you are pumping the lymph, the fluid that eliminates waste products and activates immunity.

Deepening the breath is the key to stimulating the lymph system. The second key activating the lymph is movement—contracting and releasing your muscles. The movement doesn't have to be vigorous. A big part of why gentle exercise is so spectacularly effective is that it effectively turns on the lymph system.

Shifting Out of the Adrenaline Mode

This is important, because the presence of high levels of adrenaline in the human body literally cancels the activity of the immune cells. When you leave the adrenaline bases and migrate to the choline bases, your body has shifted into the relaxation response and the rest-and-repair side of the autonomic function. In this mode, your body can produce the neurotransmitters that actually turn on the immune cells. The addition of relaxation to exercise has an positive impact on the effectiveness of the immune cells.

WALKING

Walking is one of the most overlooked forms of exercise because people think, "I walk all the time, what's so special about that?" In the 1996 surgeon general's report, walking was considered a preferred form of moderate exercise. Walking is a perfect exercise for those who are not well enough to pursue more vigorous exercise and perfect for those who have health challenges but are not drawn to more unusual forms of exercise like tai chi, Qigong, or yoga.

However, we want to point out that no form of exercise will suit everyone. Even something as universal as walking may not be a match for you in the present. If that's true, it may be a program that you can move into as your health improves. For those readers who can't use walking or who may be using a wheelchair, we would like to direct you to modified Qigong, yoga practices, or other forms of gentle exercise that can be done at home.

Those who can use walking for exercise find that it increases circulation and oxygen levels. If the walker deepens the breath, even while walking slowly, that provides an acceleration of the lymph, which is the detoxification mechanism of the system. It is also possible to modify walking so that it is coupled with deep relaxation or meditation, which activates the healing capacity of the nervous system.

Getting Started

You can walk at a variety of paces. There's slow, purposeful walking, which is a little bit more like Qigong and yoga, and brisk walking that's more like an aerobic activity. There's also race walking, which provides a strong cardiovascular stimulus. For someone who is suffering from a chronic type of disorder, remember that slow, purposeful walking still gives you all the benefits of oxygen, circulation, and stimulation, yet the beneficial by-products of the practice, that fuel or healing resource that we have discussed, are not used up through exertion in the process.

◆ *Begin slowly and build up.* *The 90-Day Fitness Program* by Mark Fenton offers an excellent approach to getting started. Walk for five minutes on the first day and then add just a minute a day. If you do that, in ten days you'll be walking for fifteen minutes, and in a month you'll be walking more than half an hour. By the end of the second month, if you wish, you could be walking an hour a day.

◆ *Build walking into your life.* Another approach to walking is to build it into your life and your routine, by making it part of the things you must do. To the degree possible, group your errands in one location, park your car, and walk. When you're going to an appointment, if you can leave a little early, park a few blocks away (you may have to anyway!) and walk. Take the stairs at work or anywhere you happen to be.

◆ *Link walking to something you enjoy doing.* If you like a spontaneous approach to life, just remember to include a good walk in your activities each day, or several short walks. If weather inspires you, take joyful walks on sunny days, romantic walks in the rain, or brisk walks in the wind. Bird watchers walk, shoppers walk, lovers walk.

◆ *Walk with a friend.* This can be one of the best ways to walk and enjoy it. You may have a buddy that you walk with on a regular basis, or friends with whom you go for long walks on the weekends, or whenever you can. Enjoy!

◆ *Track your progress.* If you value an organized way of doing things, you may want to have a routine that's predictable, and you may find it satisfying to keep a log or a journal. If your doctor says you must walk, get a pedometer so you'll know how far you're actually walking and you can celebrate your goals as you reach them.

Resources

BOOKS

Fenton, Mark. *The 90-Day Fitness Program.* Perigee, 1995. An unassuming book with a great step-by-step method (no pun intended) and a journal built in.

Iknoian, Therese. *Fitness Walking.* Human Kinetics, 1995.

Malkin, Mort. *Aerobic Walking, the Weight-Loss Exercise.* Wiley, 1995. A more vigorous approach to walking.

MAGAZINES

Walking—800-829-5585

Prevention—800-763-2531

QIGONG

Qigong (pronounced *chee-gung*) is the umbrella of all the traditions of personal improvement and mind-body fitness from the ancient Chi-

---

Just Walking around

❖

My wife, Rebecca (who also happens to be my best friend), and I have a favorite way of spending free time we call "just walking around." I may ask her on Thursday if she wants to plan something for Saturday, and she may say, "Why don't we just walk around?" That means no plan. It means we'll go for a walk and see where we end up. We could end up window shopping or at the movies, hiking on the beach, or eating at a newfound or old favorite restaurant. So just walking around is a really fantastic combination of getting good (moderate) exercise, the fun of not knowing where you're going but knowing you will be with someone you like, or just being out on your own on a surprise voyage of discovery.

nese culture. What we know about these traditions dates back to the beginning of writing in China, around 500 B.C. At that time, existing documents indicate quite clearly that the Chinese people had already been using these practices for many hundreds of years.

The fact that Qigong and tai chi (a form of Qigong) have stood the test of time demonstrates their effectiveness. These gentle fitness practices have been carefully refined over several thousand years. The practice involves the gentle movement of the body, with mindful adjustment of the posture. A primary focus is on the breath, usually to deepen and relax the breathing. At the same time, as an essential part of the practice, the mind is encouraged to move toward a state of meditation, relaxing and clearing it of details or worries.

The practice can be done literally thousands of ways. By most estimates, there are somewhere between 3,000 and 5,000 variations of Qigong. The various kinds of practice can be categorized by the degree of activity, from the completely quiescent (still practice, standing, sitting or lying down) to vigorously dynamic (slow, full-body movement or fast as in kung fu). Non-moving practices are called Qing Gong, and movement practices, Dong Gong.

The initial practice, which is done while completely still, can be lying down or sitting. To that practice, very gentle and small movements of hands, feet, and shoulders can be added. Next, as vitality improves, the practice can be done while sitting. Later, as strength is building, walking forms of Qigong can be added, logically called Walking Qigong. Tai chi is, in fact, a beautiful form of Walking Qigong. The most renowned form of Walking Qigong is called Guo Lin, named after a woman in China who had a very serious form of cancer and recovered using Qigong as a complement to her medical treatment.

What to Do When We Can't Formally Exercise

Lying-down Qigong can be very useful because when we're really unwell, we spend a good deal of time lying down. So we may think, "Well, I can't exercise—I'm in bed lying down." The Chinese would say, "No, not so, you can exercise while you're lying down." "But," you might respond, "I'm not able to move." The Chinese would answer, "External movement is the least important part of the healing exercise. Internal activity is the essence of healing exercise practice."

Guo Lin's form is one of the most common Qigong forms that is seen in the parks of China, early in the morning.

Other forms of Walking Qigong include a graceful, philosophical form associated with Taoism called the Wild Goose. Some of the more dynamic forms are called by poetic names: the Crane, Five Elements, Tendon Changing, Vitality, Intelligence. Although some forms of Qigong are highly complex and difficult to learn; others are extremely simple. For example, tai chi has 108 movements, which might take anywhere from six months to a year to learn. Whereas there are forms of Qigong that are very beneficial and can be learned in a few minutes. All forms of Qigong, from the simple to the most complex, are improved with regular practice over time.

The body of research from China on Qigong is immense; however, Chinese research techniques have not been as rigorous as those in the United States. The National Institutes of Health (NIH) has funded a number of studies on Qigong and tai chi. There have been numerous international scientific congresses on Qigong in China, Japan, Europe, and the United States. The consensus is that Qigong triggers physiological mechanisms with a positive effect on inner healing including increased oxygen delivery, enhanced immune function and elimination of waste, and improved brain chemistry.

Getting Started

If you find this practice intriguing, you'll want to get a book or a video or both. If the opportunity presents itself, take a class or seek out a private teacher. Simple Qigong practices can be learned and practiced at home. Many hospitals have begun to offer Qigong or modified tai chi as a part of their mind-body programming. The YMCA in many communities offers classes. In a growing number of communities it is possible to link up with a practice group either in the park or at the local recreation center. Some of these are offered without charge.

Books and Videos

BOOKS

Jahnke, Roger. *The Healer Within*. HarperSanFrancisco, 1997.

Cohen, Ken. *The Way of Qigong*. Ballantine Books, 1997.

MacRitchie, James. *Chi Kung: Cultivating Personal Energy*. Element Books, 1997.

VIDEO

Jahnke, Roger. *Awakening the Medicine Within.* Health Action, 1995; 800-824-4325.

YOGA

Yoga is another subtle practice which originated in India and developed as one of the practices associated with spiritual growth in the philosophy of Vedanta. Hatha yoga is one of the Eight Limbs of Yoga, which also includes breathing practices (pranayama), meditation, and activities of service (karma yoga). Patanjali's Yoga Sutras, written around 200 or 300 B.C., described yoga, so we know it had been codified by that time. Hatha yoga combines postures, movement, breath regulation, and meditation.

The essence of hatha yoga is the postures, or asanas, that poetically imitate the movements of animals and bear their names (the Cobra, the Lion, the Fish). Each posture is designed to stretch the muscles, flex the joints, and stimulate the internal organs and glands in a different part of the body. When the posture is performed, the body is gradually moved into position through a process of gentle stretching. The position is held without moving, usually for less than a minute, while breathing slowly and deeply, and then the body is returned to a position of rest, lying outstretched or standing quietly.

The postures are designed to strengthen, stretch, and tone muscles and ligaments. In modern exercise terms, yoga has come to mean the same thing as stretching; however, because of the links to the breath and mind, yoga is much more than just stretching. The practices also encourage blood circulation while stimulating the secretions of the glands, and encourage the optimal function of the internal organs. For example, the shoulder stand is thought to stimulate the thyroid gland through the gentle pressure of the chin on the throat area. The forward and the backward bend (the Fish) are designed to stretch, align, and strengthen the spinal column and surrounding muscles. A very thorough session of yoga postures can leave one with the sense of relaxation comparable to a good massage.

Getting Started

Yoga can be done with simply the guidance of a well-written book, as long as care is taken not to move too fast, stretch too far, or force the body. There are also good videos and sometimes good TV yoga classes. A live class can also be very encouraging, as long as the teacher doesn't move too fast or too aggressively. Be wary of teachers who say things like "No gain without pain." The idea is to grow into the postures and become more flexible day by day, comparable to adding a minute a day to your walking routine.

Resources

VIDEO AND AUDIOTAPES

Video: Honig, Meenakshi. *Yoga Feels Good*, Wellbeing International; 800-For-Yoga. There appear to be a wealth of yoga tapes on the market.

Audio: Mindfulness Meditation, University of Massachusetts, in conjunction with Jon Kabat-Zinn offers a set of audiotapes with hatha yoga exercises (Series 1 Tapes). The tapes can be ordered from Stress Reduction Tapes, P.O. Box 547, Lexington, MA 02420 or by checking their website at www.mindfulnesstapes.com

BOOKS

Christensen, Alice. *The American Yoga Association Beginner's Manual*. Fireside, 1997. Readers say if you want to start doing yoga, this is the book to buy.

Mehta, Silva, and Shyarn Meta. *Yoga the Iyengar Way*. Knopf, 1990.

Schiffmann, Eric. *Yoga: The Spirit and Practice of Moving Into Stillness*. Pocket Sales, 1996.

Birch, Beryl Bender. *Power Yoga: The Total Strength and Flexibility Workout*. Fireside, 1995. This is the first book about astanga yoga, a vigorous form of hatha yoga designed to build strength and stamina, used by the U.S. cycling team and the New York Road Runners.

ORGANIZATIONS

Integral Yoga, Swami Satchidananda Ashram, Buckingham, Virginia; 800-858-9642

Kripalu Retreat Center, Lenox, Massachusetts; 413-448-3224

Sivananda Yoga Society, world headquarters in Canada; 819-322-3226 or by e-mail at hq@sivananda.org

LOW-IMPACT WEIGHT TRAINING

Strength training has been found to produce spectacular benefits and can be used by people with a wide variety of needs. The practice generally involves basic exercises with or without small handheld weights, that can involve either mild or intense exertion. The program was developed by researchers from the Tufts University working with people in their eighties and nineties. The original participants were nursing home residents with severe chronic illness who were able to double their strength in just three months working with the weights! This approach to weight training has now been in development for more than fifteen years and continues to gain enthusiastic reviews. Strength training has been found to:

♦ Halt bone loss and even restore bone
♦ Improve balance
♦ Help prevent bone fractures from osteoporosis
♦ Energize
♦ Trim the body and tighten muscles
♦ Help control weight
♦ Improve flexibility
♦ Revitalize

In our culture, it is typical to think of weight training as being something that requires going to the gym and having a lot of special equipment. Clearly this practice is not about buffing up and getting big muscles. In the context of what we're discussing here, it's about using weight training with the goal of mobilizing inner resources. The extent to which you get the increase of muscle mass or muscle strength is really secondary. The most essential improvements result from doing the practices and increasing benefits for the metabolic system. These subtle but important gains include retaining calcium in the bones, stimulating the mobilization of oxygen throughout the blood and the tissues, and building stamina. Weight training also enhances your body's ability to burn fat.

Getting Started

Once you have your doctor's clearance, you may want to gradually work into a weight training program. Really take your time in building up the number of repetitions you do and in building up the amount of weight you're using. The weights used in this program include handheld heavy hands, small free weights, or weights you can strap on to your wrists and your ankles to give you a little resistance.

Some people are going to enjoy having an exercise routine or going to the gym. It can also be helpful to keep a log and track your progress. When you're getting started at the gym, you can use their weight training machines without any weight! This still provides the benefits of range of motion plus the resistance of the weight of the device itself, stimulating your circulation, providing mild stretching, and mildly accelerating your metabolism.

Strengthening the lower back and the abdominals could be one of the most important by-products of gentle exercise, because people with chronic inflammation sometimes have a loss of tone as a result of their illness. Bracing against low-grade pain could alter posture or muscle tone. When tone is lacking, it's especially important to begin moderately, to protect muscle and nerve tissue, and avoid new problems. Some gastroenterologists suggest that improving GI tone can make a significant difference in conditions such as motility problems. But it's still best to work all parts of the body, rather than just working the abdominals or the biceps.

If you find yourself craving a less structured approach to life, saying to yourself, "Why should I go to the club? I'm going to rake my backyard," it's helpful to know that both approaches are just fine. What the surgeon general reported in 1996 was that washing your car, weeding your garden, and raking your lawn are all actually mild forms of exercise that generate fitness. Enjoy!

Resources

BOOKS

Nelson, Miriam. *Strong Women Stay Young*. Bantam Books, 1997. This excellent book describes the research by Tufts University, which has revealed that people of any age and condition can use strength training, like it, and definitely benefit from it.

EQUIPMENT

Keiser Sports Health Equipment, 411 South West Avenue. Fresno, CA 93706-9952; 800-888-7009

All Pro Exercise Products, Inc., 135 Hazelwood Drive, Jericho, NY 11753; 800-735-9287

ALEXANDER TECHNIQUE

The Alexander technique is a learning process that teaches individuals to adjust the body position to maximize natural inner resources. The process was discovered when the originator, Mathias Alexander, found that by adjusting the area between the skull and the upper back, he was able to heal a chronic voice condition. Since then, millions of people with a wide variety of diagnoses have found that using this method has helped to cure their musculoskeletal problems, as well as more organ-based diseases.

When you sit or stand up straight, arrange your head so that it is atop the spine, relax the shoulders, and then breath deep, you have taken one early step in the implementing the Alexander technique. To begin working with this self-care method, look for classes at your community recreation center, local hospital, or through your health plan.

Resources

Brennan, Richard. *The Alexander Technique Manual*. Tuttle Publications, 1996.

Gelb, Michael, and Laura Huxley. *Body Learning: An Introduction to the Alexander Technique*. Henry Holt, 1996.

FELDENKRAIS METHOD

It has been discovered that many of our health challenges are aggravated or even caused by long term habits of body movement or posture. When these habits and patterns are resolved so that the body functions in the way it was originally designed to function, then aches, pains, and the symptoms of disease can be eased and even healed. The Feldenkrais method is one of the most highly regarded methods for resolving these dysfunctions (usually called neuromuscular patterns).

This health improvement process can involve individual lessons (which looks a little like a body work session) or a group instruction (which looks a little like a very gentle yoga class). The goal in both cases is to help the individual to heal old patterns of movement and posture and learn to use the body in ways that resolve pain and heal organ dysfunction.

Resources

Hanna, Thomas. *Somatics: Reawakening the Mind's Control of Movement, Flexibility, and Health*. Perseus Press, 1998.

Shafarman, Steven. *Awareness Heals: The Feldenkrais Method.* Perseus
   Press, 1997.

ISOMETRICS

Isometrics involves exercising muscles by pushing against resistance.
The advantage to isometrics is that they can be done anytime, anywhere, without special equipment, by most anyone. You'll notice that
if you press your left hand down with your right hand, pretty much
the same kind of effort is made as if you were lifting a weight with
your left hand. So one way to exercise is to use pressure from the hand
on different body parts to create the weight and resistance.

   You can do isometrics lying in bed. For example, to do bicep curls,
just press your left hand against your right hand and lift the right
hand toward your chin. Then if you want to work the triceps, take the
right hand and then press it into the left hand, and resist with the left
hand so that way you're working the right tricep. Lift your knee
toward your head while pushing downward with your hands to
strengthen the thigh.

   This form of exercise can be applied to any part of the body. It is a
very simple way to mobilize and circulate inner healing resources.

PILATES

Body Control, developed by Joseph Pilates, is the fastest-growing exercise in the world. Pilates was a frail, sickly child who became obsessed

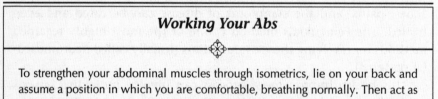

Working Your Abs

To strengthen your abdominal muscles through isometrics, lie on your back and
assume a position in which you are comfortable, breathing normally. Then act as
if you are blowing out a candle. As you do that, contract your stomach muscles,
so your belly button is moved toward your backbone. Be careful not to contract
the muscles you would normally use in doing a sit-up. Simply lie still, contracting
the inner abdominal muscles. *Hold them contracted and breathe.* The action of
the breath stretching against the muscles is what creates the exercise. Breathe in
that way, pulling your navel toward your backbone, and breathing against that
tension of the muscle. This exercise tends to strengthen the inner two layers of
muscles in the abdomen. It's also very relaxing!

—*Jerry Stine*

with physical fitness and in the process of healing himself, created an eight-point exercise program. The basic Body Control program can be done at home without special equipment. Stretching exercises, however, involve the use of specialized equipment that can be purchased or is available through classes and trainers. This technique is used by the New York City Ballet and the Cincinnati Bengals.

Resources

Pilates equipment for use in your home can be ordered through QVC Home Shopping Channel. Phone orders at 800-345-1515.

BOOKS

Robinson, Lynn, Joseph Pilates, and Gordon Thomson. *Body Control: Using Techniques Developed by Joseph H. Pilates*. Trans-Atlantic Publishing, 1988. Readers indicate this book is most ideal for people new to Pilates.

ROGER JAHNKE, O.M.D., is the author of *The Healer Within,* a practical guide to the Chinese self-healing arts known as Qigong, which include gentle exercise, breath practice, massage, and meditation. He is an internationally respected teacher and lecturer on Chinese medicine, Qigong, and tai chi; senior faculty member at the College of Traditional Chinese Medicine in Santa Barbara; and a founding board member of the National Qigong Association. He has been in the clinical practice of traditional Chinese medicine for more than twenty years. He is a consultant and lecturer on health enhancement and the integration of complementary and alternative medicine. Roger Jahnke provides workshops in tai chi, Qigong, and Chinese Medicine. He can be reached through Health Action at 805-685-4670.

The Health Action Group in Santa Barbara provides training to hospitals, clinics, and corporations nationwide on a wide range of health improvement topics. Health Action can be reached at 243 Pebble Beach, Santa Barbara, CA 93117, and by phone at 805-685-4670.

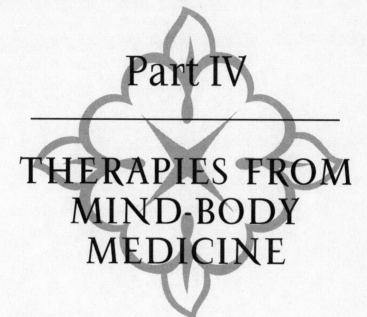

Part IV

THERAPIES FROM MIND-BODY MEDICINE

44

Quality of Life*

MICHAEL LERNER, PH.D.

❖

I am often asked, what would I do if I became seriously ill?

I don't know the answer to that question. I do not think anyone can know that unless they actually face the experience. But here are my thoughts.

I would pay a great deal of attention to the *inner healing process* that I hope a diagnosis would trigger in me. I would give careful thought to what had meaning for me *now*—what in my life I wanted to let go of and what I wanted to keep.

I would give careful thought to choosing a mainstream physician. I would be looking less for someone with wonderful empathetic skills than for someone who had a reputation for basic kindness who would also be willing to take the time I needed to answer my questions. Above all, I would be looking for someone who really stayed on top of the technical aspects of my treatment and who recognized that I was the kind of patient who wanted to share in making the decisions. I would also look for someone who was willing to stick with me if I embarked on alternative therapies.

I would use mainstream therapies that offer what seemed to me a real and meaningful chance for recovery, and I would use them with gratitude and work to augment their effectiveness. But I suspect that I would be somewhat unlikely to undertake experimental therapies or therapies with a low probability of success that were very toxic and would compromise my capacity to live as I chose.

I would use complementary therapies. My first choices would in-

*This piece was adapted from the outstanding book *Choices in Healing* by Michael Lerner, Ph.D. (Cambridge: MIT Press, 1997, 4th printing). Used by permission of MIT Press.

clude psychotherapy with a therapist experienced in work with people with chronic illness; a first-rate support group; and a healer with a good reputation. I would deepen and augment my regular nutritional program and I would strengthen my meditation and yoga practices. I would spend a lot of time in nature, walking in the woods, along the ocean, and in the mountains.

I would unquestionably use traditional Chinese medicine.

I would explore whether any of the high-tech alternative therapies appeared to have anything to offer me.

I would recognize the months or years of active effort for recovery that lay ahead. I would strive for life, for recovery, with every possible tool and resource I could find. But I would also [acknowledge that there may be realistic limits to what can be accomplished].

I would spend time with people I care a lot about, and with books, with writing, with music, with nature, and with God. I would do everything I could do that I had not yet done and did not want to leave undone. I would not waste time with old obligations or conventions, although I would seek to extricate myself from them decently. I would be off into pure life, following its lead.

I can say none of these things with certainty. How can any of us know what they would actually do?

In chronic illness, there is no single right choice for all of us, but there are surely right choices for each of us. There are no certain courses of action, but there are certainly educated and wiser choices, as opposed to uneducated ones. The skill is in the movement from ignorance toward knowledge and from knowledge toward wisdom. In wisdom, we choose what we are least likely to regret. Accepting the pain and sorrow inherent in the fate we have been given, we can seek also the beauty and the joy.

MICHAEL LERNER, PH.D., is president and founder of Commonweal (begun in 1976) and the Commonweal Cancer Help Program in Bolinas, California. He received his BA from Harvard and his Ph.D. in political science from Yale. After serving as an assistant professor at Yale, Lerner was named a founding associate of the Carnegie Council on Children. He came to California in 1972 and founded Full Circle, a residential treatment center for children with learning and behavioral disorders in Marin County. He has been named a United States–Japan leadership fellow and received a MacArthur Prize Fellowship for his contributions to public health. Michael Lerner is author of *Choices in Healing* (MIT Press, 1997).

45

Meditation: Spirit in Healing*

JON KABAT-ZINN, Ph.D.

❖

We know how our behavior and our feelings can be driven by the play of the mind's likes and dislikes, by our addictions and aversions. When you look, is it not accurate to say that your mind is constantly seeking satisfaction, making plans to ensure that things will go your way, trying to get what you want or need and at the same time trying to ward off the things you fear, the things you don't want to happen?

As a consequence of this common play of our minds, don't we all tend to fill up our days with things that just have to be done and then run around desperately trying do them all, while in the process not really enjoying much of the doing because we are too pressed for time, too rushed, too busy, too anxious? We can feel overwhelmed by our schedules, our responsibilities, and our roles at times even when every-

---

The Restless Mind

❖

In the first meditation class, each person gets a chance to say why he or she has come to the stress clinic. Last week, Linda described feeling as if a large truck were always right on her heels, driving just faster than she can walk. It was an image people could relate to; the vividness of it sent a wave of acknowledging nods and smiles through the room.

What was the truck? Her impulses, her cravings, her desires, she responded. In a word, her mind. Her mind was the truck. It was always right behind her, pushing, driving her, allowing her no rest, no peace.

---

*From *Full Catastrophe Living* by Jon Kabat-Zinn (New York: Delta, 1990). Copyright © 1990 by Jon Kabat-Zinn. Used by permission of Dell Publishing, a division of Random House, Inc.

thing we are doing is important, even when we *have* chosen to do them all.

We live immersed in a world of constant doing. Rarely are we in touch with who is doing the doing or, put otherwise, with the world of being. To get back in touch with being is not that difficult. We need only to remind ourselves to be mindful.

STOPPING

Moments of mindfulness are moments of peace and stillness, even in the midst of activity. Formal meditation practice can provide a refuge of sanity and stability that can be used to restore some balance and perspective. It can be a way of stopping the headlong momentum of all the doing and giving yourself some time to dwell in a state of deep relaxation and well-being and to remember who you are. The formal practice can give you the strength and self-knowledge to go back to the doing and do it from out of your being. Then at least a certain amount of patience and inner stillness, clarity and balance of mind, will infuse what you are doing, and the busyness and pressure will be less onerous. In fact, they might just disappear entirely.

Meditation is really a nondoing. It is the only human endeavor I know of that does not involve trying to get somewhere else, but rather, emphasizes being where you already are. Much of the time, we are so carried away by all the doing, the striving, the planning, the reacting, the busyness, that when we stop just to feel where we are, it can seem a little peculiar at first. For one thing, we tend to have little awareness of the incessant and relentless activity of our own mind and how much we are driven by it. That is not too surprising, since we seldom look dispassionately at the reactions and habits of our mind, at its fears and desires.

It takes a while to get comfortable with the richness of allowing yourself to just *be* with your mind. It's a little like meeting an old friend for the first time in years. There may be some awkwardness at first, not knowing who this person is anymore, not knowing quite how to be together. It may take some time to reestablish the bond, to refamiliarize yourselves with each other.

Ironically, although we all have minds, we seem to need to "re-mind" ourselves of who we are from time to time. If we don't, the momentum of all the doing just takes over and can have us living its agenda rather than our own, almost as if we were robots. The momentum of unbridled doing can carry us for decades, without our quite knowing that we are living our lives.

Given all the momentum behind our doing, getting ourselves to remember the preciousness of the present moment seems to require somewhat unusual and even dramatic steps. This is why we make a special time each day for formal meditation practice. It is a way of stopping, a way of "re-minding" ourselves, of nourishing the domain of being.

To make time in your life for being, for nondoing, may at first feel stilted and artificial. Until you actually get into it, it can sound like just one more "thing" to do. "Now I have to find time to meditate on top of all the obligations and stresses I already have in my life." And on one level, there is no getting around the fact that this is true.

But once you see the critical need to nourish your being, once you see the need to calm your heart and mind and find an inner balance with which to face the storms of life, your commitment to make that time a priority and the requisite discipline to make it a reality develop naturally. Making time to meditate becomes easier. After all, if you discover for yourself that it really does nourish what is deepest in you, you will certainly find a way.

THE HEART OF MEDITATION PRACTICE

We call the heart of the formal meditation practice "sitting meditation" or simply "sitting." As with breathing, sitting is not foreign to anyone. We all sit—nothing special about that. But mindful sitting is different from ordinary sitting in the same way that mindful breathing is different from ordinary breathing. The difference, of course, is your awareness.

To practice sitting, we make a special time and place for nondoing. We consciously adopt an alert and relaxed body posture so that we can feel relatively comfortable without moving, and then we reside with calm acceptance in the present without trying to fill it with anything. You may have already tried this in various exercises in which you have watched your breathing.

It helps a lot to adopt an erect and dignified posture, with your head, neck, and back aligned vertically. This allows the breath to flow most easily. It is also the physical counterpart of the inner attitudes of self-reliance, self-acceptance, and alert attention that we are cultivating.

We usually practice the sitting meditation either on a chair or on the floor. If you choose a chair, the ideal is to use one that has a straight back and that allows your feet to be flat on the floor. We often recommend that if possible you sit away from the back of the chair so that your spine is self-supporting. But if you need to, leaning against the back of the chair is also fine. If you choose to sit on the floor, do so on a firm, thick cushion that raises your buttocks off the floor three to six inches (a pillow folded over once or twice does nicely; or you can purchase a meditation cushion or *zafu* specially made for sitting.

Sitting on the floor can give you a reassuring feeling of being "grounded" and self-supporting in the meditation posture, but it is not necessary to meditate sitting on the floor or in a cross-legged posture. Ultimately it is not what you are sitting on that matters in meditation, but the sincerity of your effort.

Whether you choose the floor or a chair, posture is very important in meditation practice. It can be an outward support in cultivating an inner attitude of dignity, patience, and self-acceptance. The main points to keep in mind about your posture are to try to keep the back, neck, and head aligned in the vertical, to relax the shoulders, and to do something comfortable with your hands. Usually we place them on the knees, or we rest them in the lap with the fingers of the left hand above the fingers of the right and the tips of the thumbs just touching each other.

When we have assumed the posture we have selected, we bring our attention to our breathing. We *feel* it come in, we *feel* it go out. We dwell in the present, moment by moment, breath by breath. It sounds simple, and it is. Full awareness on the in breath, full awareness on the out breath. Letting the breath just happen, observing it, feeling all the sensations, obvious and subtle, associated with it.

It is simple, but it is not easy. You can probably sit in front of a TV set or in a car on a trip for hours without giving it a thought. But when you try sitting in your house with nothing to watch but your breath, your body, and your mind, with nothing to entertain you and no place to go, the first thing you will probably notice is that at least part of you doesn't want to stay at this for very long. After perhaps a minute or two or three or four, either the body or the mind will have had enough and will demand something else, either to shift to some other posture or to do something else entirely. This is inevitable.

It is at this point that the work of self-observation gets particularly interesting and fruitful. Normally every time the mind moves, the body follows. If the mind is restless, the body is restless. If the mind wants a drink, the body goes to the kitchen sink or the refrigerator. If the mind says, "This is boring," then before you know it, the body is up and looking around for the next thing to do to keep the mind happy. It also works the other way around. If the body feels the slightest discomfort, it will shift to be more comfortable or it will call on the mind to find something else for it to do, and again, you will be standing up literally before you know it.

If you are genuinely committed to being more peaceful and relaxed, you might wonder why it is that your mind is so quick to be bored with being with itself and why your body is so restless and uncomfortable. You might wonder what is behind your impulses to fill each moment with something; what is behind your need to be entertained whenever you have an "empty" moment, to jump up and get going, to get back to doing and being busy? What drives the body and mind to reject being still?

In practicing meditation, we don't try to answer such questions. Rather, we just observe the impulse to get up or the thoughts that come into the mind. And instead of jumping up and doing whatever the mind decides is next on the agenda, we gently but firmly bring our attention back to the belly and to the breathing and just continue to watch the breath, moment by moment. We may ponder why the mind is like this for a moment or two, but basically we are practicing accepting each moment as it is without reacting to how it is. So we keep sitting, following our breathing.

BASIC MEDITATION INSTRUCTIONS

The basic instructions for practicing the sitting meditation are very simple. We observe the breath as it flows in and out. We give full attention to the feeling of the breath as it comes in and full attention to the feeling of the breath as it goes out. And whenever we find that our attention has moved elsewhere, wherever that may be, we just note it and let go and gently escort our attention back to the breath, back to the rising and falling of our own belly.

If you have been trying it, perhaps you will have already noticed that your mind tends to move around a lot. You may have contracted with yourself to keep your attention focused on the breath no matter what. But before long, you will undoubtedly find that the mind is off someplace else . . . it has forgotten the breath, it has been drawn away.

Each time you become aware of this while you are sitting, gently bring your attention back to belly and back to your breathing, no matter what carried it away. If it moves off the breath a hundred times, then you just calmly bring it back a hundred times, as soon as you are aware of its not being on the breath.

By doing so, you are training your mind to be less reactive and more stable. You are making each moment count. You are taking each moment as it comes, not valuing any one above any other. In this way, you are cultivating your natural ability to concentrate your mind. By repeatedly bringing your attention back to the breath each time it wanders off, concentration builds and deepens, much as muscles develop by repetitively lifting weights. Working regularly with (not struggling against) the resistance of your own mind builds inner strength. At the same time you are also developing patience and practicing being nonjudgmental. You are not giving yourself a hard time because your mind left the breath. You simply and matter-of-factly return it to the breath, gently but firmly.

WORKING WITH YOUR THOUGHTS IN MEDITATION

During meditation we treat all our thoughts as if they are of equal value. We try to be aware of them when they come up and then we intentionally return our attention to the breath as the major focus of observation, *regardless of the content of the thought!* In other words, we intentionally practice letting go of each thought that attracts our attention, whether it seems important and insightful or unimportant and trivial. We just observe them as thoughts, as discrete events that appear in the field of our awareness. We are aware of them because they are there, but we intentionally decline to get caught up in the content of the thoughts during meditation, no matter how charged the content may be for us at that moment. Instead, we remind ourselves to perceive them simply as thoughts, as seemingly independently occurring events in the field of our awareness. We note their content and the amount of "charge" they have—in other words whether they are weak or strong in their power to dominate the mind at that moment. Then no matter how charged they are for us at that moment, we intentionally let go and refocus on our breathing once again and on the experience of being "in our body" as we sit.

Letting go of our thoughts, however, does not mean suppressing them. Many people hear it this way and make the mistake of thinking that meditation requires them to shut off their thinking or their feelings. They somehow hear the instructions as meaning that if they are thinking, that is "bad," or that a "good meditation" is one in which there is little or no thinking. *So it is important to emphasize that thinking is not bad nor is it even undesirable during meditation. What matters is whether you are aware of your thoughts and feelings during meditation and how you handle them. Trying to suppress them will only result in greater tension and frustration and more problems, not in calmness and peace.*

Mindfulness does not involve pushing thoughts away or walling yourself off from them to quiet your mind. We are not trying to stop our thoughts as they cascade through the mind. We are simply making room for them, observing them as thoughts, and letting them be, using the breath as our anchor or "home base" for observing, for reminding us to stay focused and calm.

By proceeding in this way, you will find that every meditation is different. Sometimes you may feel relatively calm and relaxed and undisturbed by thoughts or strong feelings. At other times, the thoughts and feelings may be so strong and recurrent that all you can do is watch them as best you can and be with your breath as much as you can in between. *Meditation is not so concerned with how much thinking is going on as it is with how much room you are making for it to take place within the field of your awareness from one moment to the next.*

These are moments of wholeness accessible to all of us. Where do they come from? Nowhere. They are here all the time. Each time you sit in an alert and dignified posture and turn your attention to your breathing, for however long, you are returning to your own wholeness, affirming your intrinsic balance of mind and body, independent of the passing state of either your mind or your body in any moment. Sitting becomes a relaxation into stillness and peace beneath the surface agitations of your mind. It is as easy as seeing and letting go, seeing and letting go, seeing and letting go.

FORMS OF MEDITATION

Sitting with the Breath

1. Continue to practice awareness of your breathing in a comfortable but erect sitting posture for at least ten minutes at least once a day.

2. Each time you notice that your mind is no longer on your

breath, just see where it is. Then let go and come back to your belly and to your breathing.

3. Over time, try extending the time you sit until you can do it for thirty minutes or more. But remember, when you are really in the present, there is no time, so clock time is not as important as your willingness to pay attention and let go from moment to moment.

Sitting with the Breath and the Body as a Whole

1. When your practice feels strong in the sense that you can maintain some continuity of attention on the breath, try expanding the field of your awareness "around" your breathing and "around" your belly to include a sense of your body as a whole as you are sitting.

Sitting with Sound

1. If you feel like it, try just listening to sound when you meditate. That does not mean listening for sounds, rather just hearing what is here to be heard, moment by moment, without judging or thinking about them. Just hear them as pure sound. And hear the silences within and between sounds as well.

2. You can practice this with music, too, hearing each note as it comes and the spaces between notes. Try breathing the sounds into your body and letting them flow out again on the out breath. Imagine that your body is transparent to sounds; that they can move in and out of your body through the pores of your skin.

Sitting with Thoughts and Feelings

1. When your attention is relatively stable on the breath, try shifting your awareness to the process of thinking itself. Let go of the breath and just watch thoughts come into and leave the field of your attention.

2. Try to perceive them as "events" in your mind.

3. Note their content and their charge while, if possible, not being drawn into thinking about them, or thinking the next thought, but just maintaining the "frame" through which you are observing the process of thought.

Sitting with Choiceless Awareness

1. Just sit. Don't hold on to anything, don't look for anything. Practice being completely open and receptive to whatever comes into the field of awareness, letting it all come and go, watching, witnessing in stillness.

JON KABAT-ZINN, PH.D., is the founder and director of the Stress Reduction Clinic at the University of Massachusetts Medical Center and Associate Professor in behavioral medicine at the University of Massachusetts Medical School. He is internationally known for his work using mindfulness meditation to help patients with chronic pain, stress, and a variety of other conditions. Numerous health professionals have trained with him and several clinics have been established that are modeled on his program. He is author of *Full Catastrophe Living: Using the Wisdom of Your Body and Mind to Face Stress, Pain, and Illness* (Delta-Dell, 1990) from which this chapter is drawn; *Wherever You Go, There You Are* (Hyperion, 1994), and a book on mindful parenting, *Everyday Blessings* (Little, Brown, 1998).

Full Catastrophe Living includes chapters on using the breath to heal, a thorough introduction to hatha yoga practice and its health benefits, walking meditation, mindfulness in daily life, stress reduction and management, working with physical and emotional pain, and improving sleep.

Practice tapes on mindfulness meditation and hatha yoga can be ordered from: Stress Reduction Tapes, PO Box 547, Lexington, MA 02420 and on the Internet at www.mindfulnesstapes.com.

46

Guided Imagery*

MARTIN ROSSMAN, M.D.

When he first came to see me for treatment, 24-year-old Jason wanted to manage his asthma better and perhaps reduce his need for medication. With that goal in mind, I taught him a simple relaxation technique. First, he relaxed the muscles in his body one at a time and imagined himself in one of his favorite places. Next, he used a more specific kind of mental imagery: envisioning his lung passages opening wide and air moving through them freely. By practicing this imagery exercise for about twenty minutes twice a day, he was able to lower his drug dosage and even went for long periods without an asthma attack.

Then, suddenly, the method stopped working. In fact, sometimes imagery made it harder for him to breathe. Because imagery had once helped him control his asthma so successfully, I suggested that we try a different type of imagery exercise to help him understand what had gone wrong.

After Jason lulled himself into a relaxed state, I advised him to allow an image to enter his mind that would offer a clue to the mystery. He began to see an agitated dwarf dressed like a Roman soldier patrolling the entrance to a tunnel. The dwarf, who called himself Romeo, said he was guarding the roads to Jason's heart. If anyone started to get too close he would close off the tunnel entrance. Jason thought the tunnel reminded him of a bronchial tube. He also pictured many such guards at the "outposts" of his bronchial tubes and saw the tubes all contract and close down in response to a threatened "invasion."

*This chapter by Dr. Rossman originally appeared in *Mind-Body Medicine,* (Yonkers, NY: Consumers' Union, 1993). It is reprinted here with the permission of the author.

After this exercise, Jason realized that the resurgence of his asthma coincided with the onset of a new romance. His intense feelings for his girlfriend so frightened him that he had been unknowingly using the asthma to keep her away. Because of his illness, he often canceled their dates. And when they were together, she spent much of the time taking care of him, though he really wanted a relationship based on mutual caring. With frustration and embarrassment, he recalled previous budding romances that had been sabotaged by flare-ups of his asthma.

Similarly, he now saw that he had unconsciously used his condition for emotional purposes during childhood. Back then, having an attack meant getting extra care from his mother and the chance to skip activities he disliked, such as gym class and trips to visit relatives.

BREAKING THE CYCLE

To break the cycle, I encouraged Jason to tell Romeo that he appreciated being protected from emotional pain, but that this vigilance was in itself causing pain and physical illness. In his mind, he told the dwarf that he felt ready to risk more intimate relationships, though he still wanted some protection. He began to imagine a series of checkpoints at different distances along the "roads" to his heart and how it felt to allow various people closer. He even envisioned issuing "security clearances" to certain individuals, including his girlfriend. This helped him experience how it felt to allow different levels of intimacy.

After that session, Jason was better able to relax and regulate his breathing. Over the next several months, his asthma did occasionally worsen, but he took those episodes as a sign to pay closer attention to his feelings, especially about his deepening romantic relationship. Within a year, his flare-ups again became rare occurrences.

TWO USES OF GUIDED IMAGERY IN HEALING

Jason's case demonstrates two major ways in which guided imagery, as this approach is called, is now used in health care. It can be used actively to help alleviate symptoms, as Jason did by envisioning his bronchial tubes widening. And it can be used receptively, "allowing" images to come to mind to help us understand the emotional meaning our symptoms may have.

The use of inner visions to help the healing process is hardly a new concept. Tibetan Buddhists have been using images in this way since the thirteenth century, if not earlier. The Buddhist approach typically involves meditating on the image of a deity in the act of healing a symptom. Shamanistic practices in cultures throughout the world have employed a similar approach. Only recently, however, has imagery been used by Western physicians and health care providers.

As a primary-care physician treating mostly patients with chronic conditions, I became interested in imagery first as a way to help alleviate my patients' suffering. Since 1972, 1 have taught imagery techniques to thousands of people. I have seen many people recover from their illnesses after using imagery, and others who have been helped by imagery to lead rewarding lives in spite of their condition.

There are still only a few carefully controlled, scientific studies to show precisely how great an impact imagery by itself can have on the body. Such studies are difficult to design and carry out, for several reasons. For one thing, imagery is often used in conjunction with other mind/body techniques such as hypnosis and simple relaxation, making it difficult to separate out the effects of the imagery alone. In addition, the "receptive" imagery techniques are so extremely individualized that it is hard to quantify their effects.

Nevertheless, a small but growing body of clinical evidence strongly suggests that imagery can help people with a wide range of physical illnesses. And some sophisticated physiological studies are pointing the way to understanding just how imagery exerts its effects.

HOW IMAGERY WORKS

The modern use of therapeutic imagery usually entails a 20- to 25-minute session that begins with a relaxation exercise to help focus attention and "center" your mind. If this doesn't adequately ward off distractions, you can also start by inducing a hypnotic state.

Although imagery is often used together with hypnosis, the two techniques are independent and complementary. Put simply, hypnosis is the induction of a particular state of mind, while imagery is an activity. It's perfectly possible to have one without the other, though the combination may be most effective.

In hypnotherapy, specific suggestions are used to relieve physical symptoms, and imagery is generally the most powerful and effective way to provide such suggestions. Rather than simply saying "Your pain is diminishing," for example, a hypnotist may ask you to imagine a painful part of your body feeling warm or going numb. (Imagery itself can also be used to induce a hypnotic state in the first place.)

During a typical session of imagery, you focus on a predetermined image designed to help you control a particular symptom (active imagery) or you allow your mind to conjure up images that give you insight into a particular problem (receptive imagery). Depending on your needs, imagery can be explored on your own, with the help of a book or audiotape, or with a therapist's guidance (see Resources).

Although science has not found the precise basis for imagery's healing abilities, we know enough to make some reasonable speculations about how it works. Visual, auditory, and tactile imagery seem to arise from the brain's cerebral cortex, the seat of higher mental functions, such as language, thinking, and problem solving. (Imagery having to do with smell or emotional experiences may arise from more primitive brain centers.)

When researchers have used a sophisticated technique called positron-emission tomography (PET) to monitor the brain during imagery exercises, they have found that the same parts of the cerebral cortex are activated whether people imagine something or actually experience it. This suggests that picturing visual images activates the optic cortex, imagining that you are listening to music arouses the auditory cortex, and conjuring up tactile sensations stimulates the sensory cortex. Thus, vivid imagery can send a message from the cerebral cortex to the lower brain centers, including the limbic system, the emotional center of the brain. From there, the message is relayed to the endocrine system and the autonomic nervous system, which can affect a range of bodily functions, including heart rate, perspiration, and blood pressure.

Many clinicians believe that the more fully you imagine something, the more "real" it seems to the brain and the greater the amount of information sent to the nervous system. This is one reason it's helpful to use as many senses as possible during guided imagery sessions. (For example, you might imagine lying on the beach, feeling the warm sand, listening to the ocean, and smelling the sea air.) While visualization is certainly the most common form of imagery, and for most people, the easiest, it's not the only one. People who have trouble visualizing may be able to relax by imagining the warmth of the sun, recalling a favorite tune, or conjuring up the aroma of brewing coffee or the taste of freshly baked bread.

THE VALUE OF IMAGERY

Three major qualities of imagery make it particularly valuable in mind/body medicine and healing: It can bring about physiological changes, provide psychological insight, and enhance emotional awareness.

Physiological Changes

Imagery has great potential to affect physiology directly. If you were consciously to try to salivate right now, you probably wouldn't be able to. But notice what happens if you imagine the scene in the exercise below. (This exercise is particularly effective if you close your eyes and have a friend read you the description aloud.)

At the end of this exercise, most people will salivate, especially from the back of the jaws—a simple illustration of imagery's ability to trigger a physiological response. But imagery can also trigger physical reactions that are more subtle than salivation and more important for health. There is preliminary evidence that imagery can have specific effects on the immune system, although the explanation for these findings remains unclear. In several experiments, researchers have looked at the physical effects of imagery combined with other relaxation and stress management techniques, such as the relaxation response, biofeedback, and progressive muscle relaxation. Although

---

An Exercise: Imagine . . .

❖

You are standing in front of a cutting board. Next to it is a good, sharp knife. Take a few moments to imagine the kitchen, the color of the countertops, the appliances, the cupboards, windows, and so on. Also notice any kitchen smells or sounds—the running of a dishwasher or the hum of a refrigerator.

Now imagine that on the board sits a plump, fresh, juicy lemon. In your mind, hold the lemon in one hand, feeling its weight and texture. Then place it back on the board and carefully cut it in half with the knife. Feel the resistance to the knife and how it gives way as the lemon splits. Notice the pale yellow of the pulp and the whiteness of the inner peel, and see whether you have cut through a seed or two. Carefully cut one of the halves in two. See where a drop or two of juice has pearled on the surface of one of the quarters. Imagine lifting this lemon wedge to your mouth, smelling the sharp fresh scent. Now bite into the sour, juicy pulp.

---

these studies did not focus narrowly on imagery, they do suggest it can contribute to a wide range of changes in such physiological functions as heart rate, blood pressure, breathing patterns, brain wave rhythms, blood flow, gastrointestinal activity, sexual arousal, and the release of various hormones and neurotransmitters.

Psychological Insight

Imagery can also help illuminate the connections between stressful circumstances and physical symptoms, where such connections exist. It does this by helping you see the big picture.

When you perceive the world as most people usually do, through logical, linear thinking, you attempt to break it down into small pieces and find the sequences that lead from one piece to the other. Logical thinking is similar to watching a train round the bend: You see one car at a time, with maybe just a little bit of the car that went before it. But imagery puts you in a balloon hundreds of feet above the track, high enough to see the entire train and several miles of track, as well as the town it came from and the city it's going to, the fields through which the train runs, and the mountain range in the distance. You grasp the whole picture and see how each of its parts is related to the rest. In much the same way, imagery can help you perceive connections between physical symptoms and emotional or stressful situations you would otherwise realize.

Here's an example. Two years ago I treated a woman who suffered from chronic arm pain that defied medical diagnosis. During an imagery exercise, she saw the pain as angle irons in her shoulders and metal bars in her arms. She said the images were hard, rigid, cold, and unyielding. When asked for other associations, she immediately thought of her grandfather, whom she had nursed for two years until he died some months before. She wept as she told me she had loved him a great deal, but hadn't been able to have the relationship she wanted with him because he was emotionally hard, cold, and rigid—the very qualities represented in the image of her pain.

I had her use imagery to create a dialogue with her grandfather. In her mind, she expressed all of her feelings to him, and he seemed to soften and thanked her for the loving care. He told her he loved her but wasn't able to express it. They embraced, and a warm feeling began to run through her arms. She had a few follow-up sessions and has been pain-free ever since. The imagery exercises helped her make the connection between her physical pain and its psychological cause, and she was finally able to heal.

Emotional Awareness

The third significant attribute of imagery is its close relationship to the emotions. You can think of the emotions as the means by which thoughts create changes in the body. Fear makes our hearts pound, grief makes us shed tears, and joy leads to laughter. But the natural ways of demonstrating emotions, especially negative ones such as anger and sadness, are often socially unacceptable and are suppressed. People may then find unhealthful outlets for such emotions, such as physical symptoms or behaviors (smoking, drinking, workaholism, and so on) that lead to health problems. Imagery is one of the quickest and most direct ways to become aware of one's emotional state and its potential effect on health. With this in mind, try the exercise below.

Take a few minutes to think about this experience, perhaps writing down some notes about it. How did you feel as you contemplated these two simple images? How much did you write? Notice that it was communicated to you in a second or two through each image. These mental pictures (in whatever sensory mode they appear) are very often worth thousands of words and are a very efficient form of information storage and recall.

HEALING THROUGH IMAGERY

Although there is little careful, well-controlled research on the medical benefits of imagery, clinical reports suggest that the technique may

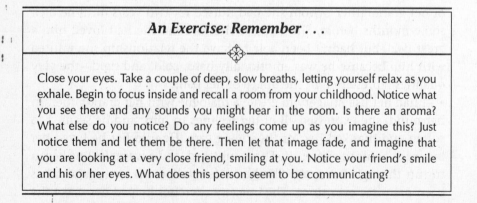

An Exercise: Remember . . .

Close your eyes. Take a couple of deep, slow breaths, letting yourself relax as you exhale. Begin to focus inside and recall a room from your childhood. Notice what you see there and any sounds you might hear in the room. Is there an aroma? What else do you notice? Do any feelings come up as you imagine this? Just notice them and let them be there. Then let that image fade, and imagine that you are looking at a very close friend, smiling at you. Notice your friend's smile and his or her eyes. What does this person seem to be communicating?

help treat a wide range of conditions, including chronic pain, allergies, high blood pressure, irregular heartbeats, autoimmune diseases, cold and flu symptoms, and stress-related gastrointestinal, reproductive, and urinary complaints. Imagery may also help speed healing after an injury, such as a sprain, strain, or broken bone.

Many of these benefits stem directly from the relaxing effects of imagery. In fact, the most common, most useful, and easiest application of imagery in health care is its use in relaxation and stress reduction. Many people find guided imagery the simplest, most natural way to relax. To get a taste of how relaxing imagery can be, try the simple, quick exercise below.

When you return to everyday reality, you're likely to feel calmer, more alert, and refreshed—as if you'd had a much longer rest. This sort of imagery is common to most relaxation techniques, from progressive muscle relaxation to various forms of meditation (see Chapter 45).

Beyond relaxation, however, active imagery is used—often together with hypnosis—to conjure up positive images designed to alleviate physical symptoms directly. In some cases, these images may have a direct physiological effect. When Jason, the man with asthma, visualized his bronchial tubes opening, he probably began breathing more slowly and deeply without quite being aware of it—changes that would be particularly beneficial for his asthma.

In other cases, imagery may have a beneficial effect on patients even though its effect on their disease can't be determined. The use of imagery in cancer therapy is a good example. In the early 1970s, radiation oncologist 0. Carl Simonton and psychologist Stephanie Simonton taught active imagery to cancer patients in the hope that it would help them fight off the disease. (A typical exercise was to imagine the

---

An Exercise: Transport Yourself . . .

❖

Keep your eyes closed while you take a few deep, easy breaths, and imagine yourself in the most peaceful, beautiful, serene place you can conjure up. Think of a time when you felt relaxed and peaceful—perhaps a walk in the park, a day on a sunny beach, or an evening at a concert—and focus intently on the sights, smells, and physical sensations associated with that event. Focus on this image for about five minutes.

immune system's cells devouring the cancer cells.) Their work received a great deal of publicity and sparked a lot of interest in imagery in general.

In the two decades since the Simontons developed their approach, no definitive, well-controlled study has been done to show whether this kind of imagery improves the overall prognosis for people with cancer. But many people find this kind of imagery helpful, even if it doesn't cure their disease. They report such benefits as relief from anxiety and pain, greater tolerance of chemotherapy or radiation therapy, and a heightened ability to cope with the illness. Imagery helps them to relax and to feel less helpless.

People with cancer or any other illness should not rely on imagery as their sole means of treatment when other, proven methods are available. Still, imagery can be a powerful aid in increasing the effectiveness of medical treatments or in helping people to endure them. Combined with relaxation techniques, imagery has helped people to tolerate such diagnostic and therapeutic procedures as magnetic resonance imaging examinations, bone marrow biopsies, and cancer chemotherapy and radiation. It can also help people prepare for surgery and recover from it.

Another role imagery plays in medical care is to put you in touch with your feelings about your illness. Imagery can be helpful in almost any medical situation that requires problem solving or decision making. By using receptive imagery to explore your emotional reactions to your medical circumstances, you may emerge with a clearer sense of how best to treat an illness or live well in spite of it. You may also better understand how your lifestyle choices may be affecting your health. If your illness is fulfilling some emotional need, coming to terms with that need may ease your physical symptoms.

Receptive imagery treatment may involve a dialogue with images representing symptoms or the illness. During receptive imagery sessions you may also wish to develop an image of your "inner adviser"—an embodiment of your inner wisdom—who can help you understand the emotional meaning of body sensations and symptoms. In my experience, this two-way use of imagery to spur communication between mind and body yields the most profound healing responses.

THE BOTTOM LINE

Depending on the severity of your problem, you may want to try using imagery on your own or with professional help. (For advice on finding

Healing and Inner Harmony Through Imagery

———⟡———

At 52, Robert suffered from chronic abdominal pain and indigestion that had been diagnosed as pancreatitis. His doctors had little to offer him but had urged him to follow a low-fat diet, which he had trouble doing. In our imagery sessions, he found an inner advisor who called himself "Moishe." Robert said he looked like a cross between his brother, Morris, and the biblical figure Moses. Moishe, like the doctors, told Robert that he would feel better and give his pancreas a chance to recover if he followed a strict low-fat diet. Robert followed Moishe's advice for several weeks and felt better than he had in years. But when he went on a trip to visit his family, he forgot about his diet. Soon after a meal at a Chinese restaurant, he had a severe episode of abdominal pain and vomiting. He tried to get back in touch with his adviser but had no success.

The next time Robert came to visit me, I guided him through a relaxation process and politely asked Moishe to come and talk with Robert again. Moishe appeared in his imagery, but stood with his head turned away and wouldn't speak. Robert asked him why he was silent, and he replied, "I don't have time to waste. If you're not going to be sincere about this, I'm not going to talk to you." Robert apologized and committed himself again to working toward better health more conscientiously.

Today, two years later, Robert feels working with his inner adviser has been one of the most helpful things he's ever learned. Not only has Moishe helped Robert with his digestive problems, but he was also of great comfort during a very difficult six-month period in which Robert lost the two people closest to him. During that time, Moishe told Robert that he was only an intermediary figure who represented his connection with God. Robert said to me, "Why deal with a middleman?" and now, in his meditations, he feels a sense of inner connection to God. Sometimes he asks questions and receives answers; other times he is satisfied just to enjoy a deep sense of peacefulness.

help see Resources.) Since imagery may change the body's requirements for medication, it may be best for you to use it under the guidance of your physician, depending on your medical condition. In any case, if you plan to begin an imagery program, it's best to set relatively small goals at first, perhaps aiming simply to learn to relax. Most people can experience relaxation with imagery in a very short time, even during the first session. Once you've mastered that, you can go on to try more complex forms of imagery.

For chronic symptoms, such as pain, you may want to begin by practicing 15 to 20 minutes twice a day for three weeks. This is usually enough to see if the imagery is helpful. For receptive imagery, it often takes two or three sessions with an experienced therapist or instructor to get initial results. It may take longer if you are working on your own or with self-help tapes.

If you use active imagery, keep a daily journal in which you estimate your symptoms' severity day to day. Over several weeks, this will help you determine whether the imagery is having an effect. Similarly, if you are using receptive imagery, it can be helpful to keep a journal of your experiences with imagery, as well as your dreams and emotional reactions.

Until more careful research is done, we don't really know imagery's potential or limitations as a healing tool. Some people seem to respond to it remarkably well, while others don't. Many factors, from your physical condition to your inner resolve, may affect the treatment's success. Experimenting with imagery, however, is easy, safe, and inexpensive. All it takes is the time and willingness to unlock the power of your imagination.

47

Self-Care*

TOM FERGUSON, M.D.

❖

We don't mean to imply that *everybody* should have a self-care plan. If things are going well for you, if you are satisfied with the present pattern of your life and not particularly interested in making changes at the moment, good for you. Keep it up. These guidelines are for those who are already interested in making some gentle changes.

Second, remember that the advice that follows has proved useful for some people. They are ideas to try, not commandments.

Third, the goal-setting exercise that accompanies this article is just that—an exercise. It gives you an opportunity to define and state a commitment you would like to make to yourself. This is a commitment to yourself, not an irrevocable promise sealed in blood. Think of it as an opportunity to "try on" some new behavior patterns. You are free to go back and revise your goals at any time.

TEN GUIDELINES FOR DEVELOPING A PERSONAL SELF-CARE PLAN

1. *Choose a goal that turns you on.* Build on strengths. Cultivate excitement. Starve problems and feed solutions. If you are a smoker and the idea of a regular running program appeals to you, you might find yourself quitting cigarettes about the time your program really steps up. If you have a problem with weight control and you've always been intrigued by meditation, a daily meditation session might be more useful than a whole stack of diet books. Goals that enrich your

*An earlier version of this article by Dr. Ferguson appeared online at www.healthonline.com and is included courtesy of the author.

life are usually more successful—and are certainly a lot more fun—than goals that deprive you of something.

2. *Start by just paying attention.* An excellent way to start an exercise program is to buy a pedometer—a small, watch-sized instrument that hangs from your belt and records the number of steps you take (available from running, sporting goods, and backpacking stores) and chart the total miles you walk each day. A good way to start an eating program is to write down everything you eat for a period of time. To start a smoking program, write down where and when and why you smoke each cigarette. Pay close attention to the ways that other people support desired or undesired behavior in the area you have chosen. Do family members insist on offering you high-calorie goodies? Does everyone else at work light up right after lunch? Don't try to change anything yet, just pay close attention.

3. *Check out your available resources.* Start with your own personal resources. Were you an athlete in high school? If so, maybe you can reconnect with some of the habits and practices that kept you in shape back then. Do you love to cook? Maybe you would enjoy developing some nutritious natural-food recipes. Is there a musical instrument or an art or craft that once meant a lot to you? Reconnecting with these areas of interest might be a way to further your own process of self-integration. Have you always had a dream of being a dancer? A painter? A writer? This may be an opportunity to develop these interests.

What individuals and groups in your community would be the best resources in your chosen area? Who already knows about what you want to know? Are there support groups in your chosen area (Weight Watchers, Alcoholics Anonymous, women's consciousness-raising groups?) Do you have friends who have lost weight, who are runners or meditators? What are the best publications in the area you have chosen?

4. *Brainstorm many possible goals before narrowing them down to one.* If you want to start an exercise program, you might start by brainstorming such goals as swimming the English Channel, walking cross-country across America, running a marathon, running five miles a day, joining (or organizing) a weekly fun run or running support group, running in place for five minutes before your shower each morning, riding your bike to work, taking the stairs instead of the elevator, or taking a fifteen-minute walk after lunch three times a week. Be creative. Feel free to be completely unrealistic. Think of goals that would be fun. Remember you are just brainstorming. Find your own way to

do it. Maybe the best way for you to start an exercise program would be to get a dog and take it for a walk once or twice a day.

5. *Design freedom into your goals.* "I will allow myself to take work breaks to do yoga whenever I feel like it." "I will go to bed early in order to give myself some quiet time in the morning before breakfast." "I will leave one Sunday a month free to be alone in the woods." "When I go running, I will let myself dance, skip, stop to look at a bird or a flower, or do anything I feel like." These are some goals with built-in freedom.

6. *Support yourself.* Pay close attention to your successes and the benefits deriving from your new practices. Celebrate your victories. "I ran a whole half-mile today without stopping!" "Doing yoga sure makes my back and shoulders feel good." Think of rewards you might give yourself for reaching short-term and long-term goals. (A hot bath after an evening run, a massage after logging your first hundred miles, dinner and a movie after completing a creative project.)

7. *Ask the support of others, and support them for supporting you.* Pick your support person (or people) carefully. Pick people who accept you as you are, who make you feel good about yourself when you are with them. Tell them that you're working on developing your own self-care plan—you might even show them this article—and ask if they'd be willing to be your support person for the goal you've chosen. Tell them the kinds of things they could do to help support you. Be as specific as you can. Here are some examples: "Serve me smaller portions." "Bicycle along with me sometimes when I go running." "Come with me to the first meeting of a self-help group [or self-care class or workshop]."

The way to get the best support from a friend is to support her or him for supporting you. "I really appreciated it that you took care of the kids so that I could play my flute." "It was really a help for you to take me into the medical library and show me how to look things up for myself." "It was wonderful when you said every time I wanted a cigarette you'd give me a kiss instead." "I really love it when you compliment me for the weight I'm losing."

You might also want to consider creating your own imaginary support person. A good description of one way to go about doing this can be found in the book *At a Journal Workshop* by Ira Progoff. A written dialogue with your own body and a dialogue with an interior wisdom figure are described.

8. *Create a supportive environment.* It may be easier to change your environment than to change your behavior. The easiest way to control

your eating is at the place you buy your food. If you have high calorie, low nutrition foods around, they'll probably end up being eaten. What goes into your shopping cart goes into your family's bodies. If you're trying to cut down on caffeine, try mixing your present brand of coffee half-and-half with decaffeinated coffee. Trouble overeating? Put your scale next to your refrigerator. And if your new, smaller portions look too tiny, buy smaller plates. If you're exploring yoga, massage, or meditation, try putting aside a special part of the house—or a special room—for these practices. Does soaking in hot water help you relax? Consider putting in a bigger bathtub. Having trouble finding a good place to run? Join other runners in a campaign for a community running path

9. *Be aware of feedback and be open to modifying your goal.* How does your new practice make your body feel? How does your awareness change? If you have a cold and are reading about the physiology of colds and taking vitamin C, how does that feel, compared with the way you used to cope with colds? How does making certain changes in your diet affect the way you feel about mealtime? At what times of day do you find yourself using your new relaxation skills?

Be aware of negative feedback, too. If you've given a chosen practice a good try and it's just not working, give yourself a vacation and reevaluate. Are you trying for too much too fast? Go back to the paying attention and brainstorming stage. You haven't failed; you've gained some useful information. Go back through the goal-setting exercise. Or if it seems right, give yourself a vacation from goal-setting for a while.

10. *Remember that your ultimate goal is to discover practices that allow you to experience and develop your own uniqueness.* There are two approaches to developing a self-care plan. Method number one is to imagine the ideal way you think you should be or would like to be. You then focus your attention on all the ways you fail to live up to that ideal. Method number one is a very effective way of making yourself miserable.

Method number two is to begin by just tasting your own being, becoming aware of your own body without comparing it to anything or anyone. When you taste a good wine, if you are comparing it to another wine or to how an ideal wine would taste, you will not be able to fully taste the wine you are drinking. If you are reading a book or watching a movie and are too involved in criticizing the plot or analyzing the style, chances are you won't be able to enjoy the story.

It may be that the most important part of developing a self-care plan is not the things you start doing, but the things you stop doing, a sort of psychological housecleaning, getting rid of some things you don't need any more. So the best of luck in working toward your own tailor-made self-care plan. And remember that it is you who must be the tailor.

Worksheet for Developing a Personal Self-Care Plan

My main area of interest (such as exercise, weight loss, or coping with an illness):

_____

My main personal strengths and resources in this area:

_____

_____

The best resources for me in this area (people, groups, classes, books, etc.):

_____

_____

Some activities and goals I might choose to help me explore this area (brainstorm!):

_____

_____

I would like to choose an initial activity that I could complete in about days/weeks/months:

_____

_____

Within this time limit, the goal I'd most like to set for myself is:

_____

_____

Some small rewards I will give myself for making progress toward this goal:

_____

_____

A big reward I will give myself for reaching my goal:

_____

_____

The people I will ask for support in working toward this goal:

_____

_____

I will contact my support person on _____ (date) to bring them up to date on my explorations in this area:

_____

_____

My commitment, again, is to accomplish the following activities between now and the following date:

_____

_____

On that date I will give my support person a report on my explorations in this area.

SIGNATURE: _____ TODAY'S DATE _____

SOURCE: Tom Ferguson, M.D., Austin, Texas, and HealthWorld Online: www.health world.com

---

Tom Ferguson, M.D., is editor and publisher of the industry newsletter *The Ferguson Report: The Newsletter of Consumer Health Informatics and Online Health.* With a medical degree from Yale University School of Medicine, he is a senior associate of the Center for Clinical Computing at Harvard Medical School and an adjunct associate professor of health informatics at the University of Texas Medical Sciences Center, Houston. He founded the journal *Medical Self-Care* and the *SelfCare Catalog,* and has been medical editor for *The Whole Earth Catalog* and a contributor to the book for Bill Moyers's series on mind/body medicine. He is the author of a dozen books on consumer health and his latest, *Health Online: How to Find Health Information, Support Groups and Self-Help Communities in Cyberspace,* was recently published by Addison-Wesley. Dr. Ferguson is also a consultant to many of the leading companies in the emerging online health industry.

Dr. Ferguson can be reached at doctom@doctom.com. or by calling his assistant in Austin at 512-282-9917.

48

Getting the Support You Need

LEN SAPUTO, M.D.,
and NANCY FAASS, M.S.W., M.P.H.

❖

"No one lives by bread, work, or medication alone . . . To flourish as an individual, it is necessary to have certain goods in our lives. Just as we need [good nutrition] to be physically healthy, there are values we must have to live well. Experiences of truth, beauty, justice, order, richness, playfulness, and meaningfulness are all food for the soul."

—JOHN SHUMAN, 1998

Many chronic digestive disorders carry with them profound life challenges, as well as obvious physical constraints. Their treatment can make us dependent on the support of health care professionals, as well as on our families and friends. Our lifestyle may become radically altered. The cost of therapy can be devastating. And our relationships may be severely tested.

We're all different, yet we're all looking for the same thing. The question is, How can we be loved for who we are? How can you get support if you have chronic illness? This is one of the toughest issues in our society—or any society. And GI illness may be life threatening or simply a nuisance. Your strategy depends on the needs of your situation. You want something that works and is emotionally satisfying, yet doesn't detract from you or anyone else. If you feel challenged, then you're being a realist.

WHAT THE RESEARCH SUGGESTS

◆ *Support matters.* A major study in New York confirmed what we all have suspected—people do better with support. Researchers tracked the progress of more than 700 people with serious illness and found that coping and improvement paralleled the adequacy of social support from family, friends, and others in their lives, even after all the variables were taken into account.

◆ *The sicker you are, the harder it may be to get support.* If you're really sick and you've been having trouble getting the kind of support you'd like to have, don't blame yourself. Because that seems to be the way it is. (This is what researchers have confirmed. Even children get less support if their illness is involved or lengthy. If this is a problem for kids, clearly it's difficult for adults too.)

◆ *It doesn't matter how many people a person has, it's the quality of support you get that is important.* (Rejoice in the support you *do* have.)

◆ *It's not easy to get support. One of the reasons support groups have evolved is because people aren't always there for each other.* There are many illnesses that tend to dim our charisma, when people need support the most. The programs of Dean Ornish have demonstrated that having support and a sense of community is an important part of healing.

DEVELOP A DIVERSE SUPPORT SYSTEM

If our needs are intense, it is important to have a support system that includes a number of people in a variety of roles: family and friends, perhaps volunteers or people whom we hire for assistance. Religious groups are frequently a good source of assistance. Nurses, physicians, and many other health care professionals are all potential resources to provide support that can help us to heal. If we need help on a daily basis, it may require setting up a network that we design to fit our own unique situation.

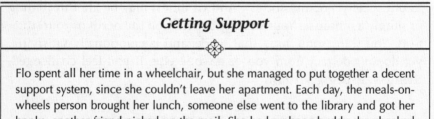

Getting Support

Flo spent all her time in a wheelchair, but she managed to put together a decent support system, since she couldn't leave her apartment. Each day, the meals-on-wheels person brought her lunch, someone else went to the library and got her books, another friend picked up the mail. She had a phone buddy she checked on and friends she talked on the phone with each day, and she visited with her daughter each week.

Getting Support

⬦

Marguerite's situation was equally challenging. At 90, she was totally house-bound in her cottage. She was able to remain at home through the support of her bridge group. She had a daily visitor, and then once a week the whole group came for a pleasant afternoon of bridge and brought her groceries for the week.

USING ILLNESS TO HEAL YOUR LIFE

If one has to go through all the trauma of chronic illness, it might as well become an opportunity for growth and change.

The Meaning of Disease: Personal Transformation

When we are ill, we want to get well. We don't enjoy being sick. Our most immediate concern is to secure relief from our symptoms and to be "cured" of our illness. We want to operate with a perfect body and to feel good. We seek out health care practitioners who promise to deliver these services and highly value their work. There is nothing wrong with this approach, and it has obvious potential value.

It is also possible to look at the meaning of illness in the context of who we are as unique individuals, determine what the illness represents in our whole life story, and prosper from the journey through it.

Like Pain, Illness Can Be a Signal

Like pain, illness may be a sign that something is deeply wrong in our life. Just as we usually take pain seriously (and are often sorry if we happen to ignore it), so we may regard illness as a sign that change is needed. Indigenous healers traditionally viewed illness as the reflection of psychological or social dysfunction that has resulted in physical and mental problems.

CHANGE = TRANSFORMATION

In the tradition of the shaman, the purpose of treatment is to restore the intactness or wholeness of the individual within the context of all aspects of their entire life. Healing is revered as a sacred journey within.

Changing Our Values

Illness may bring us back to the fundamental values of life, the importance of the people in our lives, and the spiritual aspects of life. When we're sick, we tend to become more oriented toward fundamental things. We realize the temporary nature of the material side. Illness can play an important role by awakening us to our spiritual purpose. We are reminded of the signficance of our relationships.

Transforming Our External Environment

At times the demands of illness also provide the impetus to make external changes, to find new and practical solutions to basic issues in our life. This may mean changing our environment. It may be necessary to get rid of a toxic relationships, make a career change, or move to another area. It may mean working as a freelancer or consultant, starting up an at-home business, or involving yourself in meaningful volunteer work with an organization you feel is making a worthwhile difference. It could involve refining a skill you've always wanted to use (fine woodworking, making clothes for homeless children, or taking up calligraphy). It may mean taking the vacation you've always dreamed of, just to get away for a while to catch your breath. Or it could mean developing almost any aspect of your life in a genuinely meaningful way.

Giving Is Easier than You May Think

No matter what your situation, there's always a little something you can do to help others. If you're housebound, perhaps it's phone work—calling latchkey kids to make sure they're all right, visiting with a housebound senior on the phone each day, or getting out the vote. You may have a skill you can donate—editing the newsletter of an organization you believe in, organizing a neglected project for them, or doing some Internet research. That glow that comes when you've done something worth doing can actually boost your immune response.

The Joy of Giving

❖

Lenore had a problem, but it didn't slow her down for a minute. She was afflicted with spinal scoliosis to such a degree it made her frame bent and twisted. Lenore was so gracious, so attractive, bubbly, and positive, that in her presence you immediately forgot about her disability and became swept into her interesting and engaging world. Lenore was a giver. Although she was well past 70, she spent her days shepherding women older and frailer than she to pleasant events—bridge, the theater, choral music, and volunteer work.

Twice, Lenore had cared for much older friends with extended convalescences, in each case for more than two years. She shared her spacious apartment with them, putting them up in the study, cooking and caring for them. This capacity to give may have been the source of her boundless energy and the meaningful purpose in her life.

Healing through Laughter

Being ill can be depressing. Being depressed can aggravate our illness by suppressing the immune system. And this is compounded further by the fact that it is often difficult to sleep. In addition, we may not be able to exercise, which can lead to deepening depression. Anything that can help us lift our spirits is healing.

The healing effect of laughter and positive emotional states has been found to enhance the immune system. Norman Cousins, in his book *Anatomy of an Illness*, described how he used laughter and nutritional therapy to heal from a totally debilitating condition. You may find his experience inspiring and decide to build into your life people and activities that delight you; for example, reading something humorous each day and spending time with friends who are upbeat. Since Dr. Cousins' initial work, the use of guided imagery, hypnotherapy, and a variety of meditative states has also been shown to have a powerful beneficial effect. Our state of mind has a strong influence on our body, and its ability to heal.

The Healing Power of Touch

Touch is a basic human need. Infants who don't receive touch may not survive or don't develop normally. We need human contact even more when we are ill. In addition to the soothing aspect of touch, it

The Healing Power of Laughter and Touch

❖

Edmund was in the hospital for 99 days (longer than Noah's flood!). For ninety days he was in traction—requiring the patience of both Noah and Job. Inspired by Norman Cousins, he developed a routine that helped him keep his sanity. Every day he rented a humorous movie and spent time reading comedies and uplifting books. He had a massage every evening and also had his barber stop by once a week to keep him trimmed and groomed.

can unlock painful memories stored in the muscles and tissues of our body, through treatment called somatic therapy. We've all heard of how the mind affects the body through psychosomatic illness. This can work in reverse as well: treating the body can heal the mind. There are a variety of body-work techniques that can not only make us feel physically and mentally nourished, but can do a lot to help our "mind-body" to heal. Mind-body medicine has become a popular approach over the past decade, and therapies like Alexander, Feldenkrais, craniosacral therapy, and many others have been documented to heal the mind-body through manipulation of the body.

The Healing Side of Nature

We have a sacred relationship with nature. In our own individual way, we are an integral part of its collective wholeness. Nature, too, offers a sacred relationship with us. When we accept this invitation, our relationship deepens. Connecting with nature can be very healing—it can be as simple as a walk by a river or smelling the fresh forest rain. These experiences bring us more in tune with our consciousness and spirit. They help us to remember that we are part of all that is, and that it is very nourishing.

Gardening

Activities such as gardening may have profound and lasting effects on body, mind, and soul. In many great religious traditions, gardening is considered a healing and spiritual practice—think of the herb gardens of the European monasteries and the rock gardens of the Asian monasteries. Very simple, very beautiful, yet not elaborate. This is something that can be created without great expense. There are many easy, pleasing ways to garden—for example, organic vegetable gardening using the French-intensive method is done in containers, ideal for patios or balconies. Something as basic as pots of herbs lining the windowsill can bring pleasure and provide healing herbs.

Nourish Yourself with Music

Great music, poetry and art also have the ability to bring us into harmony with nature. The language of tones, rhythm, and form allow us to deeply and simultaneously communicate within ourselves, and with each other. This resonance creates a sense of unity that can be not only awesome but truly healing. The messages of great composers and artists can transcend the conscious mind, reach us at a soul level, bringing us into more perfect balance. We have all experienced this remarkable phenomenon. The music that nourishes our soul may vary from Bach to African drumming, from choral music to world music.

Creating a Healing Space through Art

The other side of creativity is the opportunity to use our own creative expression. This can put us in touch with intense psychological and creative energy, and enable us to tap a deep vein of power difficult to describe. The medium could be anything that is meaningful, anything we enjoy and do well at. The possibilities are endless. If we are ingenious in choosing our medium, money need not be an issue.

In *The Psychology of Chronic Illness*, Robert Shuman, an insightful psychologist who battles multiple sclerosis, suggests that "art can bring the possibility of healing to those living with illness. One pur-

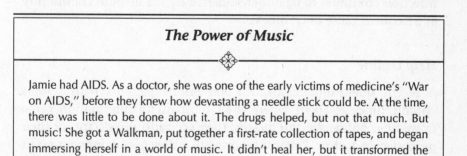

The Power of Music

Jamie had AIDS. As a doctor, she was one of the early victims of medicine's "War on AIDS," before they knew how devastating a needle stick could be. At the time, there was little to be done about it. The drugs helped, but not that much. But music! She got a Walkman, put together a first-rate collection of tapes, and began immersing herself in a world of music. It didn't heal her, but it transformed the quality of her life.

pose of art is to give form to that which is unspeakable, to render coherent the shattered and broken. Just as illness can [negate] experience, art can give it both spirit and flesh. Art is a medicine for the suffering we call illness."

Support Groups

Getting support has also been a problem for people with conditions such as cancer and AIDS. Over the past twenty years, resources for support within these communities have become quite well developed, perhaps because of the life-threatening nature of the illnesses. This has given birth to the highly successful medical support group movement that exists in this country. These groups are often highly valued by patients and praised by researchers for their life-enhancing benefits. The groups seek to provide the emotional and spiritual support that is so important in battling chronic illness, to retain what is most meaningful in life. Some of the support groups are offered to participants with a range of physical conditions, intended for anyone with serious illness, rather than just one diagnosis.

Support is valuable, but be sure the information you receive is current and correct. Beware that some groups unknowingly perpetuate misinformation about the nature of GI illness and the treatments available. For example, for decades stomach ulcers were thought to be caused by stress. We now know that in many cases they are due to a bacteria, *H. pylori*. It wasn't until an Australian researcher proved the link with the bacteria that medical opinion began to change. There are still many other GI conditions that are consistently misdiagnosed. This is a rapidly changing field with new research that has led to new understandings of the nature of GI conditions. Generally, the role of microbial infection continues to be underestimated by the medical community as a frequent cause of GI illness.

Help Online

A recent questionnaire asked 1,000 online patients with serious chronic illnesses about where their most useful information came from: their online support groups, their specialist physicians, or their primary care doctors. Patients reported that they found online support groups most useful in ten of the twelve dimensions studied. The most impressive take-home lesson was that these online self-helpers who often felt overwhelmed, isolated, and discouraged found that Internet resources provided a place where they felt welcomed, valued, and understood.

PRACTICAL MATTERS

♦ *If your needs are intense, consider seeking the help of a volunteer.* Don't overlook or turn down access to volunteer help, because many of the people who are drawn to volunteering are really beautiful people, and it may be that you can get a very special and precious kind of support in that way. Not every volunteer is ideal, however. Others may want to help but may be unable to provide what you really need. Usually you will intuitively know the ones who can be helpful from those who cannot. Follow your inner guidance.

♦ *Take offers of help seriously. At least consider them.*

♦ *Consider the value of a good case manager.* If you have access to social services and can find a case manager, it could help you assemble a support system or team. You have to either have money to hire a good case manager (they really do exist) or find a social worker within the system who can help you get linked up. Luck is also a factor in all this.

If you happen to have chronic illness, do consider getting support from the system. The social work literature says that the role of a good case manager is "the reconstruction and management of social support networks that have been altered or damaged due to illness or inability to cope with chronic illness. Concerns about the efficacy of specific models [and approaches] are not as important as the internal linkages built within each model and the external ties to other institutions and social service organizations forged as a way of synthetically rebuilding a client's social network" (Pescosolido and others, 1995).

♦ *Don't be shy to seek assistance.* A Swedish study found that people with chronic illness could typically manage at home as long as they had the periodic assistance of a home aide to help with basic chores and errands.

♦ *Be mindful of where and how you seek support.* Don't join the wrong group or stay in a bad relationship, thinking that it's necessary for your survival. The stress could further weaken your immune defenses.

The Needs of Children

Clearly, children need support just as adults do. The research found that teenagers with chronic illness tend to get less support than small children and that teenagers do better if they have support from peers as well as parents.

Girls tend to have more positive relations than boys. This was the conclusion of a series of seventy interviews with adolescents. Although boys (and men) benefit from support just as much as girls (and women), boys may be less likely to have supports in place or to ask for the assistance they need.

Obviously grandparents can play an important role in providing support to children with special needs. Grandparents have been found in many studies to provide support that complemented that of the immediate family and continued to provide help longer than any other relative. When there are grandparents in the picture who can be helpful, be sure to include them in the planning process to the degree they desire.

THE OPPORTUNITY FOR SPIRITUAL TRANSFORMATION

Illness can be looked at as more than physical disability and psychological challenge. It can be seen as an opportunity for spiritual transformation. This is not always easy. Many of us may not feel inclined to engage in this side of our life. In fact, we may even be angered by the suggestion. We may become totally consumed with "putting out the fire" created by the illness, with little energy to search out spiritual transformation! And we may be kept busy just holding on to the shreds of our former life. Most of us consider it asking a lot to make spiritual transformations when we are well!

If there is meaningful interconnectedness of everything in the Cosmos, then there is meaning for illness, too. Illness can be viewed from a deeper perspective that considers more than physical misfortune and psychological challenge. It relates to who we are, and is considered in the context of our entire life story and how our life interrelates with the Cosmos. It can be valued as a transformative opportunity that presents the possibility of evolving further on our spiritual path. This is what "healing" is about. Even though curing the body and healing the soul are not the same, they can occur simultaneously, and are not mutually exclusive.

RELATIONSHIPS

When we are ill, restoring our lost dignity and self-respect as human beings is of the utmost importance. Our relationship with ourselves, with those we love, and with God can be mercilessly challenged. We may have difficulty maintaining these vital nourishing relationships at the very time when we need them most.

Here's what the research has to say about chronic illness, support, and relationships:

♦ *When you have chronic illness and you're in a close relationship, you probably notice (again) that there are advantages and limits to partner relationships.* If the relationship has a strong foundation, you may do better than those without a support system. If there have been problems with communication, illness may amplify them.

♦ *The quality of the relationship in general probably has an impact on the illness.* If it's a strong relationship with good communication, a person has a better shot at dealing with chronic illness more effectively.

♦ *On the other hand, toxic relationships can make healing more difficult.* Stress can play a major role in suppressing immune function, so these issues are relevant to the healing process.

♦ *Chronic illness can place tremendous stress on a marriage.* In general, the divorce rate averages about 50 percent. In families where there is a child with chronic illness or a disability, the divorce rate runs about 70 percent. If you find yourself on the losing side of this equation, step back and then move on. Sometimes these apparent losses are a turning point toward a better life.

♦ *Looking for support? Take a second look.* If you are not getting the support you need from your family and friends, take one more look and see if there is anyone you may have overlooked who could be helpful. You may find that there is a relationship that would work if you adjusted it a little.

On the other hand, sometimes a relationship is simply unworkable. It's like beating your head against a wall. But sometimes you can shift an aspect of the situation and restore the relationship. It's important to know when to make the effort and when to conserve your energy.

♦ *Love can only be found if it is looked for.* Look for practical places to invest your energy. Look for people who could be available to you and be supportive. They may not be the people in your life with whom you are closest. But notice where the investment of your energy pays off.

◆ *Diversify.* We rarely get all our needs met by one person. Sometimes putting together a support system is most successful if we rely on different people to meet different essential needs. This may avoid burning out any one person in his or her attempts to be helpful.

◆ *When our physical capacity is compromised by chronic illness, our need for nourishing human relationships becomes especially apparent.* At these times we may be less able to care for our own needs and may also be less able to satisfy the needs of our friends and family. Unfortunately, fulfilling these needs may be a critically important aspect of maintaining some of these nurturing relationships, and as a consequence, they may disintegrate at the very time that we need them the most.

◆ *Illness can be viewed as a functional "stress test" that measures the strength of our relationships.* No one can predict how a relationship will weather the challenges imposed by chronic disease. We do the best we can, and should not be judged by our choices. It is possible for us to continue to learn about improving our relationships. This is our responsibility as human beings.

Doctors report that sometimes a health crisis is the very time when a relationship disintegrates. In some cases, the physically "healthier" partner leaves the relationship. But the one who is ill still has to get on with his or her life and overcome any guilt about what has been left behind. At that point, there is often an opportunity for spiritual and personal growth without the limitations of the prior relationship. This may be the point at which true healing can begin. In addition, it may provide an opportunity to clear old psychological baggage and emotional habits that may have kept us from relying on our own inner strength. Sometimes the life that follows has higher quality than the earlier existence.

Accessing Healing Relationships

Our personal challenge when we are chronically ill is to make changes within ourselves that can empower us to continue to obtain what we need from our relationships. It is risky, and may be wishful thinking, to assume that those around us will change. Ideally, in our deepest and most meaningful relationships, we are loved for who we are, unconditionally, and not just for what we can do or give. For many people, there are a few relationships that survive the test of illness. These become exceptionally precious.

Jean Shinoda Bolen, M.D., describes the transformation in our value system that frequently develops from the impact of serious illness in our lives. In this context, we transcend a self-centered and materialistic orientation to one oriented to bringing love into our relationships.

The Relationship Between Patient and Healer

While the practices of indigenous healers have not been very sophisticated, their strategies leave both the patient and practitioner with a sense of satisfaction and connection. In these systems, patients are not looked upon just as a set of symptoms to be treated with a bag of tools. "Being with" a patient supersedes "doing to" them.

Part of the change in your own life may involve finding a health care practitioner who you feel can be more understanding of your situation, or seeking out alternatives that are more congruent with who you are and more compatible with your unique needs. Many people have more than one health care practitioner, supplementing their care with a second therapy such as acupuncture.

Throughout history our ancestors have viewed healing as the return to wholeness. The abstract nature of wholeness makes it a concept that can be difficult to fully appreciate. From a personal perspective, wholeness focuses on our human experience, independent from nature. There is obviously great value in the fulfillment of our individual destiny. However, from a broader point of view, wholeness is all-inclusive and relates to our interconnectedness with the entire Cosmos. Achieving wholeness from this greater perspective is part of the conscious awakening that our culture is now beginning to experience. In the final analysis, healing is about wholeness, and wholeness is about remembering to live centered in love.

49

Support Groups*

REBECCA McLEAN

❖

Humans are social creatures. It's our nature to want to interact and support one another. Groups formed around a common goal or challenge can bring us together for strength and unity. Group members can draw on each other's strengths and celebrate our growth and victories. And the group can help us to hold a positive vision in times of challenge.

A review of the research on social support in the journal *Science* cited sixty-two studies showing that supportive relationships had a positive effect on recovery from chronic illness, infectious diseases, and surgery. Social connection was also shown to improve immune response and heart function. These studies indicate that we tend to function more optimistically when we're supported in a positive environment, connecting in a meaningful way with others.

If you have chronic digestive illness, particularly if it's severe, you may find that you're having difficulty getting the long-term support you need from family and friends. In that case, a support group could be helpful. If you find a group where you feel respected and heard, group support can be deeply meaningful.

THE POWER OF GROUP PROCESS

Many of the participants of groups I've facilitated say they found the support group process was a life-changing process for them, and that meeting weekly with the group, they felt their lives changed at an

*This chapter is adapted from material that appears in *The Circle of Life* workbook, created by Rebecca McLean. Reprinted courtesy of the author and Health Action, Santa Barbara, CA.

The Healing Power of Support

Brent joined one of our support groups because he had ulcers and he was finding that his medications were no longer working for him. Brent tended to become highly stressed at work, which was making his ulcers even worse. In the group, we went through an assessment process and looked at everyone's strengths and needs. He discovered his strengths were in exercise and relationships. When we explored the places where people wanted to make changes, he felt he was in a rut in his job and needed help with his ulcer diet. First we evaluated his diet, which revealed that he drank a lot of coffee and ate junk food. He was pouring coffee acids into his very sensitive stomach!

His initial action step was to gradually remove coffee from his diet and replace refined foods with more whole grains, like oats and brown rice and also steamed vegetables. He also realized he was bored with his job and that he drank coffee to feel stimulated. He wanted a better position that would use more of his talents and hold his interest.

His action steps involved going back to college three nights a week to meet the education requirements he needed to get a better job. Once he reduced the stress, his ulcer symptoms began to diminish almost immediately, as he decreased the physical stressor (coffee) and the mental stressor (feeling stuck in an unsatisfying job).

Gradually, the ulcers began resolving and Brent got a new job. He no longer needs sick days, doctor's visits, or medication. Through the self-inquiry process, Brent found his medical problem was being made worse by diet and work stress. Clarifying the problem and taking personal action not only helped to heal his ulcer, it changed his whole life.

accelerated rate. In addition, group participants say they discovered that their primary source of healing lies within themselves. Many of these groups have continued for years after people were in remission, changing the group's identity to "life support" groups!

A nine-year study published in *The American Journal of Epidemiology* on social networks reported that people with the lowest number of social ties were two to three times as likely to get sick as those with more social connectedness. A series of studies of weekly support groups by psychiatrist David Spiegel, M.D., at Stanford University demonstrated that women with breast cancer who participated in these groups lived twice as long as those who did not. His extensively documented research shows that health support groups create effective, measurable positive health outcomes.

Working within a group can support the process of improvement. A group can provide expanded resources for information, feedback, coping skills, experiences, testimonials, accountability, and support. It can help us grow and improve both by encouraging us and challenging us to stretch.

THE POWER OF SELF-INQUIRY

Self-inquiry is a master key that opens the door to the discovery of the inner self. Self-inquiry initiates a profound process of awareness. There is a saying: "If you are aware, you are halfway there!"

In the support group work, we have found that people often experience great relief simply by identifying their challenges. Without clarity, a person can feel powerless and directionless. Self-inquiry consists of posing questions for ourselves and carrying on an inner dialogue. This creates an opportunity to review all that we have learned, read, experienced or intuited regarding the issue. By consciously inquiring within, we often find we have more information than we have realized. Asking questions of ourselves enhances insight, consciousness, and clarity.

This process can create a kind of self-awareness and is also useful in assessing medical issues. We can use self-inquiry to evaluate what we're doing that improves our health, and identify those things that may be moving us in the wrong direction, whether they involve food choices, stress, or whatever. It can help us sort out our level of improvement and whether we need to seek additional medical resources, collect more health information, seek alternative approaches, or implement new heath strategies. It's also important to identify periods when no progress is being made and new solutions are needed.

THE POWER OF TESTIMONIAL:
TELLING AND HEARING STORIES

We're so incredibly influenced by each other and our stories that the power of testimony is big medicine. When people share how they've implemented self-care practices in their lives or were able to discontinue a damaging behavior, it proves that it can be done. It proves that someone who is no greater than ourselves has been able to achieve a breakthrough.

When someone expresses real insight on how they're getting their life to work, our ears get bigger and our listening deepens! When we see someone with challenges similar to our own making good lifestyle choices and feeling better, there's an automatic sense of inspiration. It gives us the courage and permission to take action ourselves. When we see someone having a breakthrough with their health, their relationships, or in some other area, it reminds us that this possibility is available to us as well. We are each other's mirrors.

We see evidence of the effectiveness of shared experience in the many thousands of success stories from Alcoholics Anonymous. The strength of this movement is built on the power of sharing. Another example of highly effective informal support is the Chinese Cancer Recovery Society, which has millions of members who meet in small groups in parks throughout China. The format of their gatherings includes self-healing practices such as Qigong, having tea together, sharing stories of recovery, and laughter! The impact of the gatherings on members is remarkable.

THE POWER OF FOCUSED ACTION

An action taken at the right time can mean the difference between easy and impossible. Deciding to quit smoking on the day before your income tax audit may be bad timing. But quitting smoking might be better when the audit is over and you can go cycling to occupy your hands and exercise your lungs. Deciding to start walking every day may be bad timing if it's January in Chicago. But walking outside every day in late April in Chicago is perfect.

It's also helpful for most people to remember that an action step can be broken into smaller, more attainable steps. Taking one small step in the direction of achieving a goal is a setup for success! While we realize this most of the time, when we are mired in chronic illness, the burdens can be overwhelming—physical, medical, financial, social, family, relationships, logistics, and quality of life. This may be the time to use this stepwise action approach.

Weight loss is a good example. The goal of losing 25 pounds can be daunting, but if it's broken down into 52 weekly steps, it's much easier to approach. That's less than half a pound a week. Then, rather than trying to do it all by dieting, divide up the process. Part of the half pound can come off from eating the right foods, part from exercise and part by using positive affirmations. Some can be taken off through breathing exercises that accelerate your metabolism, and some from drinking herb teas that improve digestion. That's five different strategies to address the half a pound a week. Stepwise goals reduce problems down to human scale.

THE POWER OF AFFIRMATION

When we acknowledge the barriers we face, it may become easier to create strategies for overcoming them. We may find our own attitudes, behaviors, and negative internal dialogue are slowing our progress. It's important to be sure we're not self-saboteurs or that someone else in our life isn't unconsciously sabotaging us. One of the most powerful tools for eliminating this internal negativity is the use of positive self-messages, also known as affirmations. Replacing negative self-talk with positive affirmations creates new possibilities and breakthroughs.

Research has demonstrated that carefully constructed affirmations cause shifts in the internal chemistry of the body, particularly brain chemistry and immune function. Dr. Candace Pert, a respected research scientist at the National Institutes of Health, has said: "The body is the outward manifestation of the mind." Simply stated, an affirmative thought or attitude neutralizes a negative thought. Acknowledging the barriers to the fulfillment of your goal can help you to create the affirmations and actions that may ultimately clear the negative energy.

THE POWER OF ACCOUNTABILITY

Accountability helps to sharpen the awareness of how we live our lives and how to better manage our time. Accountability, in a safe environment, can have a profound effect on our ability to set more realistic goals and action steps. Accountability gives us support and motivation to keep our commitments to our goals, priorities, and purpose. The objective is to practice external accountability in order to develop a more internalized accountability to oneself.

HOW SUPPORT GROUPS WORK

The goal of the group process is to provide support for participants and give them the opportunity to realize what they need to heal faster. So when we first meet, we talk about what it is that everyone wants from the group and what it is that they need in their life in terms of support. The groups start with a self-inquiry process. I use a diagram I call the Circle of Life, which has twelve major components of life—including self-care, stress mastery, relationship, finances, spirituality, work, and life purpose. First we just look at our lives and evaluate the areas that are strong and those that need support. What do you need? Do you need tools or skills or information or emotional support?

When a person isn't well, it's as if there's a drain on our life energy. It's like being in a boat with holes in it. You know that your goal is to get well, so you have a clear destination, but you sense that there's a leak. Sometimes it's a slow leak, but when it becomes a big hole, you feel yourself sinking. So you want to find out what is leaking your energy. And sometimes just having an illness itself is a big energy drain, because it takes tremendous energy for the body to heal itself and to cope. Stress may even be one of the causes of the illness. Being closely involved with someone who is extremely negative tends to deepen an illness. So we look at relationships and also identify sources of support.

This assessment process is important. A lot of times when we're not well, we tend to feel overwhelmed by everything. So we ask, Where is the drain? What's draining your life force, your energy, your power, your motivation? And what will shift the balance? What strengthens your joy, your health, your peace of mind, your self-acceptance? What supports you? We look at all the different aspects of one's life to see where we need to put the energy.

A GOOD SUPPORT GROUP—A SAFE PLACE

It can be nurturing to take part in a support group, where you know other people are having some very similar experiences and where there's no judgment. That's one of the most essential requirements—that you feel you're in a safe environment. The group must be a place where people understand because they're going through a similar experience. When you have safety, there's the potential for healing—there's always healing where we feel comfortable because then we're not using energy to override our emotions, we're not overextending ourselves, and we're not trying to prove anything. We can just be really real.

STEPS TOWARD HEALING

The main focus of the group is to acknowledge what's happening in each person's life and where they need support.

1. *First, there's a time of self-inquiry and self-evaluation,* looking at your whole life, to ask what gives you energy, what drains your energy. We want to start sealing up the leaks in the boat.

2. *After the inquiry process, we move forward by focusing on our strengths.* When you're sick, sometimes that becomes your identity, who you feel you are as a person. And of course that's not the essential you. Even if people are experiencing a major health challenge, they still have their gifts and their strengths. So each person begins their involvement in the group by sharing his or her greatest strengths—they may have a spiritual focus or know a lot about nutrition or have a strong sense of life purpose. By connecting with each other's strengths, we also realize the resources that each member brings to the group, that we can learn and grow from.

3. *At that point, each person decides where he or she needs support.*

4. *Then we will draw on the strengths we've seen in each of us, to provide support in areas where people need it.*

THE CIRCLE OF LIFE

The Circle of Life is the name we have chosen for our approach to the support group process. We use a diagram of a circle that reflects all of the basic aspects of life as a tool for the self-assessment of strengths and needs. The circle serves as a kind of reminder we can come back to, that shows us where we're making progress and where we still need more resources and support.

The Circle of Life can be used in a number of ways:

◆ *In a group setting,* the circle is the gathering of participants, the group or team, that cooperates to improve and support each other. In this context, the circle is the offspring of the ancient council circle or the meeting of the clan. It is also an expression of the breakthrough models for collaboration, such as quality circles that are being implemented in corporate settings.

◆ *As a self-improvement method,* the circle is representative of the Circle of Life process, the actual method which can be used by individuals, partners, or groups to encourage continuous personal improvement, cycle after cycle.

◆ *As a visual image, which can be used in a process of self-inquiry* to assess where we are in each of the major aspects of our lives.

The Circle represents twelve of the primary areas of our existence, focusing on:

Nutrition

Exercise and fitness

Self-mastery

Self-care

Relationships and communication

Work and career

Financial health

Play and creativity

Environmental responsibility

Emotional life

Life purpose, service, and contribution

Spirituality and intuition

At the end of the chapter is a copy of the Circle of Life Assessment. We encourage you to photocopy it and explore the value of the Circle as a self-assessment tool.

HOW TO USE THIS TOOL

The Circle of Life can be used in a stepwise journey by assessing where we are, setting goals, and taking action. When we revisit the Circle, we have a chance to celebrate successes and set new goals. The process offers an opportunity to:

- ◆ Decide on your goals.
- ◆ Clarify and refine the goals.
- ◆ Acknowledge the physical problems, situations, barriers, and communication issues that may keep you from attaining your goals.
- ◆ Design powerful positive affirmations (self-talk) that help clear barriers.
- ◆ Select measurable, attainable action steps.
- ◆ Design your action steps, breaking them down to the right size and pace, to guarantee successful outcomes and gradual but assured improvement.
- ◆ Set up accountability by stating your action step to the group or to another person.

The breakthrough secret of the Circle of Life process is remembering that when a goal is broken down into small, realistic action steps and time frames, it may be transformed from a challenging possibility to a manageable probability. And the strength gained from the group, from the circle of support, is literally a joining of energy—an opportunity to share group energy.

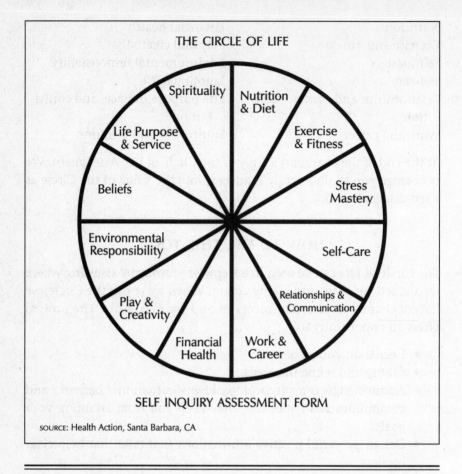

THE CIRCLE OF LIFE

Spirituality

Nutrition & Diet

Life Purpose & Service

Exercise & Fitness

Beliefs

Stress Mastery

Environmental Responsibility

Self-Care

Play & Creativity

Relationships & Communication

Financial Health

Work & Career

SELF INQUIRY ASSESSMENT FORM

SOURCE: Health Action, Santa Barbara, CA

REBECCA MCLEAN works as a facilitator, one-on-one or with small groups, using the Circle of Life process to improve quality of life and enhance healing; she counsels clients and groups in-person and also has phone clients from across the country.

Ms. McLean provides training to agencies, hospitals, churches, and corporations on the support group process and gives workshops on how to facilitate a group, expand existing programs, and how to initiate new groups. She can be reached at rjahnke@west.net or through Health Action in Santa Barbara at 805-685-4670.

50

Resources Online*

TOM FERGUSON, M.D.

❖

A new generation of online medical computing systems is becoming available to serve the public as well as doctors. Experts have recently predicted that these new systems will become an important part of our current effort to reinvent health care.

The self-care movement goes back at least to the early 1970s. What is different today is that we are seeing the emergence of a whole new generation of electronic tools that will make it considerably easier to do what only the most dedicated and diligent could do before. A growing number of resources are developing in the exciting new field of medical computing. Consumer Health Informatics (CHI) is the study and development of a new breed of computer and telecommunication systems designed to be used by the broad public. It now seems clear that later generations of these systems will allow us to build a new information health care system around the health-savvy, health-responsible individual layperson.

System demos at recent Informatics meetings have included a home-health workstation for people with AIDS (the CHESS program); an interactive system that helps men with enlarged prostates decide whether to have surgery (the Dartmouth-Sony series of decision-support video disks); a psychological spreadsheet for people experiencing high-stress life events (the Therapeutic Learning Program); a personal health information system for home use (HealthDesk); a voice mail-based self-help network (Talknet); consumer-initiated literature searches of the medical literature; and a wide variety of dial-up health-

*An earlier version of this article appeared in *The Millennium Whole Earth Catalog* and online at www.healthonline.com and is included courtesy of the author.

oriented bulletin board systems (BBSs). Increasingly useful and accessible health forums and real-time support groups are now available on:

- ◆ Commercial computer networks
- ◆ Internet mailing lists
- ◆ Internet newsgroups
- ◆ Web pages

The hands-on program demos at meetings on Informatics have made those attending feel as if we'd been catapulted five or ten years into our common heath care future. Also proposed or in development are consumer-provider e-mail/voice mail links, patient interfaces for computerized medical records, and a variety of online and interactive self-help and home-health networks, databases, bulletin boards, and other resources.

Many of the highly animated discussions at recent meetings have been interrupted by stunned silences as we bumped up against some of the long-term consequences of these emerging systems. As health information flow becomes widely available to all, we are beginning to see the medical equivalent of the coming down of the "Berlin Wall" that once separated lay health care from professional medicine. We are realizing that our widely held assumptions will no longer do.

- ◆ We can no longer safely ignore our own health until we have a breakdown experience, then count on the doctor to bail us out.
- ◆ Medicine is no longer considered something only doctors can know about. We need to provide our citizens with the tools, skills, information, and support they need to play new roles in the emerging new health care systems.

The industrial age "map" of health care, developed nearly a century ago, divided health care into three categories:

- ◆ Primary care—front-line health care professionals, typically doctors
- ◆ Secondary care—community hospitals and specialists
- ◆ Tertiary-care—academic medical centers

The whole realm of lay medicine was literally left off the map. Thus we have habitually overlooked (and often actively discouraged the use of) our biggest health resource of all—the self-help capacities of each individual to prevent and manage some of our own health problems.

These new information systems will help us reconnect self-help and self-care with professional medical care. In this emerging new information age, health care will actively involve the health-aware consumer, the concerned, supportive family member, the neighborhood helper, the corporate wellness professional, the online self-help group coordinator, the newsgroup coordinator, the web masters, and perhaps other key players yet to evolve, all working in cooperation with a new generation of supportive health professionals. Self-help groups and networks are a perfect supplement to professional services in an era of intense cost controls. The empowerment of health consumers means that consumers will now increasingly be seen not only as problems but also as resources for health care. There is a rich culture of lay medicine, most evident in active self-help groups and networks.

There are many important ways that professionals can help promote and work with self-help groups and networks, everything from providing referrals to being a guest speaker or serving as a group adviser. In the long term, one of the important contributions of professionals will be to facilitate the formation of new groups.

Clinicians are in a perfect position to start new groups and networks and to encourage the people with whom they come in contact to find or form their own support networks to help them deal with their problems. According to Edward J. Madara, executive director of the American Self-Help Clearinghouse, one out of three self-help groups was started with some help from a professional. Professionals are in a perfect position to identify and link people who have the potential to start a self-help network. To do so, the professional has to adopt a slightly different role from the traditional role—that is, the role of facilitator or consultant, to empower laypeople who are taking a greater degree of responsibility for their own health.

Those unfamiliar with online communications may have their doubts as to whether such keyboard contact with a group of strangers would have much meaning. Let me assure you that from my own experience and that of thousands of avid online networkers, these support group e-mail buddies can quickly become the most important relationships in one's life. What we're talking about here is the growth of electronic self-help communities.

Who are the best candidates for such online groups? People who are computer savvy, people who are already connected to the Internet or one of the commercial services, or people who are information workers. Online groups also appeal to people who have trouble attending face-to-face meetings because they have a rare disease; there are not enough self-helpers in the area; they might have physical limitations that make it difficult to travel to local self-help groups; and they might be busy and not have the time.

A number of self-help organizations have already gone online. Others are in the process of doing so. Current examples include the NPWA-Link, a computerized AIDS bulletin board developed and run by the National Association of People with AIDS in Washington, D.C. There is an active forum on Prodigy run by the Crohn's Disease and Colitis Foundation of America. Other related examples include the WID-Net developed by the World Institute on Disability, the New Parents Network, and several different networks for chronic fatigue syndrome. America Online and CompuServe both have active self-help forums. And America Online recently added a special self-help section run by the National Alliance for the Mentally Ill. The Cleveland Freenet offers an online health clinic, health fairs, and health education. Such locally based networks are a natural breeding ground for locally oriented self-help groups.

Whether they take place online or face-to-face, self-help groups and networks are an important vehicle by which people with health problems and other special concerns can empower themselves to take charge of their own problems. Such networks can help build proactive communities and can help people solve problems on a personal, local, and national level.

51

The Healer Within*

ROGER JAHNKE, O.M.D.

❖

"The marvelous pharmacy that was designed by nature and placed into our being by the universal architect produces most of the medicines that we need."

—NORMAN COUSINS, editor, inventor

Your body, in cooperation with your mind and spirit, is marvelously blessed with miraculous self-healing abilities. The body is the temple of your life. Mind and spirit are the dwellers within the temple. Mind and spirit maintain the temple. Mind's intelligence and spirit's inspiration vitalize and quicken the body. These three together—body, mind, and spirit—cooperate to produce the most profound medicine ever known in the history of the human race, right within you.

OUR BODY'S NATURAL ABILITY TO HEAL

Injuries or illnesses heal naturally when self-healing resources are operating optimally. If you cut yourself, the wound heals automatically. When you have a sprain or bruise, it heals automatically. A broken bone must be set correctly by the doctor, but then nature heals it spontaneously. The famous sixteenth-century physician Ambroise Paré said, "I administered the treatment, but nature provided the cure."

I had a personal experience of this early in my own life. Through a series of sports accidents, one of my front teeth was broken off to half its length. While the planning for a cap for the tooth was in process, the tooth actually began to grow. Over six months, this tooth grew past its normal size until it was as long as the other, unbroken front

---

The Power of the Healer Within

⟡

Margaret was diagnosed with chronic lymphocytic leukemia in 1987. This condition involves an abnormal increase of white blood cells and is considered to be a kind of cancer, because it is characterized by uncontrolled and unnatural cell growth. Her doctor informed her that this type of leukemia generally worsens slowly and that there was no medical treatment that would retard the progression of the disorder. He indicated that medical treatment, including chemotherapy and radiation, would be available when complications became a problem, typically swollen lymph nodes, an enlarged spleen, or restricted breathing.

Relieved to know that the progress of the disease would be slow and alarmed that there was no medical solution, Margaret began to explore alternative strategies for health enhancement. She looked into nutritional and herbal support and began to practice some self-healing methods. Twelve years later, Margaret continues to do well.

---

tooth. Some unexplained interaction of forces and elements caused this healing event to occur. Science cannot explain much of what causes what we call healing. The "original cause" of healing, health, life itself, and the entire universe remain fundamentally unexplained. In ancient China, this "original cause" is known as "mystery."

An inside joke in medical circles reflects on the healing power of nature: "With a doctor's expert care, you should be better in a week, but without access to the marvels of modern medicine, your recovery will require at least seven days." With or without a physician, with or without medical intervention, the natural medicine that we produce—our healer within—is working to heal us and sustain our health.

This remarkable gift belongs to every person from birth. A wonderous self-healing mechanism has been built into us by the architect of the universe from the beginning of all life. Unfortunately, most people have not known about this gift; it has been a secret. Freeing the potential of self-healing in your own life and sharing it with your family and community will have marvelous effects.

When our natural healing ability does not function automatically, something is terribly wrong. Our spontaneous self-healing resources have become damaged or disordered. So one important aspect of healing is removing any blockages to the functioning of the immune system and restoring it to maximum capacity, while providing the nutritional raw materials the body needs to heal.

Margaret's Story, in Her Own Words

After I was diagnosed with leukemia, I began to refine my diet, use vitamin and herbal supplements, and became more focused with my exercise and self-care practices. An inner, almost spiritual kind of intuition directed me. I felt that anything I would do to increase my health generally would slow the progress of the disease. My physician did not confirm this idea, but it felt right to me. I had gained tremendous support from prayer and the study material from my church over the years, so I deepened my spiritual practice as well.

I was always a healthy person overall, so I didn't really expect to feel much different. I did have a sense of well-being, particularly when I did my self-healing practices. My lab tests showed that the leukemia was progressing slowly. But the doctor seemed pleased that the white cell count was stable. Apparently the leukemia was progressing even slower than he had expected.

Recently, I had a blood check and my white and red cell counts had returned almost to normal. Two separate doctors commented that knowing my case, they would not have expected to see such readings this many years after the diagnosis. I take that as a very encouraging sign.

I feel my case is a great testimony to three things that should be added to the benefits of modern medicine. First, I was amazed at how I felt immediate benefit from the increase of prayer from my family. It was very notable to me and boosted my faith. Second, I feel sure that nutrition and herbal tonics have helped me to recover my energy after chemotherapy. Third, throughout this whole experience I have faithfully applied self-healing practices every day (gentle exercise, breathing practices, Qigong) and felt the power of their assistance all along the way.

I also very definitely benefited from radiation treatments. And my daily self-healing practice and my spiritual practice are the rock on which I have built my recovery and mental calm. The healing capacity within seems to complement and reinforce the medicine from outside.

We are entering a time when the secrets of healing will become the property of the many, rather than the few. You are now part of this extraordinary and historic moment. Like the secret of fire, centuries ago, knowledge of the art of healing will become available to the many. The keepers of the secrets of healing have made a profound discovery—that the essential resources for healing, which are naturally occurring within each individual, can be activated purposefully at no cost. The importance of this knowledge can be compared to the discovery of fire. For many thousands of years, the human race lacked the power of fire. Eventually, a powerful few gained the secret of fire, dramatically changing the course of human history. Keepers of the secret of how to produce fire had tremedous authority. Then, in an extraordinary historical moment, fire became the property of the many, rather than that of the few. Now anyone can ask for matches at the corner store and have fire at no cost.

Formerly, we lived in a world where the only solution to medical problems was thought to require physicians, hospitals, medicines, and tremendous expense. Now we know that the best, easiest, and least expensive cure is *first* to rehabilitate the automatic healing capacity through self-healing methods. This involves simple self-healing practices, such as focusing on the breath, applying self-massage, gently moving the body, and deeply relaxing to restore the natural balance between the body, mind, and spirit.

In mild cases, these self-healing methods may replace the need for medication, when there is stress headache, occasional constipation, colds and flus, aches and pains, insomnia, and anxiety. Even when medicine becomes necessary, self-healing methods complement and support the treatment.

Many techniques and methods for self-healing are quite ancient. Spontaneous self-healing ability is not a dramatic new scientific discovery. Nor is it a New Age phenomenon. There are stories of deep conviction in the early Judeo-Christian traditions regarding the healing resources that we have within ourselves. In China and India, as well as in Africa, ancient America, Australia, and Europe, rich traditions of self-care and self-healing have existed since long before written history. One of the first things I learned about in the study of traditional Chinese medicine was Qi (Chi), which is the name for the medicine within. The process of cultivating the medicine within is called Qigong (Chi Kung).

For decades, we in the modern Western world have believed that medical science would invent better medicines and healing procedures than those automatically born within us. Given that cancer, heart disease, stroke, and diabetes remain terrifying realities throughout our communities, we now know that the promise of medical science has limits. Exciting new scientific research and clinical experience show, however, that the most profound medicine is produced naturally within us.

Research of the U.S. Department of Health and Human Services, represented in the *Healthy People 2000* report, states that over 70 percent of all disease is preventable (DHHS, 1991). *The New England Journal of Medicine* reported that eight out of nine deaths occur from preventable causes (Fries, Koop, 1993). In 1996, the Office of the Surgeon General confirmed that simple, mild exercise significantly decreases the risk of many serious diseases (DHHS, 1996). Of adults, 60 percent were found to be insufficiently active and 25 percent were found to be completely inactive. It was found that simply increasing physical activity a small amount has a powerful fitness-enhancing and disease-reducing effect.

It is obvious that self-care and prevention are preferable to medical intervention. Even our own folk traditions—the wisdom of our grandmothers—insists that "an ounce of prevention is better than a pound of cure" and "a stitch in time saves nine." When we take steps to sustain and enhance the mysterious "healer within," medical intervention is necessary less often. Even in cases where health has been lost and where pain and disease have set in, self-care can lead to dramatic recovery.

Think of it: If 70 percent of each medical dollar were saved through self-reliance and prevention, the U.S. annual medical bill of nearly $1 trillion could be cut by $700 billion! Even cutting it by two-thirds would free up $500 billion a year. Imagine the kind of society we could live in if we intelligently applied an additional $500 billion each year to education, the repair of roads and bridges, research, and the renewal of our communities.

The naturally occurring self-healing ability of your own body, mind, and spirit is your greatest healing resource. This means that you, not someone else, but *you* can reduce your risk of disease. If you have lost your health and have become challenged by a disease or illness, this means that you can contribute to your own healing. You can use this healing power as part of any healing process, including the efforts you make in cooperation with your physician to speed your recovery.

This also means that your best health insurance is to be sure that all of the self-healing mechanisms within you are operating optimally. This does not suggest that physicians will no longer be needed. Nor does it suggest that the medical advances of the last one hundred years are any less remarkable. But it does mean that our physicians' time could be used more effectively in dealing with the 30 percent of health problems that are *not* preventable. And when it is necessary to have expert medical care, we can work as partners with our physicians and therapists by purposefully stimulating our own precious gift of self-healing.

SPONTANEOUS REMISSION

Spontaneous remission is the phrase typically used in the medical literature to describe cases in which a disease is cured or resolved but no one understands how. In the decades to come, the mechanism for spontaneous remission will be vigorously explored and will probably be better understood. For now, it is not so important how it happens; it is just enlightening that it does happen.

When doctors acknowledge that a cure has occurred and then acknowledge that they don't know how, it is possible that internal healing resources have been spontaneously activated to cause the cure. In the 1980s, the Institute of Noetic Sciences decided to explore the remission concept as a possible strategy to confirm the human capacity for self-healing. Brendan O'Regan, then the vice president of research, began a systematic exploration of the medical literature for references to remission. To everyone's amazement he found an immense number of references: three thousand articles from over 860 medical journals in twenty languages. Some of the articles discussed hundreds of cases, so the overall number of cases actually reported in the literature turned out to be in the many thousands.

"We have many cases of remission (one-fifth of all cases) with no medical intervention at all. These are the purest ones, the ones that give us the strongest evidence that there is an extraordinary self-repair system lying dormant within us." (O'Regan, 1995) This historic analysis of the "remission" literature from the Institute of Noetic Sciences is a powerful confirmation of the healer within.

THE ESSENCE OF SELF-HEALING

"The physician who teaches people to sustain their health is the superior physician. The physician who waits to treat people until after their health is lost is considered to be inferior. This is like waiting until one's family is starving to begin to plant seeds in the garden."
—*Yellow Emperor's Classic on Internal Medicine,* 500 B.C.

Three areas, all based on personal choice and personal action, maximize the activity of our naturally occurring self-healing capability. The first is our choice of attitudes and mental influences. When we choose to think, believe, and act from a position of power, refusing to be a victim of circumstances, the healer within is automatically strengthened. When we refuse to live under the influence of worry and doubt, the internal medicine is enriched.

The second area of choice is lifestyle: nutrition, exercise, rest, relationships, finances, work, spiritual practice, play, water intake, avoidance of alcohol and cigarettes, and so on. From moment to moment, each of us personally elects whether to enhance or sabotage the healer within, through our behaviors and personal choices. In my practice of acupuncture and Chinese medicine, I have found that the people who don't take care of themselves—who dislike their work, don't take time to play, or have poor self-esteem and communication skills are typically the most difficult patients to treat successfully. In such cases, the acupuncture often activates the healer within, but then the person's life situation tends to neutralize the self-healing capacity.

The third area of choice is personal self-care, the practice of self-healing and health enhancement methods. Self-care involves gentle movement (such as Qigong or yoga), essential breathing practices, hand and foot massage (as in reflexology), and deep relaxation and meditation practices. These are tools for improving, sustaining, and ensuring the function of the healer within. Self-care practices, positive attitude, and proactive lifestyle complement and enhance each other. I predict that these three areas—attitudes, lifestyle, and self-care—will be the foundation on which health care and healing are built in the twenty-first century.

When these aspects of personal choice keep health and healing active in a person's life, they have less need to go to a clinic or hospital. When the healer within is strong and efficient, self-healing can progress. Empowered by knowledge and inspiration to take action, each individual becomes the principal source of health, healing, and mastery of stress in their own life.

The effects of attitude, lifestyle, and self-care are noticeable in people's lives. It is fairly obvious when an individual is under the influence of self-doubt, poor nutrition, and a lack of exercise. It is equally obvious when an individual is influenced by enthusiasm, purposeful work, and the regular practice of health enhancement methods. The first person is typically exhausted and frustrated, the other radiant and energetic. One is a victim, the other a leader and a role model. One is part of the problem, the other part of the solution.

To accelerate our naturally occurring healing capability is actually quite easy. Once we replace the idea that health improvement comes from external sources with the knowledge that healing can come from the healer within, the practice of self-healing methods is simply logical.

> There must be some primal force,
> but it is impossible to find.
> I believe it exists, but cannot see it.
> I see its results, I can even feel it,
> But it has no form.
> —Chang T'su, philosopher,
> poet, fourth century B.C.

52

The Proactive Patient

NANCY FAASS, M.S.W., M.P.H.

DECIDING ON YOUR NEXT STEP

In order to get well, it's important to identify what you need:

- Is it a diagnosis or more information?
- A second opinion on your treatment or pending surgery?
- Do you need a plan for self-monitoring to find out what's working and what isn't?
- Do you have a complicated routine and need support to carry it out?

WORK WITH A GOOD PROFESSIONAL

Even doctors don't treat themselves. Seek out someone who is knowledgeable and highly informed. You want someone who understands your condition, through experience, training, and also intuitively.

It's important that you work with a practitioner with whom you have a meaningful dialogue—who listens to you, answers questions, offers advice, and discusses options. It is essential to work cooperatively with him or her in sorting out your problem. It is the interplay, the feedback between their creativity and yours, that may actually heal you.

They must know the generalities of your condition—the therapies used to treat it and the typical response. But it's utterly impossible for them to predict how your particular body will respond. Since they can't be with you every hour of every day, and you probably couldn't afford it if they had the time, you become their eyes. It will be up to you to observe your responses, to see when the shifts toward healing

Can You Afford to Turn Your Back on Digestive Illness?

—◈—

Once there was a great man who was loved by millions for the beautiful music he created. He had friends all over the world and an adoring wife, with whom he was very close. One day he came home, walked up the stairs to his room, closed the door, and did not come down for a year. His wife pleaded with him (through the door) to return to his work, to join her for dinner. She reminded him that his audiences missed him. But the man could not be dissuaded. A year later, he resumed his work and his family life, and pronounced himself cured of the illness so frustrating, so humiliating, he would not even discuss it—digestive disease.

Does this story have a familiar ring? Have you ever wished you had the resources to simply close the door on life because you, too, have digestive illness?

If so, you are not alone. Sixty million Americans suffer with digestive disease, according to the National Institutes of Health. Some researchers suggest a total as high as 120 million people a year, in the United States alone. Worldwide, about 3 million people die each year from GI infection and diarrhea-related conditions. A large number of them are children.

For many, digestive illness can be so limiting that they become unable to work, to socialize, or to carry on the simplest activities of the day, to do things most of us have so taken for granted. Even in their mildest form, digestive disorders are confining. Imagine something important that you want to accomplish and then imagine trying to do it *well* while suffering from diarrhea or constipation. Could you deliver a speech effectively? Negotiate a contract powerfully? Get your work done rapidly? Could you flirt? Have fun at the beach . . . or anywhere.

Yet digestive illness is beyond the range of polite social discourse—and therefore an illness for which it can be difficult to rally support. If you broke your arm, you could get tremendous sympathy and encouragement. Everyone would ask what happened, sign your cast, offer you advice, and wish you well. And next week, they would want to know how you were doing. In contrast, it's difficult to imagine, for example, discussing a colonoscopy, even with family members. And for some people, these issues are so taboo, they would literally rather die than discuss these issues with their doctor.

If you have chronic digestive illness, this book was written for you. Our goal is to provide you with all the important new resources—safe, effective, relevant— that are now available in integrative medicine and coming into the fore. Soon, we expect that nutritional medicine (healing through nutrition) will be broadly available, and your own family doctor or internist will be using the new lab testing and nutrients for your healing.

But your illness is *now*, limiting each day as the clock ticks away. So we want to place these resources at your disposal, for your consideration. We wish you well.

occur. Find ways to record what is needed to measure change in your condition—keep a log, a food diary, or a journal. You must be the one to watch for downturns and report on how you turned them around, or how aspects of your illness refused to be remedied. It's important to catch a problem soon after you begin to slide away from health, to keep you on a healing path.

STATE YOUR OWN TRUTH

Tactfully, politely, state your own truth, your perceptions, your experience. Create an alliance with your doctor and become a powerful team—go for a balance between respecting your doctor's advice and not abandoning what you believe to be true from your own experience.

If you have approached your relationship with your doctor or practitioner in this spirit, and it isn't working, you may want to bring along a patient advocate on your next office visit or bring your partner or your best friend. If that doesn't change the dynamic, it's time to seek a second opinion.

THINGS YOU CAN DO FOR YOURSELF

You have to *want* to get well—no one else can make that commitment for you. Be as realistic as you can, because denial will cheat you of the information you need to heal. Never give up hope. Positive thoughts can be healing and despair may aggravate your condition.

♦ *Become highly self-observant.* To the degree that you can, come out of denial so you can accurately discern what's going on with your body and your situation. This can be harder than it sounds. As much as you can, reconnect with your body so that you can feel where there's pain and when things aren't working. This information is vital to the healing process.

♦ *Educate yourself.* Make use of books, the Internet, Medline, your public library, and the medical library, as well as the media.

♦ *Get copies of your own records.* Legally you have a right to them. Remember that ultimately you will experience the impact of all medical decisions about your care far more than anyone else involved.

♦ *Ask for what you need.* Advocate for yourself impartially, as objectively as possible. Be assertive but not aggressive. Take good care of yourself.

GET A SECOND OPINION—FROM ANOTHER POINT OF VIEW

Integrative medicine is based on the same scientific information used in mainstream medicine. The same science forms the basis for understanding and diagnosing illness. The therapies are frequently different. They are milder and more natural, and therefore slower acting, often involving healing stimulated by nutrition and herbs.

The emphasis is also different; it involves another way of looking at the same information. One example is that in treating GI illness, practitioners of complementary medicine place more emphasis on treating GI disorders due to bacteria, yeast, parasites, and viruses. It continues to surprise us that this emphasis should come from the alternative side, since Western medicine is based on an understanding of pathogenic microbes and the use of antibiotic (antibacterial) medications. Yet mainstream labs and doctors continue to overlook the issue of infection and consider it simply a problem of underdeveloped countries, rather than a frequent aspect of digestive illness in our crowded big cities.

Complementary practitioners also focus on supporting the immune system. This means providing the raw materials the body needs to heal—good nutrition and nutritional supplements, clean air, water, and food, rest and relaxation, and gentle exercise.

Restoring the proper functioning of the organs and cells is a primary strategy of functional medicine, by removing irritants and allergenic foods, and restoring GI processes using nutritional supplements. Acupuncture unblocks the energy and circulation in the body and stimulates the vital force. Homeopathy also focuses on stimulating the vital force, using minute doses of nontoxic remedies.

When to get a second opinion? If you find that you're not getting well, or if your doctor is scheduling you for major surgery and you're not sure that's what you want, get a second opinion from a doctor who practices integrative medicine—nutritional, functional, orthomolecular, or naturopathic medicine. To find an alternative physician, check the resource section for organizations that provide practitioner referrals:

- ◆ The American College for the Advancement of Medicine (nutritional medicine)
- ◆ The American Academy of Environmental Medicine
- ◆ The Broda Barnes Foundation (particularly for glandular and thyroid problems)

- Bastyr University (for trained naturopaths)
- Health-Comm International (for practitioners of functional medicine)
- The Society for Orthomolecular Health-Medicine (nutritional medicine)

YOU DON'T HAVE TO HAVE A FIRM DIAGNOSIS TO BEGIN HEALING

This is the value of functional testing, which looks at impaired function rather than damaged tissue and pathology. This emphasis on function makes it possible to intervene much earlier in the disease process. Nutrition, acupuncture, and homeopathy can also promote healing in situations in which the diagnosis is unknown. As you know from this book, there are many other excellent strategies for healing and many excellent resources.

PROCEED CAREFULLY, SENSIBLY

This is true of everything you do. If you want to take an herb, begin slowly and check with your practitioner. Are you taking a drug? Again, be mindful. Check with your pharmacist to avoid multidrug interactions. Use informed judgment, common sense, an open mind, and healthy skepticism in all you do.

MAKE PEACE WITH YOUR ILLNESS

Love your body; respect all the parts and functions of you, even when they don't seem glamorous. If you can, take high pleasure in the food you eat, respect the importance of disposing of spent food. Appreciate the intricacies of your body, value the importance of your stomach acid and mucus, and all the other seemingly mundane miracles that make your life possible each day. These are the mechanisms through which your body works. Respect and honor them.

Remember that you are your own best advocate.

> *If I am not for myself, then who will be for me?*
> *If I am for myself alone, then what am I?*
> *If not now, when?*
>
> —Hillel

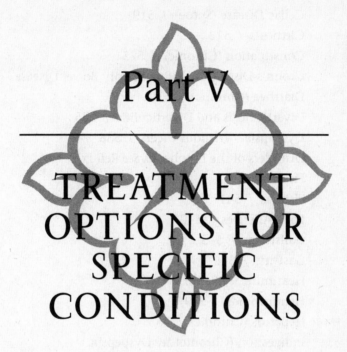

Part V

TREATMENT OPTIONS FOR SPECIFIC CONDITIONS

TRENT NICHOLS, M.D.

Cancer of the Colon / 511

Cancer of the Pancreas *See* Pancreatic Cancer.

Candida / 515

Celiac Disease (Sprue) / 519

Cirrhosis / 522

Constipation (Chronic) / 525

Crohn's Disease *See* Inflammatory Bowel Disease.

Diarrhea (Chronic) / 530

Diverticulosis and Diverticulitis / 535

Dyspepsia—Without Ulcers / 538

Disorders of the Esophagus *See* Reflux.

Fissures / 541

Fistulas / 541

Food Allergies / 542

Gallstones / 543

Gastritis / 546

Heartburn *See* Reflux.

Hemorrhoids / 549

Hepatitis (Chronic) / 553

Indigestion (Chronic) *See* Dyspepsia.

Inflammatory Bowel Disease (IBD)
    and Crohn's Disease / 555

Irritable Bowel Syndrome (IBS) / 561

Lactose Intolerance / 566

Liver Disease / 567

Malabsorption / 571

Pancreatic Cancer / 574

Pancreatitis / 575

Parasites/Parasitic Infection *See* Chapter 21.

Pruritus Ani / 578

Reflux and Heartburn—GERD / 579

Strictures and Structural Conditions / 585

Ulcers / Ulcer Disease / 588

Ulcerative Colitis *See* Inflammatory Bowel Disease.

Viral Bowel Disease *See* Chapter 22.

CANCER of the COLON

Malignant tumor of the large intestine. A malignant growth that invades surrounding tissue, may spread throughout the body, and is likely to reoccur after attempted removal and can be fatal.

CAUSES

The incidence of gastrointestinal cancer has been associated with diets high in fat and sugar and low in fiber. In societies that traditionally have a low incidence of colon cancer, such as the Japanese, it has been found that when people begin to eat a westernized diet of refined foods and high fat, the prevalence of colon cancer increases and becomes comparable to industrial nations with diets of refined foods.

Increased fat intake has been found to be a factor because fats are subject to free radical damage. Saturated fats stimulate at least one gene that promotes inflammatory messengers (prostaglandins) shown to initiate the cancer process.

Certain illnesses tend to be associated with increased risk for colon cancer:

- IBD (Irritable bowel disease)
- Ulcerative colitis of more than ten years' duration
- Crohn's disease
- Inflammation that lasts for an extended period of time
- Genetic factors
- Breast cancer
- Obesity, inactivity, and constipation
- The presence of polyps. Patients with many polyps have such a high rate of colon cancer that by age 30, almost all have diagnosed colon cancer. The two primary medical interventions for this condition have been colon removal at a young age or the use of a drug (Sulindac) that inhibits the production of an overly reactive immune response by the prostaglandins. Aspirin also decreases the risk of colon cancer. To minimize GI bleeding, a safer therapy uses a newer product, Cox-2 inhibitors—check with your pharmacist.

People with constipation and slower colonic transit time are more prone to colon cancer. Therefore, take constipation seriously and seek professional help if you find this condition has lasted for more than one month.

EARLY DETECTION

Routine screening for polyps is an excellent preventive measure and should include direct examination of the colon. Polyps are benign nubbins that grow in the colon. The development of cancer is believed to occur about ten years after polyps begin developing. If the polyps are removed, the potential for cancer is decreased. Therefore, routine screening and periodic polyp removal are important. This is early intervention, which to date has the support of only about half the medical community.

Hemoccult blood testing of the stool looks for hidden blood in the stool. Given the increased risk of colon cancer, particularly in the young, this should be done yearly after age 20. However, this test is not always totally accurate. If there is a family history of colon or breast cancer or if there is a positive result on the test for blood in the stool, colonoscopy should be performed, and then periodic screenings should be begun.

Flexible Sigmoidoscopy is another useful form of monitoring, done every three years from age 40 on. This provides direct examination of the lower two feet of the colon and should be done for both men and women. This can be performed by your primary care physician.

EARLY INTERVENTION—SIGNS AND SYMPTOMS

- Rectal bleeding or blood in stool
- Abdominal pain
- Weight loss
- Iron deficiency anemia

TESTING

- Stool test for undetected blood (fecal occult blood test—Hemoccult)
- Sigmoidoscopy
- Barium double-contrast enema (X-ray)
- Colonoscopy
- Virtual colonoscopy (a new CT scan X-ray of the colon, enhanced by computer analysis)
- Blood tests for those who have a history of colon cancer. Testing for carcinoma embryonic antigen (CEA) can reveal an antigen that is a by-product of active cancer.

COMPLEMENTARY TESTING

The AMAS Test is a blood test with a very high degree of accuracy that reflects the presence of an antibody found to be elevated in most patients with active malignancies. It can be ordered by your doctor from Oncolab in Boston at 800-922-8378.

MAINSTREAM TREATMENT

Prevention and early intervention are still the most important aspects of treatment. The removal of polyps usually interrupts the cancer sequence. Most polyps are initially benign. If polyps are detected early enough, abdominal surgery can be prevented. Polyps are usually removed with a wire snare and cautery during colonoscopy, so this kind of surgery usually doesn't require an incision. In cases where the polyp is too large or the malignancy is too advanced to be removed by snare, surgery through an incision in the abdominal wall is necessary and removal of a section of the bowel is indicated. This procedure, called resection, is used to treat 50 percent of colon cancer; the other 50 percent require adjunct chemotherapy, or in the future will be treated with immunological therapy. Radiation is not generally helpful except in cases of anal-rectal carcinoma (anorectal). One of the more promising forms of chemotherapy appears to be the drug Campostar.

Surveillance with yearly colonoscopies are essential for those in remission. This is really important to prevent reoccurrences or new cancers.

COMPLEMENTARY TREATMENT

In individual cases, nutritional therapy has been found useful and is reported by some complementary practitioners to be have been effective in specific cases. Even for people undergoing conventional treatment, excellent nutrition can offer a significant benefit by supporting the body.

Resources for integrative treatment include the Cancer Treatment Centers of America in Zion, Illinois; Tulsa, Oklahoma; and other cities. These centers have perhaps the broadest experience in this area. They use mainstream approaches such as surgery, radiation, and chemotherapy. They complement these therapies with the use of nutrition, guided imagery, massage, and behavioral therapy.

Other respected centers that use nutrition and alternative therapies include the Block Center, in Evanston, Illinois, and the Geffen Cancer Center, in Vero Beach, Florida. Some patients have excellent experience with this approach, and in other cases the cancer could not be halted, but for some of these, quality of life is improved. Clearly, no therapy works for everyone.

Some of the specific alternative therapy programs that have been also used include the Gerson diet, the Kelly method used by Dr. Nicholas Gonzales in New York City, and the macrobiotic diet as described by Michio Kushi.

Vitamin therapy has been a promising component of nutritional treatment. Specific nutrients found to be important in prevention include vitamins C, D, and E, and the minerals calcium, selenium, and other trace minerals. Research has found that cancer prevention (for example lung cancer in smokers) has not been effective when a single nutrient alone was used in supplement form. Therefore, we highly recommend the full complement of vitamins and minerals from natural sources. Since we are all affected by stress and pollution, most people benefit from supplemental nutrients.

Two highly useful books on this topic are *The Definitive Guide to Cancer* by the Burton Goldberg Group (Future Medicine Press, 1997) and *Choices in Healing* by Michael Lerner (MIT Press, 1997).

TREATMENT IN DEVELOPMENT

◆ Toxins from the bacteria pseudomonas have been used in combination with antibodies in tumor therapy in some cases; this treatment has been evaluated by the National Cancer Institute (NCI). You can call the NCI and get information on new research and new clinical trials. This information is also available on the World Wide Web at www.nih.gov on the page for NCI.

◆ Urso, used in the treatment of gallstones, has also been found to prevent colon cancer; this substance, used in Chinese medicine, is derived from bear bile. It is now available in prescription form under the names Urso or Actigall. Urso tends to decrease secondary bile salts, which are potentially carcinogenic to the body.

◆ Anti-angiogenesis is a mechanism that contains the spread of cancer, decreasing the metastases of tumors by cutting down on the blood supply to the tumor.

PREVENTION

◆ Exercise
◆ Not smoking
◆ Avoid sugar and fat, and eat fewer calories
◆ Increase intestinal motility with fiber, fruits, and vegetables or motility enhancers such as cellulose (FiberCon), bentonite, or aloe vera in capsule form

♦ The use of probiotics to promote motility and decrease inflammation

Take any inflammatory condition seriously.

PREVENTIVE DIET

For general prevention, good nutrition has been proven to be essential. A preventive diet should include fiber and antioxidants from both fresh foods and a good quality supplement. Flaxseed oil as a supplement and for salads (an omega-3 oil), and olive oil (a monounsaturate) can be helpful in preventing the stimulation of the body chemicals that cause inflammation (prostaglandins). Calcium supplements are also preventive, by apparently toning down the genetic mutation that can play a role in cancer (K-*ras*). Antioxidants in general have an important preventive effect that has been proven. Be sure to take antioxidants and trace minerals either individually or in a formula that includes copper, zinc, manganese and selenium.

Avoid diets that are low in calcium and vitamin D, high in phosphates (such as sodas), and high in fat. Regular aspirin use can help prevent polyps, but is known to cause leaky gut and GI bleeding (ask your pharmacist for Cox-2 inhibitors as an alternative). B complex vitamins are extremely important in minimizing the production of the metabolite homocysteine, which is also carcinogenic. Alkalinize your diet through salads and low starch vegetables, alkaline water, and liquid chlorophyll (DeSoussa's). (See Chapter 32—First Aid for Inflammation).

CANCER of the PANCREAS
See Pancreatic Cancer.

CANDIDA
Candida is a form of yeast normally found in the digestive tract that can overgrow and become too numerous in the intestines. This is a species of yeast-like fungi; the most frequently occurring species is *Candida albicans*. It can be pathogenic when it becomes too populous, crowding out the beneficial bacteria. This overgrowth can be caused by prolonged use of antibiotics, the use of steroids (prednisone), taking birth control pills, severe infection, or major immunosuppression (such as in AIDS).

The most frequently seen symptoms of candida include fatigue, irritability when hungry, headache, depression, brain fog, bloating and gas, diarrhea, constipation, itchy bottom or vagina, urinary frequency, sore throat and mouth, severe athlete's foot or fungal toenails, chemical sensitivity, cravings for sugar or alcohol, and food sensitivity.

CAUSES

♦ Antibiotic therapy—one of the most frequent causes
♦ In women, elevated hormones due to pregnancy, hormone supplementation, or birth control pills
♦ Use of prednisone or other immunosuppressant medication
♦ Depressed immune function in combination with a highly sweet and starchy diet
♦ Frequent exposure to a high mold environment
♦ Parasitic infection
♦ In conjunction with AIDS, Candida is particularly prevalent.

There is now medical coding for candidiasis of the colon, which indicates that candida is now recognized as a cause of illness throughout the body. Until this time, it was viewed as a disorder primarily of the esophagus and the vagina only. Doctors are now beginning to view it as a legitimate health condition throughout the rest of the body.

Yeast in the digestive tract can produce toxins that can make you ill in a variety of ways. They also produce alcohol as a by-product in the process of breaking down starches (which can cause brain fog and intoxication). They can promote an increase in pathogenic enzymes (called proteolytic or protein-digesting enzymes) that allows the candida to invade the tissue elsewhere in the body, as is often seen in cases of AIDS and other conditions of immunosuppression. The journal *Medical Hypothesis* has reported on research suggesting that chronic candidiasis can be associated with chronic fatigue syndrome.

DIAGNOSIS AND TESTING

Stool testing under the microscope or a culture sample in which the yeast is grown (for example, a 24-day culture). Species include *Candida albicans* and *Candida glabrata*. Microscopic exam of stool produces information on the type of candida (whether the infection is due to dividing forms, which are considered more disease producing and pathogenic than non-dividing forms).

Some labs report the yeast and also test the yeast to see which antifungals and herbs destroy it (sensitivity testing).

Many commercial and hospital labs do not consider yeast to be a problem and do not report it on stool exams.

MAINSTREAM TREATMENT

♦ Nystatin is the number one therapy, the most frequently used antifungal, which is available in capsules, liquid, powder, gels, and a troche (a lozenge).

♦ Diflucan (fluconazole) is very useful but expensive.

♦ Nizoral (ketoconazole) can be useful but may have accompanying liver toxicity. There are some people who have a yeast condition that is resistant to all the previously mentioned drugs. For these, the risks of ketoconazole may be worth it. Before beginning this medication, consider getting the functional medicine liver detox test. It is also recommended that you get a liver enzyme profile periodically during the therapy to be sure the drug is not causing damage. An additional treatment option for those with resistant yeast is miconozole, available only from compounding pharmacies. (See Appendix Resources section for information on compounding pharmacies.) Major systemic treatment that supports immune function could be helpful; ask a physician practicing functional/nutritional medicine about such treatment.

COMPLEMENTARY TREATMENTS

HERBS: Herbs alternated with drug therapy or used individually:

♦ Available from the health food store—garlic oil in capsule form or fresh; oil of oregano; *Pseudo winteracolorata*; grapefruit seed extract (Nutritibiotic); berberine (barberry extract); pau d'arco; tea tree oil. General immune stimulants include echinacea and goldenseal.

♦ From physicians' offices and compounding pharmacies—Tanalbit; SF-722 (undecylenic acid) by Thorne in capsules and topical form; combination formulas such as AC Formula by Pure Encapsulations; gentian violet used as topical; and Candacin by Metagenics.

♦ From Chinese medicine—Ganoderma, also called Ling-Zhi (ling-shi), is a mushroom imported from China, which tends to removes toxins, may stimulate immunity, and seems to have antibacterial and antifungal properties.

DIET

A diet very low in refined carbohydrates with no sugar is key in gaining control of this condition. Avoid foods with fermented content such as vinegar or pickles. Refer to *The Yeast Connection* by William Crook, *The Body Ecology Diet,* 5th ed., by Donna Gates (B.E.D. Publications, 1996) and *Depression Cured at Last* by Sherry Rogers.

All these authors recommend staying off antibiotics and predisone to the degree possible, staying off sweets and starches (simple carbohydrates such as sugar, pastas, and breads), and eating complex carbohydrates in moderation. Avoid any product that contains brewer's yeast or baker's yeast, and minimize other fermented products. Avoid sodas and fruit juice; instead, develop the taste for spring or mineral water, lemon water (hot or cool), and herb tea (hot, iced, or even room temperature).

NUTRIENTS

Take probiotic supplements to restore the friendly flora. This is key. Treatment is not meant to totally rid the body of candida—this is impossible. Rather, the goal is to keep the flora in balance and avoid overgrowth. Probiotics, periodically taken, can help maintain this balance. This is important, because yeast can become pathogenic when they overgrow.

Blood sugar and insulin swings tend to be associated with yeast conditions, in part because of deficiencies in the trace minerals chromium and vanadium. These two minerals can be supplemented in capsule form as chromium and vanadyl sulfate and can help with insulin sensitivity and insulin resistance. If there is a significant overgrowth, also supplement trace minerals and/or ask your doctor to measure trace mineral levels, prescribe supplements, and monitor them. Mineral testing is available from National Medical Laboratories or Pantox Laboratories through a prescription from your doctor. Antioxidant vitamins A, C, and E are important, as well as alpha-lipoic acid (which is a metabolic antioxidant).

Risk factors: Diabetics tend to be more prone to yeast overgrowth because of the tendency for high blood sugar. Some people who consume too much alcohol may actually have alcohol cravings driven by the yeast. People who eat a highly sweet or starchy diet, with lots of yeast products may have a greater tendency to yeast. Soft drinks and commercial fruit juice are also high in sugar.

COMPLEMENTARY THERAPIES

♦ *Acupuncture* can enhance immune function and assist the body to fight off the overgrowth of yeast and then keep the yeast population in balance. EPD therapy also appears to be useful against yeast and fungal sensitivities.

♦ *Mind-body therapies* can help to keep stress at a minimum by allowing your immune system to recoup and cope with the overgrowth.

◆ *Allergy testing:* In Germany, allergy testing and general evaluation is performed using a small noninvasive electronic acupuncture instrument, Voll electrodermal skin testing, also called bio-resonance therapy. This therapy is used to determine overgrowth of pathogenic bacteria and yeast, allergies, deficiencies in nutrients, and to determine the value of particular treatments. It measures the resonance at the acupuncture points. Then the practitioner either treats the meridians or uses homeopathy or herbs, based on the feedback received.

CELIAC DISEASE (Sprue)

Celiac disease, also known as celiac sprue, is a chronic problem of malabsorption that results from an allergic response to gluten, which is a protein found in wheat. Sprue leads to malabsorption and a deficiency of nutrients. This is due to the shrinkage and destruction of the structures in the GI lining that absorb nutrients from our food—the microvilli and later the villi on the lining of the small intestine. This condition also usually causes diarrhea.

Sprue is a condition that is frequently overlooked or misdiagnosed. Sprue often occurs as a latent condition and is found in about 25 percent of diabetics. This is a genetic disorder that is inherited, common in Ireland and northwestern Europe. It is rare among Asians, people of Jewish heritage, and African Americans. Sprue occurs in about 4 to 5 percent of the population; latent sprue (hidden gluten allergy) may be as frequent as 10 percent. It is frequently associated with blood group O and occasionally in type A blood.

Problems due to sprue actually occur at the level of the cell. Research has found that sugar residues (lectins) on the cell surface selectively bind the microscopic particles of wheat that are toxic (gliadin fractions). This explains why extremely tiny amounts of wheat or gluten can set off this condition. Avoiding sprue symptoms means far more than just avoiding bread or even wheat. It means not eating any prepared or processed food to which wheat or gluten have been added. It is important to keep a strict diet because a number of more serious illnesses can occur as the result of an untreated sprue condition.

ASSOCIATED DISEASES

There are a large number of associated conditions. Of these, the most common is Type I diabetes. Neurological disorders that can also result from the malnutrition of sprue include peripheral neuropathy, abnormal myelinization of the spinal cord, and night blindness. In rare cases, encephalopathy can occur—a toxic brain syndrome due to sprue and B vitamin deficiency which can lead to coma, because insufficient nutrient absorption is taking place. Other serious complications that can occur in rare cases include increased incidence of lymphocytic cancer. Incidents of hypocalcemia have also been reported (tetany), as well as increased incidence of fractures and collapsed vertebrae.

SYMPTOMS

Typical symptoms include chronic diarrhea, abdominal pain, gas, bloating, and other signs of malabsorption, weakness, weight loss, failure to thrive, and chronic sensitivity to starches and foods that contain grains. In 10 percent of people with sprue, a bumpy itchy rash occurs (dermatitis herpetiformis). Sprue can also cause infertility or delayed menarche, chronic fatigue, anorexia, frequent bruising due to vitamin K deficiency, and many conditions related to malabsorption, such as anemia.

Children with sprue develop a characteristic appearance, with thin, wasted extremities, a bloated abdominal area, and loose stools. Low levels of vitamins D and K can lead to softening of the bones (osteomalacia). Protein malabsorption can lead to loss of muscle mass, weakness, and generally impaired development. Lactase deficiency can be associated. Sprue causes the most extreme form of leaky gut. Testing shows that when particles are released in a sprue condition, the lining of the GI tract is so damaged that extremely large molecules leak through. This can cause all the symptoms associated with leaky gut syndrome (see Chapter 7 on the syndrome).

CAUSES

Celiac disease is caused by a specific antibody (the antigliadin antibody). It is often linked to other autoimmune disorders and may be linked to the overstimulation of the T cells and the immune system in general. The offending substance is wheat protein, which contains gluten components (glutamine and gliadin). Other grains besides wheat that contain gluten include barley, rye and oats. For some, rice and corn are tolerated staples.

This is typically an inherited autoimmune disorder. Sprue is associated with specific genetic patterns and tissue types. If the gene for sprue is present the immune system can be overstimulated by gluten in the diet. This can bring on sprue symptoms and a destructive immune response can occur. For those with the gene, this may occur after exposure to a virus.

TESTING

◆ Testing for the gliadin antibody should be considered a general screen, especially whenever any of the symptoms of this destructive and easy-to-correct condition are present. This test is most stable in blood (serum).

◆ The most highly sensitive blood test for this condition is the antiendomyseal antibody.

◆ Testing for 24- or 72-hour fecal fat is a measurement of all the fat in the stool over a one-hour period to determine the level of fat absorption.

◆ Small bowel biopsy is still helpful in order to observe the lack of villi under the microscope. This exam is also performed at the three-month follow-up to check on the progress of healing.

MAINSTREAM AND COMPLEMENTARY TREATMENT

Diet Therapy

Working carefully with a dietitian can be exceptionally helpful, using diet diaries and other approaches to help track food intake and symptoms. Nutritional counseling is vital, because overcoming this condition requires reading every label, even on apparently innocent products such as chewing gum, medications, and vitamins. The diet for sprue requires careful monitoring for life. The good news is that when patients stick to the diet, no other therapy is usually needed, and they typically do very well. However, patients who cheat on their diet continue to suffer and need the assistance of a dietitian.

Some patients may also need steroids (prednisone). Nutritional supplements can be beneficial in many cases, such as the peptide preparation Seacure and the amino acid L-glutamine, as well as vitamins, enzymes, and other nutrients.

A whole food gluten-free diet is the most important single factor in treating this condition. On a gluten-free diet, eliminate all wheat, oats, barley, and related grains. Rebiopsy to see if the villi are growing back. Once the patient is off the offending foods, the villi should return, along with the restoration of many functions.

Patients who don't respond to these therapies may require the elimination of all food containing amylopectin (all carbohydrates containing disaccharides, eliminating sugar, starch, lactose, and all the grains). Foods not permitted include wheat, barley, corn, rye, oats, rice, buckwheat, millet, triticales, bulgur wheat and wheat germ, spelt, potatoes, yams, parsnips, chick peas, bean sprouts, soybeans, mung beans, fava beans, garbanzo beans, amaranth flour, quinoa, or even cottonseed grain substitutes, and seaweed. See *Breaking the Vicious Cycle* by Elaine Gottschall (Kirkton Press, 1994), which also contains delicious recipes.

Supplements

♦ *Nutritional therapy* also involves probiotics, L-glutamine, bromelaine.
♦ An enzyme supplement (preferrably a plant-based enzyme formula that includes protease and amylase) to support digestion until healing is well progressed.
♦ Permavite powder from Allergy Research Group (see appendix); also trace minerals, folic acid, Vitamins A, B complex, B_6, gamma-orazinol, Robert's formula, and Seacure.
♦ *Herbs* include DGL, nettles, and aloe vera (liquid or gel).

COMPLEMENTARY THERAPIES

Complementary therapies include acupuncture and in some cases EPD allergy therapy (see Chapter 38). To allow the body to heal fully, also consider the usefulness of stress management and gentle exercise, as well as Reiki or massage therapy.

On a gluten-free diet, symptoms typically abate in six months, and some people see major improvement in three to four months. The most important actions are getting an accurate diagnosis and then avoiding all wheat products.

CIRRHOSIS

Also see the section on Liver Disease.

Cirrhosis is a chronic liver disorder involving damage to liver cells and scarring of liver tissue (fibrotic tissue), decreased blood flow, and the development of abnormal nodules that interfere with liver function. Symptoms include jaundice, ascites (the accumulation of fluid in the body cavity), and eventually liver failure.

MAJOR CAUSES

♦ *Alcoholism.* Among people with alcohol addiction, almost half eventually develop cirrhosis. Both genetics and lifestyle appear to be factors in the development of this condition. Women have a greater susceptibility to this condition because their livers are smaller.

♦ *Chemical and drug overload* can overwork the liver's capacity causing scarring.

♦ *Viral hepatitis* B and C, chronic active hepatitis, and autoimmune hepatitis.

◆ *Autoimmune conditions* include biliary cirrhosis, which can result from bile duct obstruction, and sarcoidosis, a condition that resembles tuberculosis which can cause cirrhosis.

◆ *Genetic factors* also play a role in cirrhosis, such as excess deposits of the mineral copper in the liver (Wilson's disease); excess iron deposits in the liver; an enzyme that inhibits the protein trypsin, sometimes causing cirrhosis and respiratory disease (alpha-antitrypsin deficiency); cystic fibrosis, which can cause enzyme deficiencies leading to cirrhosis; and glycogen storage disease, a rare inherited condition.

◆ *Heart failure* can cause blood to pool in the liver; this congestion can cause cirrhosis

PHYSICAL FINDINGS
◆ Enlargement of the parotid gland in the cheek
◆ Weight loss and muscle atrophy
◆ Weakness, fatigue
◆ DuPuytren—contractures of the palm or reddening of the palm
◆ Arterial spiders—red marks on face or chest and neck
◆ Enlarged breasts in males (gynecomastia) because cirrhosis changes the metabolism and affects hormone levels, increasing estrogen and decreasing testosterone
◆ Diminutia—chest and pubic hair are decreased in males, again due to the hormonal imbalance

TESTING
◆ Early intervention is possible through alternative functional testing—the liver detox profile (See Chapter 17).
◆ Conventional liver test (which assesses enzyme levels) and looks for elevated transaminase, bilirubin, and a decrease of albumin in the blood
◆ Antibody tests for hepatitis B and C
◆ ANA Test (antinuclear antibody) for autoimmune hepatitis, which untreated can cause cirrhosis
◆ AMA Test (antimitochondrial antibodies) for antibodies associated with biliary cirrhosis (in about 90 percent of cases)
◆ Serum iron levels—test for elevated levels of iron in the liver (hemochromatosis)
◆ Ultrasound can demonstrate nodules in the liver
◆ CT scan can confirm diagnosis by recording density of the scar tissue

- Liver biopsies tend to be accurate in 98 percent of cases when done by laparoscopy but tend to be too expensive and invasive
- Needle biopsy (without laparoscopy) is about 75 percent accurate

MAINSTREAM TREATMENT

- Rest and repair—avoid all toxins such as drugs, alcohol, and chemical exposure
- Drug and alcohol abstinence
- Hemochromatosis can be treated by extensive blood draws to decrease the iron load
- Wilson's Disease—penicillamine removes copper by chelating it, drawing it out of the liver
- Autoimmune conditions are treated with corticosteroids or nutritional medicine
- Biliary cirrhosis is treated with bile salts such as Urso and Actigall with or without the addition of the drug methotrexate to calm the immune system
- Colchicine, used for gout, has been found helpful in alcoholic cirrhosis because it helps reduce scar tissue
- Liver transplantation is effective in 70 percent to 80 percent of cases
- Unfortunately, there are often not enough livers to go around

ALTERNATIVE TREATMENTS

Nutrition amd Vitamins

- Good nutrition is essential—a diet lower in fat, high in protein (70 to 90 grams protein daily) and complex carbohydrates
- Antioxidants
- SAM—S-adenosyl-methionine, a specific biochemical that acts as a powerful free-radical squelcher, particularly useful for liver disease and related conditions.
- The amino acid family of nutrients
- Decrease copper in copper-excess forms of cirrhosis
- Be sure to avoid supplements that contain iron in iron-excess forms of cirrhosis

Herbs

Herbs applied in the treatment of alcoholism include:

- Silymarin (milk thistle) is known as a potent liver healer
- Dandelion
- Chinese herbs such as schizandra, especially for hepatitis B and C

- Systemic Formulas—L-Liver and also Systemic Forumula #5 which acts as a stabilizer
- Turmeric is a secondary herb (less potent but helpful)

(See also Chapter 37 on herbs. Check the section on liver-support herbs.)

COMPLEMENTARY THERAPIES
- Acupuncture
- For detailed treatment information, see the section in this appendix on Liver Disease, with additional information on supplements, acupuncture, detoxification, chelation therapy, and new treatments.

RESOURCES
Bland, Jeffery, *The 20-Day Rejuvenation Diet Program* (Keats, 1997). This book provides insight into liver function and its role as one of the most important organs of the body, including recent research, and information on how to optimize liver function.

CONSTIPATION (Chronic)

Constipation is defined as a decrease in the frequency of bowel movements accompanied by prolonged or difficult passage of stool. It is a symptom complex, not a disease. In other words, it is a dysfunction of the body and can be caused by a number of diseases or imbalances.

There is no rule for the optimal number of daily or weekly bowel movements. However, for research criteria, two or fewer bowel movements a week are considered constipation.

MAINSTREAM DIAGNOSIS AND TESTING
- Obstructions from colon cancer or stricture must be ruled out through examination by colonoscopy or barium enema. The minimal direct exam should include the lower sigmoid colon by sigmoidoscopy.
- Colonic transit time is a useful supplementary test. (See chapter 14 for further information.)
- Since low thyroid production can be a cause of chronic constipation, lab testing of blood for thyroid status is a useful initial screening.
- Stool analysis. Sometimes stool volume and frequency can be measured, especially in hospitals. The stool can be weighed and the moisture calculated.
- Evaluations using the pelvic floor EMG, which uses a sensor to

provide information on the dynamics of the colon as well as the sphincter relaxation and pelvic floor function.

♦ A defogram is a special type of X-ray that records a bowel movement, also called a defecatory exam. The video-proctogram is an X-ray video that provides information on the workings of the lower colon. It can measure the anal-rectal angle, sphincter contraction, and the activity of the muscles used in evacuation.

♦ Physicians who suspect laxative overuse sometimes order a stool exam to detect the presence of laxative preparations. A stool evaluation with phenolphthalein is a dye test that can detect the presence of Ex-Lax. Magnesium from milk of magnesia is measured in a blood sample. To save time and money, be honest with your doctor about your habits and whether you use laxatives. That way you can work together to solve your problem.

COMPLEMENTARY TESTING

Problems from Infection

Constipation can also accompany infection by parasites, bacteria, or yeast. In a survey performed by Leo Galland, M.D., in his New York City practice, of 100 patients with giardia, 40 percent indicated constipation with no diarrhea as a symptom.

♦ *Antibody testing* for parasites, yeast, or bacterial overgrowth by a simple test in saliva or blood (Immunosciences Lab).

♦ *Stool testing for parasites*, bacteria (both aerobic and anaerobic), or yeast overgrowth by a lab that specializes in this type of testing. Stool testing should be performed by a lab that has the special expertise necessary for good detection such as a university lab or a private lab such as Diagnostic Labs.

♦ *The comprehensive diagnostic stool analysis* (CDSA), based on stool samples, provides a profile of fat absorption and bacterial flora. It also rules out parasites and includes information to some extent on how well food is and is not digested.

♦ *Testing for the overgrowth of bacteria* through chemical markers called organic acids (Great Plains Lab and Metametrix). (See also Chapter 21 on microbes and bad bugs.)

Nutritional Deficiencies

♦ *Profile of nutrient status* to detect any major deficiencies that might be causing constipation. Vitamins Diagnostics and Body-Bio, both in New Jersey, are respected labs. (See Resources.)

♦ *Magnesium-calcium levels.* Inadequate levels of magnesium in the body can also cause constipation. Therefore testing for low magnesium levels is an important initial evaluation. Elevated calcium levels can also be a cause of constipation. Testing is performed on blood.

MAINSTREAM AND COMPLEMENTARY TREATMENTS

Treatment primarily consists of increasing liquids and increasing fiber. Both mainstream and complementary practitioners favor these solutions. Note that both medical traditions also identify laxative overuse as a problem (over-the-counter products *and* herbs).

Diet Therapy

Liquids should not be sweet; fruit juices should be kept to a minimum and diluted half with clear water. Best choices include spring or mineral water, lemon water (hot or cold), herbal tea (hot or iced).

Fibers include soluble fibers, such as:

♦ Psyllium seed (available in health food stores under a variety of brand names and in drugstores as Metamucil (which typically contains added sweetener). Psyllium is helpful to some, but even as a fine powder, can cause problems if there are allergies or major inflammation.

♦ Wheat bran is helpful to some because of its iron content, but too rough for those with inflammation, and potentially harmful to those with celiac disease, an allergy to wheat protein.

♦ Oat bran and baby oat bran are favored by some, and known as a reducer of cholesterol, but will cause reactions in those with overgrowth of bacteria, yeast, or parasites and carbohydrates intolerance.

♦ Flaxseeds can provide a good source of fiber. They can be used in several ways: sprinkled on food, they have a nutty flavor (try about two tablespoons); they can be eaten in the morning as a kind of aromatic cereal—pour boiling water over two to four tablespoons of the seeds, cover, and let steep for about five minutes. If whole flax are too irritating, the seeds can be ground into a powder that can be added to juice, milk, or food—whatever is tolerated. If inflammation is extreme, try a more mucilaginous substance such as slippery elm or aloe vera.

♦ Cellulose is a nonsoluble fiber helpful in some cases. In pharmacies, available as FiberCon and from nutrient companies, found in Permavite (which contains cellulose and a formula of supportive nutrients) available from Allergy Research Group.

MAINSTREAM TREATMENTS

Medications and therapeutics include:

♦ Betalactulose (Chronulac), an absorbable sugar that promotes bowel movements. Available by prescription only.

♦ Calcium polycarbophil (Equalactin) holds liquid in a sponge-like action that encourages motility; it also increases hydration of the stool.

♦ Magnesium can be useful, including milk of magnesia. Magnesium chloride is also available in an enteric-coated tablet as Slow Mag. Magnesium stimulates muscle contraction and peristalsis throughout the intestines and hydrates the stool.

♦ There is prokinetic medication that stimulates the smooth muscles of the colon by stimulating the serotonin receptors in the GI tract (Procalopride). Propulsid also stimulates the serotonin receptors.

SURGERY

♦ Sometimes surgery is performed in cases of severe constipation, which we call colonic inertia, when there is really no motility of colon. Some patients have had to have subtotal or total colectomy. We are hoping that in the future, this type of treatment can be avoided through magnetic therapy and other forms of noninvasive systemic therapy.

♦ Sphincterotomy involves the removal of a strip of the muscle from the lower sphincter when there is an outlet obstruction problem, which can be diagnosed with the radiopaque markers and EMG tests. This surgery removes a centimeter-wide bit of muscle from the upper sphincter and 8 centimeters from the distal rectum.

♦ Impaction can require a nonsurgical medical procedure in the emergency room. Be sure to monitor a tendency toward constipation and see the doctor before things get this serious.

COMPLEMENTARY TREATMENTS

Nutritional and Herbal Supplements

♦ Fiber is essential. Include fresh fruits and vegetables, but monitor for carbohydrate intolerance.

♦ Alkalinize the body. A salad a day can provide additional wholesome fiber. If inflammation is a problem, try butter lettuce or juice your vegetables). (See Chapter 30 for more on alkaline diets.)

♦ Increase *omega-3 fatty acids* (*flaxseeds or flax meal*), make the effort to get off laxatives, and retrain the bowel. Flaxseeds can be ground in a coffee grinder to create a powdered meal or prepared by steeping covered in boiling water for five minutes.

◆ Avoid frequent use of senna or cascara sagrada because they tend to lead to laxative abuse.

◆ *Aloe vera* as a laxative can be quite helpful, in capsule form. Try two at bedtime. Some people respond to the juice or gel.

◆ *Yellow dock* is a mild herbal laxative that can also be used in combination with aloe vera. Consider all laxatives temporary measures.

◆ *Magnesium* is useful, but in high doses is known to cause "a precipitous cleanse"—the very rapid propulsion of the stool when it finally works, which can be unpredictable and as much as six hours later, so use it at a time when you don't need to leave home. This is also true of cascara sagrada.

◆ Sometimes a lot of *vitamin C* can be useful. Vitamin C can be taken in high doses of up to 10 grams a day. Taking vitamin C "to bowel tolerance" means taking 1,000 or 2,000 mg every two hours until diarrhea occurs. That indicates the maximum dose. At that point, scale back from that dose and try it at the more moderate level for several days to determine if symptoms improve. Do not remain on these high doses indefinitely due to the occasional potential of kidney stones.

◆ *MSM (methyl-sulfonyl-methane)* works well for constipation in some cases; this is a mild mineral supplement of a sulfur derivative in capsule form.

◆ *Slippery elm* is a soothing natural fiber somewhat like flaxseed that creates a gelatin-like substance and encourages motility; available in capsules or bulk.

◆ *Bentonite clay* can be helpful for periodic cleanses. As it moves through the body, it mechanically absorbs material from the lining of the GI tract, so it is believed to draw and remove some of the bacteria or parasites adhering to the GI lining. However, it also absorbs minerals, so it should not be used for more than a month at a time. Sonne #7 is a highly respected brand of bentonite. Important: Be sure to take enough liquid with it, or constipation could become worsened and it could even cause impaction.

◆ *Take probiotics.* Better bowel flora increases motility. Types of flora that seem to provide a good response include: *Lactobacillus acidophilus* (DDS strain by Natren); bifidobacteria, and soil-based protolytic bacteria (Prime Defense). After antibiotics, consider taking the beneficial yeast *Saccharomyces boulardii*. Optimally, take one container of probiotics supplements and then have your stool reanalyzed with a CDSA.

Colonics and Enemas

Some people will need periodic enema therapy, but we do not recommend it indefinitely. Enemas mean that natural function has not resumed. If there is infection present, reinfection can occur and can also be spread to other members of the household when they come in contact with microscopic remnants of fecal matter.

Sometimes people really do feel benefit from a colonic session. However, periodically, people are infected through colonic therapy. Since the procedure is quite invasive for a nonsurgical treatment, it is important that cleanliness be paramount and that disposable speculums and tubing be used.

Conventional medicine uses a liquid preparation to clear the colon in preparation for GI examinations. These liquids can be taken as an emergency measure. They are called CoLyte and GoLytely and are available from pharmacies with a prescription from your doctor. They can be used with the monitoring of your physician until normal function returns. They can also be taken during a detoxification regimen.

COMPLEMENTARY THERAPIES

♦ *EMG biofeedback* and pelvic flow retraining.

♦ *Gentle exercise* such as Qigong, tai chi, and yoga. Exercise with machines that work the abdominal muscles (the abs) or gentle crunches with knees bent to protect the back and sciatic nerves. Walking is useful, although surprisingly it does not help everyone.

♦ *Acupuncture*

♦ *Energy work* on the abdomen for irritable bowel. Abdominal massage can be used in some cases if it helps. If not, explore other therapies.

♦ *Magnetic therapy* can be used, in which one wears a large magnet (the back flex) on the abdomen or sleeps on a magnetic sleep pad.

CROHN'S DISEASE

See Inflammatory Bowel Disease (IBD).

DIARRHEA (Chronic)

An abnormally frequent discharge of semi-solid or fluid fecal matter from the bowel. Diarrhea is a symptom rather than a specific disease. It can result from deranged motility or from infection by bacteria or parasites or from chronic inflammation. Diarrhea can cause additional problems such as the malabsorption of nutrients and the inability to absorb water from the colon.

CAUSES

◆ *Bacteria* can trigger diarrhea; offenders include toxigenic *E. coli,* salmonella, shigella, campylobacter, staphylococcus, and *Clostridium difficile.* These bacterial infections are often described as food poisoning.

◆ *Following antibiotics,* an overgrowth of yeast or toxic bacteria can cause diarrhea.

◆ *Viruses* include rotavirus, Norwalk agent, and *Enteric adenovirus,* which often accompanies colds, with symptoms that resemble flu.

◆ *Parasitic infections*—microscopic parasites that can cause infection include giardia, amoebas such as *E. histolytica* and *D. fragilis,* cryptosporidium, cyclospora, microspora, and *Blastocystis hominis.*

◆ *Travelers diarrhea*—parasitic infections and bacteria such as toxigenic *E. coli* and cholera can cause diarrhea in travelers to foreign countries where sanitation and food preparation may expose travelers to pathogens, particularly those for which no immunity has been developed. Tropical pathogens tend to be more virulent and harmful than those of temperate climates. This actually occurs frequently here in the U.S. as well.

◆ *Marine toxins*—ciguatera toxins in fish poisoning from jack fish, mackerel, and other sources.

◆ *Tuberculosis* can affect the GI tract through raw, unpasteurized milk.

◆ *Changes in the intestinal tract due to surgery*—removal of a portion of the small or large bowel or intestinal bypass.

Diarrheal infections are typically contracted through food, water, or fecal/oral transmission from food handlers; from people in contact with stool such as day care workers; transmission in school or institutional settings; from eating spoiled food (don't keep any food longer than two to three days); and from intimate contact with someone who already has an infection.

SYMPTOMS

◆ *Watery diarrhea,* abdominal cramping, heavy fatigue/malaise, fever.

◆ *Bloody diarrhea* can be caused by amoebas, campylobacter, salmonella, shigella, and toxigenic *E. coli*. If you have bloody diarrhea, see a doctor as soon as possible.

In general, diarrhea tends to be self-limiting. Self-medicate if diarrhea is not bloody, your temperature is below 102, and your immunity is strong. Keep fluids up and replace electrolyes: Pedialyte, available in most drugstores, is a good source. If diarrhea persists beyond seven days, be sure to see a doctor.

DIAGNOSIS

◆ *Antibody testing* can be exceptionally helpful (see Immunosciences Lab in the Resources at the end of the book).

◆ *Stool cultures*. Three samples are best, each taken 48 hours apart. Many labs are not trained in the detection of these microbes. Send to a university lab or a lab with specialized expertise such as Diagnostic Labs (see Resources).

Stool cultures should include testing for yeast, which can play a role in diarrhea. Patients with heavy overgrowth of yeast tend to develop toxigenic diarrhea and may have ongoing inflammation. In severe chronic cases, colonoscopic or sigmoidoscopic exam with biopsy is necessary to identify the inflammation.

MAINSTREAM TREATMENTS

◆ *Rest*. In severe cases of diarrhea, it may become essential to rest the gut with parenteral intravenous nutrition.

◆ *Medications*. Antibiotics can be given for persistent diarrhea to eradicate pathogens: ciprofloxin (Cipro), ampicillin (Amoxicillin), or other broad-spectrum antibiotics, as well as metronidazole (Flagyl). Calcium polycarbophil (Equalactin) is used for loose but not watery diarrhea. The choice of medication is based on either:

—Sensitivity testing in the lab (which identifies the drugs that will destroy the pathogen)
—A review of the current medical literature on Medline to identify the medications currently successful against a particular microbe, compared with your history of response to drugs.

◆ *Drugs to slow motility*. Imodium or Lomotil are sometimes used to slow motility and decrease water secretion, but they should not be used until *after* you have had a stool culture. The diarrhea is the body's way of washing pathogens out of the GI tract. Slowing motility when there is a pathogenic infection blocks the body's way to remove the pathogen. Slowing motility can prolong the infection.

♦ *Antitoxin drugs.* The medications Questran or cholestyramine are drugs that bind the toxins produced by pathogens such as *C. difficile.* Drugs are currently in development for the toxins produced by cholera bacteria and toxigenic *E. coli.*

♦ *Oral gamma globulin.* Immune antibodies are found in preparations from the health food store such as colostrum and in UltraFlora Plus available from Metagenics (a concentrate of globulin protein from whey, lactobacillus NCFM strain, bifidobacteria, FOS, and rice malto-dextrin). These preparations may be used in cases of diarrhea from infectious agents because they interfere with adherence of the microbe to the GI wall.

COMPLEMENTARY TREATMENT

Remove the cause:

♦ *Remove any pathogenic microbes (bacteria, yeast, parasites).*

♦ *Remove any foods from the diet that may be causing an allergy,* sensitivity, or intolerance or which are difficult to digest or absorb. (See Chapters 8 and 20 on allergies.)

♦ As a rule, stop dairy products and wheat. If diarrhea or sensitivities continue, seek comprehensive allergy testing. With a dairy allergy, diarrhea can sometimes wash away the source of lactase, the enzyme that digests milk. In some cases, the enzymes to digest milk don't return, or at least not immediately. With a wheat allergy or celiac disease, diarrhea can be a primary symptom.

Replace digestants:

♦ *Replace digestants whose secretion may have been slowed by the presence of the pathogen, such as digestive enzymes,* which can be supplemented through a multiple enzyme formula. It may also be necessary to supplement hydrochloric acid production with betaine hydrochloride. If impairment is significant, a useful strategy is to support pancreatic function with pancreas glandulars. Another secretion that can become depleted over time includes intrinsic factor (a protein essential for the absorption of vitamin B_{12}).

Restore flora:

♦ *Restore beneficial flora (particularly acidophilus).* Good bacteria include acidophilus, bifidobacteria, *Saccharomyces boulardii* (a beneficial yeast available from Pure Encapsulation and Thorne). Real cultured yogurt tends to be good (for example, the brand Brown Cow, which includes bifidus cultures).

Repair:

Repair refers to nutritional support for healing and regenerating the GI mucosa. A list of beneficial nutrients follows; select those most relevant to your needs or work with your physician in designing an individualized program in response to testing for deficiencies.

♦ Vitamin A or beta-carotene for the differentiation, growth and function of the GI lining.

♦ A good multivitamin.

♦ Vitamin B_5 (pantothenic acid), which stimulates protein synthesis.

♦ Vitamin C helps in collagen formation.

♦ Vitamin E (alpha-tocopherol), an important antioxidant, essential to the integrity of GI mucosal cell membranes.

♦ Zinc is involved in enzyme function, in the structure of cell membranes, and in replication of cells, so it's important in the repair of the GI lining and works with vitamin A.

♦ Trace minerals to minimize inflammation.

♦ Pepto-Bismol (the mineral bismuth) or the generic version helps prevent bacteria from adhering to the wall of the gut—taken 20 minutes before meals.

♦ L-glutamine, an amino acid, is the preferred fuel for the small intestinal lining cells (enterocytes); include trace minerals as cofactors to optimize the L-glutamine.

♦ Inulin in capsule form stimulates the production of butyrate by the friendly flora. Inulin has an insulin-like activity, that helps the transfer of glucose across the cell membrane.

♦ Butyrate nourishes the lining cells of the large intestine (colonocytes).

♦ Short-chain fatty acids (omega-3s) flaxseed and cod-liver oils act as anti-inflammatories.

♦ Omega-6s—black currant seed oil, borage, and primrose cut down on inflammation. (See information on fatty acids, Chapter 25).

♦ Glutathione, taken with the precursors N-acetyl cysteine and cysteine, which all provide molecular fuel for detoxification pathways.

♦ Bioactive peptides like Seacure help with the rebuilding process.

♦ UltraClear Sustain, which is rice based, to provide additional nourishment while minimizing allergic responses.

♦ Colostrum supplement. If you are milk-tolerant, colostrum is a supplement that contains anti-toxigenic antibodies (IgG) extracted from cow's milk. If well tolerated, this product tends to speed healing.

HERBS

Anti-inflammatory herbs that are mild and mucilaginous include aloe vera, slippery elm, and flaxseeds (ground). They may supplement the mucus action of the gut. Products that contain pectin also promote mucous action, firm the stool, and provide soluble fiber. Primary herbs helpful with diarrhea include: ginger (in capsules, liquid tincture, or tea), garlic, oil of oregano (in capsules), black tea (for its astringent properties), dried oak bark (use in powdered form, as a tea), fenugreek, and psyllium. Secondary herbs include red raspberry leaf, bayberry root bark, goldenseal and cinnamon in small doses, geranium root, carob, chamomile, and marshmallow root.

COMPLEMENTARY THERAPIES

♦ *Homeopathic treatment* is well documented to be a significant strategy against diarrhea, and has been successful even against cholera. If you are extremely or chronically ill and want to use homeopathy, have the remedy prescribed for you by a well-trained homeopathic physician. This is especially important if your fever is over 102°, if you have bloody diarrhea, or your condition has persisted more than seven days. If the episode seems mild, give your vital force a boost with one of these noninvasive remedies (see Chapter 41). However, should your symptoms grow worse or persist, be sure to call your doctor immediately.

♦ *Acupuncture*, if you can leave home.

DIVERTICULOSIS AND DIVERTICULITIS

Diverticulosis consists of pockets that occur in the wall of the colon, in which the wall is stretched and bubbled due to a rupture (herniated tissue). It occurs primarily in the descending colon (the sigmoid), which is on the left side of the body.

When the muscle of the colon wall is weakened, the pressure can produce a hernia in the wall of the gut, particularly in places where the blood vessels penetrate through the muscular wall. This has been found to be due to imbalanced pressure in the colon, which can result from a diet low in fiber.

Diverticulitis occurs when there is infection and inflammation in the pockets or herniated sacs.

Half the U.S. population over 40 have one of these conditions. They are diseases of Western civilization, believed to be due to the refined diet of industrial nations, low in fiber and high in sugars. It has been observed that people in non-Western cultures eating a high fiber diet have no incidence of this disease.

CAUSES

This condition can result from poor diet and also is associated with processes that occur in the body due to aging. As we age, there is a change in the ecology of the gut bacteria, with a loss of the beneficial bacteria (lactobacillus and bifidobacteria). As a result, when refined sugar and starches are eaten, an overgrowth of harmful bacteria can occur. This can cause an increase in bloating and gas, which raises the pressure in the colon.

Pancreatic enzymes also decrease as we age, so that starches and sugars are digested less efficiently, another contributor to bloating, gas, and increased pressure. Decline in good quality collagen can occur with aging or poor nutrition. Note that many people have both irritable bowel and low-grade diverticulitis. Delayed food allergies may be an element in triggering diverticular spasm. Not drinking enough fluid is another factor.

SYMPTOMS

Diverticulosis often causes no symptoms whatsoever. Nonspecific complaints can be associated with it, such as gas, constipation or diarrhea, abdominal pain, or bloating.

Diverticulitis occurs when there is a high degree of inflammation. Features of this inflammation may include detectable pain, occasionally a fever or bleeding and a change in bowel habits. Testing will show a high sedimentation rate, a reflection of the level of active antibodies in the bloodstream and therefore the degree of inflammation. Sometimes this can produce the symptoms of appendicitis, called left-sided appendicitis.

Divericulitis with bleeding should be considered a medical emergency.

TESTING

+ Testing for sedimentation rate
+ CBC—a white blood count to check for the presence of infection and other markers of illness
+ A physical exam to check for tenderness in the abdomen
+ Other testing may include the barium enema, a CT scan, or a colon-

oscopy. Note to doctors: In the barium enema process, Swedish research has found that methyl-cellulose enemas are more useful in the diagnosis of diverticulosis.

◆ Helical CT scans offer increased sensitivity in the detection of inflammation.

MAINSTREAM TREATMENTS

◆ Antibiotics such as Cipro and Flagyl are given orally if the condition is mild or intravenously if it is severe. There may be a need to be treated with nystatin afterward. It is essential that all antibiotic therapies are followed with probiotics taken for several weeks.

◆ When there is recurrent or frequent diverticulosis, a partial colectomy may be indicated, especially in cases where there is continual bleeding or when the condition is severe and the patient is not responding to treatment. Provide support to the immune system and IV antibiotics before considering surgery.

◆ For mild conditions, antispasmodic drugs such as hycosamine sulfate (Levsin-SL) or dicyclomine (Bentyl) have been found helpful.

DIET

Eliminate sugar and other refined sweeteners and starches that might feed bacteria (such as pastas, bread, potatoes, and corn). The earlier approach to this condition was to eliminate high fiber foods that might get caught in the diverticular pockets, such as seeds, corn, and nuts. However, we now recommend a high fiber diet, which does not appear to trigger the inflammation because it does not feed the harmful bacteria. In addition, be sure to drink enough water (at least 6 to 8 glasses a day) so that stool does not become too dry, which could then become caught in the diverticular pockets.

NUTRIENTS

For inflammation, consider the use of:

◆ Trace minerals (zinc, copper, manganese, and magnesium can become significantly depleted)
◆ Vitamin C and the other antioxidants
◆ A multiple-enzyme product, plus additional bromalin
◆ Cod-liver oil or fish oil (in lemon flavor or in capsules) contains vitamin A (also DHA and EPA)
◆ UltraClear Sustain, a powdered low-allergenic dietary supplement from Metagenics
◆ Butyrate, an essential fatty acid and an effective colon fuel

- Inulin helps the body produce butyrate (found in Jerusalem artichokes)
- Butyrate enemas have been effective and can be obtained from a compounding pharmacy (see Resources)

HERBAL REMEDIES
- Alternative therapies to control the inflammation include herbal combinations that decrease the harmful gut bacteria, such as Microdex (from Metagenics)
- Aloe vera (juice, capsules, or gel meant for internal use) as an anti-inflammatory; slippery elm; psyllium; powdered flax meal (but not the whole seed); Seacure; or garlic oil in capsules
- In mild to moderate cases, antispasmodic herbs such as peppermint, spearmint, deglycrrhizinated licorice (DGL), and hawthorn may also be helpful
- In some cases, curcumin

COMPLEMENTARY THERAPIES
- *Massage.* Visceral manipulation seems helpful in painful types of diverticulosis; this can be done by a physical therapist. Shirley Trickett recommends solar plexus massage in her book *The Irritable Bowel Syndrome and Diverticulosis: A Self-Help Plan* (Thorsons, 1990, pp. 106–107). Chi ne sang is a helpful form of visceral massage. Both approaches should be focused on maintaining peristalsis.
- *Exercise.* Use yoga, gentle exercise, or walking to keep the peristalsis moving.
- *Stress reduction.* Hypnosis and self-hypnosis and other stress reduction techniques are helpful, because of the inflammatory nature of this condition.
- *Acupuncture* has been specifically used for both diverticulosis and diverticulitis. Specific points for diverticulosis and diverticulitis, especially in the mild form, are included in textbooks on acupressure and acupuncture. In mild cases, self-applied acupressure can be used or Acu-Stim can be performed with a small electromagnetic unit. The Solitens is a medical device that can be ordered with a prescription from a physician, from Nikken—888-264-5536—order #1322. A good guiding text is K. Serizawa, *Tsubo*, 2nd ed. (Japan Publications, 1995).

DYSPEPSIA—Without Ulcers

This diagnosis describes any upper GI conditions that typically include indigestion or heartburn and ulcer-like symptoms without evidence of an ulcer. In nonulcerative dyspepsia, there is no localized inflammation or ulcerated crater visible in an endoscopic exam. This condition may be the equivalent of irritable bowel syndrome in the upper digestive tract; there is no clear cause but there is evidence of dysfunction. Nonulcerative dyspepsia is also called NUD. Symptoms include belching, bloating, pain, or discomfort after eating. Dyspepsia may be a catch-all category for a number of frequently occurring subtle conditions.

DIAGNOSIS

This disease is defined by ruling out organic disease. Likewise, this diagnosis is applied if no reflux of the esophagus and no *H. pylori* infection are detected. Previously, *H. pylori* infection was suspected to be the cause, but recent studies have shown that treating this form of dyspepsia as if it were an *H. pylori* infection produced no improvement.

CONVENTIONAL TESTING

♦ *A viral infection* of the intestinal tract can cause a motility disorder. Symptoms of diarrhea, flatulence, bloating, or other GI symptoms may follow the infection. Titers for antibody response to the virus can confirm this (Immunosciences Lab).

♦ *Acid levels* are tested to rule out hyperacidity and peptic ulcer disease. A gastric capsule or nasogastric tube can measure the acidity (pH) with a pH meter.

♦ *Abnormal gastric pacemaker evaluated by EGG.* Nonulcer dyspepsia may be a motility disorder of the stomach in some cases. A study of nonulcerative dyspepsia by Ken Koch, M.D., at Penn State Medical Center in which this author participated involved the following: An electrogastrogram (an EGG, the equivalent of an EKG of the stomach) was used to evaluate patients with symptoms of nausea or bloating. It was found that these patients often had an abnormal gastric cycle. There is normally a housekeeping rhythm of the stomach of 3 cycles per minute. These are electrical and muscular waves that help the digestion and churning of food into smaller particles. In these patients there were often cycles that were too slow (1 to 2 cycles per minute) or too rapid (6 to 10 per minute). Therapy for this consisted of low-dose cisapride (Propulsid), a prokinetic medication of 5 mg to stimulate stomach motility. Diabetic patients with delayed emptying were given doses of 10 to 20 mg.

♦ *Small bowel motility study* at a tertiary care or major medical center may be required in some patients.

FUNCTIONAL TESTING

◆ *Flora balance.* Any motility disorder changes the flora balance, which can also affect the intestinal transit. Check through a comprehensive diagnostic stool analysis (see Chapter 17).

◆ *Bacterial overgrowth* of pathogenic organisms can also occur following antibiotic therapy or steroid therapy. This can be confirmed by testing for Organic Acids, which evaluates the by-products of the bacteria. Available from Metametrix Laboratories or Great Plains Lab.

◆ *Liver detox panel* may also detect the presence of an increased toxic load on the liver from the gut, causing chronic depletion from the effort of detoxification (see Chapter 17).

MAINSTREAM TREATMENT

◆ Low-dose cisapride (Propulsid)
◆ Multiple small meals
◆ Stress reduction
◆ Anti-nausea medications

NUTRITIONAL THERAPY

◆ *Remove infection* by microbes (typically with prescription medication in combination with or alternating with herbal remedies.

◆ *Detect and remove any offending allergic foods* through careful self-monitoring for reactivity or blood testing for allergies.

◆ *Replace digestants.*

◆ *Restore flora.*

◆ *Repair GI lining* with nutrients and anti-inflammatories.

◆ Nutrients include pyridoxal phosphate, a form of vitamin B_6, found to help with nausea; be sure to take a vitamin B complex supplement as well.

◆ Include a balance of vitamins, minerals, and magnesium.

◆ Pepto-Bismol (bismuth) may be helpful in cases where there is an undetected *H. pylori* infection.

◆ Herbs that might help include: peppermint; licorice and DGL; aloe for inflammation; ginger for nausea; slippery elm.

COMPLEMENTARY THERAPIES

◆ *Acupuncture* can be used to treat nausea and possibly normalize the gastric pacemaker rate.

◆ *Magnet therapy* uses a strip over the pacemaker area of the stomach that entrains the rate and normalizes pacemaker function.

◆ *Stress reduction* to allow the immune system to participate in healing, including yoga, hypnotherapy, biofeedback, exercise, and music therapy. These can be helpful as stress reducers, which can bring about indirect improvement, since stress makes everything worse.

DISORDERS of the ESOPHAGUS

See Reflux.

FISSURES

A fissure is a cut in the skin lining the anal canal, usually in the internal portion of the canal, but occasionally in the anal opening. Its symptoms are pain and bleeding, in some cases following constipation.

Possible causes for fissures include anal trauma or extreme constipation with large stools that tear the skin. Chronic anal fissures are another class; when they persist more than a month, this indicates a problem of increased sphincter pressure, which implies the need for surgical treatment.

DIAGNOSIS

Anoscopy can find the tear in the bottom of the anal area. However, often examination under anesthesia is necessary. Anal-rectal manometry (EMG) can be used to measure pressure in the case of sphincter problems.

MEDICAL TREATMENT

- ◆ Warm sitz baths
- ◆ Astringents
- ◆ Ointments
- ◆ Topical low-dose nitroglycerin to relieve spasm of muscle
- ◆ Stool softeners
- ◆ Injection therapy
- ◆ Cauterizing the area with silver nitrate stick (performed by a physician as an office procedure)
- ◆ Chronic fissures may require a surgical excision to remove a portion of the sphincter muscle (sphincterotomy).

HERBAL THERAPY

For mild cases, take gotu cola or aloe vera, in conjunction with medical treatment.

FISTULAS

One or more tracts that drain from the anal canal. Fistulas most often occur in Crohn's disease, but can also be due to trauma, syphilis,

TB, radiation therapy, anal cancer, chlamydial infection, or anaerobic bacterial infection. Symptoms include drainage of pus from the area.

MEDICAL TREATMENT

- Surgical incision and drainage
- For Crohn's disease, treatment with metronidazole or Infliximab (which contains tumor necrosis antibodies, in a treatment targeted at the immune system) and requires an intravenous infusion, which is costly.
- Cases of chlamydia are treated with Bactrim.

HERBAL THERAPY

Treatment is with cleansing herbs, including gotu cola, aloe vera, chaparral (now off the restricted list) or red clover, goldenseal (not to be taken for more than three weeks at a time).

FOOD ALLERGIES

(See also Chapters 8 and 20 on Allergies.)

Symptoms can be virtually anything, and may include headaches, irritability, inappropriate weight gain, aching joints, diarrhea, or abdominal complaints.

DIAGNOSIS

- Elimination Diet
- IgG food allergy testing for delayed symptoms
- IgE testing for immediate food allergy

TREATMENT

- Remove the allergen, replace digestants, restore flora, repair the GI tract.
- *Medication:* Cromolyn sodium (Gastrochrom) can be taken before meals to block the release of histamine (from the mast cells, which are immune-reactive cells).
- *Supplements:* Bioflavonoids such as quercetin, vitamin C, and proanthanols such as grape seed tend to reduce allergic reactivity. MSM tends to decrease histamine release, the cause of many allergic symptoms.

COMPLEMENTARY THERAPIES

- *EPD allergy therapy* (see Chapter 38.) Additional information is available through the American EPD Society, in Sante Fe, New Mexico, at 505-983-8890.

◆ *NAET therapy.* In *The NAET Guidebook*, Debi Nambudripad, Ph.D., discusses applied kinesiology for use in allergy elimination. This is a specialized approach most often used by acupuncturists, which involves using acupuncture and acupressure.

◆ *Hyposensitization,* also known as provocative neutralization.

◆ *Homeopathy* can be helpful in treating allergies if it is provided by a knowledgeable practitioner.

GALLSTONES

The gallbladder is the reservoir for bile, which is a natural solvent within the body that helps to emulsify fat and digest it. Bile is a body chemical made from cholesterol that links with fat to assist in its transport from the digestive tract through the bloodstream into the cells for absorption.

The bile can clump into solid, stone-like formations that may lodge within the bile ducts, either as gallstones or as a sludge-like material that can interfere with the functioning of the gallbladder. An acute inflammation of the gallbladder (cholecystitis) can result due to the blockage and sometimes requires immediate surgery. In addition, when there is defective functioning, the gallbladder doesn't empty as well. This means there is poorer digestion of fats due to insufficient bile secretion.

INCIDENCE AND RISK FACTORS

◆ Rare under age 20.

◆ A gene has been identified that makes people more susceptible to gallbladder disease.

◆ Northern Europeans may have a higher incidence.

◆ Gallstones occur primarily in females, especially those that have been pregnant.

◆ Gallstones seem to accompany obesity.

◆ Rapid weight loss, particularly in previously obese women, puts them at higher risk.

◆ Those who consume a high fat diet have the highest incidence. This is because consuming a high fat diet saturates the bile, making it more likely to form stones. Example: In the Pima Indian peoples of California, 70 percent have gallstones, because of heredity and a diet high in saturated fats and starches. However, Pima Indians in Mexico, who are similar genetically, have a low incidence due to the difference in diet. Heredity is not destiny.

◆ Bacteria is implicated in the development of gallstones. They apparently can initiate the core formation of the stone, called the nidus.

◆ A gallstone with a different chemical makeup than that typically found in gallbladder conditions is associated with sickle-cell anemia and hemolytic anemia. This form is not cholesterol-based.

SIGNS AND SYMPTOMS

◆ Abdominal pain in the upper right area of the abdomen under the liver. The pain can radiate around to the back, especially the right shoulder blade. The pain is associated with eating fatty foods. Sometimes it may be just a dull ache or bloating after meals.

◆ Attacks of severe pain, with blockage, fever, and jaundice, can occur due to blocking of the bile ducts into the gut.

◆ Problems with motility of the bile duct and the gallbladder may be the issue, a condition which may be improved by taking drugs or nutrients that promote motility, such as magnesium or olive oil taken in small amounts to avoid a rapid gallbladder flush and a lodged stone.

◆ No symptoms—about half of the patients with gallstones will have no symptoms (are asymptomatic) and will be diagnosed through a routine screening.

◆ When there is long-standing untreated gallbladder inflammation, gallbladder cancer can occur.

DIAGNOSIS

◆ *Ultrasound* of the gallbladder has been the standard for several decades.

◆ *The biliary scan* is a scan using a radioactive material that is then excreted from the liver into the gallbladder. This test can be useful in diagnosis when the ultrasound does not show a gallstone but the symptoms are present. The scan measures emptying time using a hormone called CCK, which empties the gallbladder. Doctors also monitor for pain during the test as a symptom. This delay in emptying is often misinterpreted as a symptom of gallbladder disease, especially in cases of irritable bowel syndrome. The customary solution is the removal of the gallbladder, only to have the symptoms return in a month or two. If gallbladder removal is recommended based on delayed emptying, we encourage you to seek a second opinion from a gastroenterologist.

◆ *ERCP* is a multifaceted procedure involving the endoscope and an injection of dye into the gallbladder, which makes it possible to detect gallstones in the ducts. If stones are detected, it is possible to open the ducts surgically to remove the stone.

SURGERY

◆ Surgery is now frequently used to remove the gallbladder (cholecystectomy). Laparoscopic removal of the gallbladder is the most frequently performed procedure. This surgery is delicate and complicated and should be performed by a surgeon highly familiar with this specific operation. After laparoscopy, stones may recur in the remaining ducts. At that point, the ERCP procedure can later be used to remove stones, using endoscopy for stone extraction.

◆ The disadvantages to removing the gallbladder are that bile salts are no longer concentrated in the gallbladder so they can cause a bile diarrhea. When bile comes directly out of the liver, the small intestine must adapt, which it eventually does. Postsyndrome diarrhea can last for six to twelve months after surgery. Of those who have their gallbladder removed, 25 percent will have some symptoms following surgery. Questran is a bile resin that may help with diarrhea.

◆ Post-cholecystectomy syndrome can often trigger or worsen irritable bowel syndrome.

◆ Alternative surgical treatment—Lithotripsy is a treatment infrequently done in certain cases, in which sound waves are used to smash the gallstone, while the patient is under anesthesia, similar to the procedure for kidney stones.

MEDICATION

Urso and Actigall are the two primary drugs used in gallbladder therapy. Surgery is a more frequently used option because drug therapy can take up to two years and not fully dissolve all the stones. Small amounts of Urso (bear bile from Chinese medicine) or aspirin have been found to protect against the development of gallstones, by reducing the saturation of the bile.

COMPLEMENTARY TREATMENTS

Naturopaths do a gallbladder flush typically using olive oil. This approach appears to work better for sludge or in very moderate cases. If you haven't had a scan and don't know the size of the stone, don't do an olive oil gallbladder flush because the stone could be released and then lodged in one of the ducts of the system, requiring emergency surgery.

NUTRIENTS

◆ The appropriate diet is one with low fat and high fiber
◆ Vitamin C and other major antioxidants

- As a preventive, low dose aspirin has been found to reduce the incidence of stones
- Phosphatidyl-choline; choline and inositol
- Magnesium sulfate; trace minerals, but if there is jaundice, avoid supplements with copper
- Pancreatic enzymes, particularly lipase, which digests fats
- Gallbladder flush using olive oil—*have a scan first* and have the flush performed under a doctor's supervision

HERBS

- Silymarin is highly recommended
- Red beet (fresh or powdered in capsules)
- Pancreatin (pancreatic enzymes to promote digestion)
- Peppermint, alfalfa, ginger, fennel
- L.V.R. is also a very helpful herbal combination from Pure Encapsulation
- Dandelion root leaf can be used as a mild diuretic
- Bladderwrack is moderately helpful with weight loss
- Compounded fennel and wild yam can be very useful in combating flatulence

HORMONES

In women, this condition is often associated with hormone changes in midlife or pregnancy. If this is a major problem, get your hormone levels checked, particularly by a physician who practices nutritional medicine or is knowledgeable about herbs and nutrition to address both issues at once.

COMPLEMENTARY THERAPIES

- *Acupuncture* therapy involves a specific gallbladder meridian that can be stimulated for treatment.
- *Homeopathy* does not dissolve stones, but can help with the symptoms.

GASTRITIS

Gastritis is defined as an inflammation of the stomach lining, and it can either be acute or occur as a long-term chronic condition.

CAUSES

- *Helicobacter pylori* bacteria
- A decrease in the number of cells that produce essential digestive

acids (associated with autoimmune conditions and the presence of overly reactive T cells)
♦ Drug-associated sensitivity to nonsteroidal anti-inflammatory drugs (NSAIDs) or arthritis drugs
♦ Cause unknown (idiopathic)

This condition is fairly common, seems to accompany aging, and occurs in almost 4 percent of those aged 21 to 30 and in more than 16 percent of those over 70. Some facts to consider:

♦ Autoimmune gastritis is strongly associated with genetic predisposition.
♦ Gastritis is more common in patients of Scandinavian origin.
♦ *H. pylori* infection can cause thinning of the stomach lining (atrophy) and the loss of acid-producing cells. This predisposes people to gastric cancer later in life.

SYMPTOMS
♦ Bloating, bad taste in the mouth, poor digestion, diarrhea; in some cases, no symptoms
♦ Pernicious anemia (vitamin B_{12} deficiency) or megaloblastic anemia (a type of anemia in which the red cells become enlarged and are more fragile)
♦ Vitiligo (skin discoloration) is sometimes associated with autoimmune gastritis
♦ Flatulence
♦ Chronic fatigue
♦ Stroke (in the central nervous system). Malabsorption is associated with gastritis and low acid production. The nutrient deficiencies (such as vitamin B_{12}) that result from malabsorption can ultimately lead to stroke. This is especially true if elevated homocysteine levels also occur (due to inadequate vitamin B_6 and folic acid, malabsorption, or genetic abnormalities). Vitamin B_{12} levels may also decrease when there is bacterial overgrowth. The use of antibiotics can be helpful in correcting bacterial overgrowth.
♦ Untreated chronic vitamin B_{12} deficiency from pernicious anemia can cause major cognitive problems, mental confusion, and disorientation. If this goes untreated, it can lead to demyelinization of the spinal cord, which causes significant sensory, motor, and neurological problems.

DIAGNOSIS

♦ Endoscopy of the stomach reveals the appearance of the stomach wall; in gastritis, it may appear thin or inflamed.

♦ Multiple biopsies can also demonstrate the presence of inflammation when gastritis is present. In the early stages of gastritis, metaplasia occurs, involving the transformation of the stomach lining cells into another, less functional type of cell. When this occurs, gastric glands lose their function and are no longer able to produce hydrochloric acid, which is essential for digestion. In addition, intestinal lining cells invade the stomach region. This can be a precancerous condition.

♦ Measurement of acidity. A nasogastric tube is swallowed and a hormone (pentagastrin) is injected to stimulate acid and the pH is measured.

♦ In most cases of autoimmune-related gastritis, the body develops an antibody targeted against the acid-producing cells of the stomach. Tests are available that can detect this antibody.

♦ Another test is available that identifies the antibody erroneously targeted against intrinsic factor (the essential body chemical needed for the absorption of vitamin B_{12}). The antibody that attacks intrinsic factor is usually present in autoimmune gastritis.

♦ Testing for vitamin B_{12} levels in serum.

♦ Testing for pepsinogen 1, a peptide that rises in patients lacking the hormone that stimulates essential acid secretion (gastrin).

TREATMENT OF GASTRITIS CAUSED BY *H. PYLORI* OR AUTOIMMUNE CONDITIONS

♦ Replace acid with a betaine hydrochloride supplement

♦ *H. pylori* is treated with antibiotics and proton pump inhibitors to eradicate the infection.

♦ Vitamin B_{12} by injection or sublingual tablets or drops

TREATMENT OF GASTRITIS RESULTING FROM NSAIDS OR ARTHRITIS MEDICATION

Superficial erosions occur in the stomach lining. This condition is treated by:

♦ Reducing acid with H2 blockers

♦ Avoiding NSAIDs or arthritis medication

♦ Taking Cytotec, a medication that acts as a protection against the erosion of the gastric lining, and can be taken in combination with the NSAIDs or arthritis medication

NUTRITIONAL THERAPIES
- Juice therapy (cabbage juice)
- Aloe vera
- DGL (deglycyrrhizinated licorice)
- Bitters or gentian to stimulate acid production
- Betaine HCl

DIET
- Individualize diet
- Consult *Eat Right 4 Your Type*, Peter D'Adamo, Putnam, 1996
- Try mono-meals (eating a single food at a sitting, which tends to be more digestible) taken over the course of day
- Testing for food allergy or the elimination diet (see Chapter 20)
- Vitamins. Low hydrochloric acid means poor absorption; therefore all vitamins and minerals need to be supplemented

HERBS
- Peppermint oil, turkey rhubarb root, fresh goldenseal (not to be taken for more than three weeks at a time), vegetable glycerin, fennel seed
- Rice bran oil may normalize production of gastric acid; slippery elm eases inflammation; marshmallow root is soothing; butter burdock root is an antispasmodic

COMPLEMENTARY THERAPIES
- *Acupuncture*
- *Homeopathics*
- *Massage and energy work:* solar plexus massage, Reiki, Qigong
- *Soothing therapies* to supplement other treatment: aromatherapy, music therapy (the Mozart effect—relaxation promotes digestive secretions)
- *Limit exercise.* Note that active exercise *cuts back* on acid secretions

HEARTBURN
See Reflux.

HEMORRHOIDS
Hemorrhoids are enlarged and protruding blood vessels in the anal area, with weakened prolapsed walls, either inside the anal canal or outside in the tissue surrounding the anus.

Typical symptoms include bleeding or blood in the stool. Swelling or protrusion of the hemorrhoids can occur. Clotted external hemorrhoids are very painful, and can cause swelling and discomfort when sitting.

Possible causes include overactivity or a motility disorder such as diarrhea or constipation. The internal sphincter muscle can spasm in abnormal muscle contractions and aggrevate a potential condition. Persistence of congenital hemorrhoidal bands can also be a factor.

Collagen problems can also play a role, and may occur during pregnancy, from heavy lifting, from sitting a lot, due to a vitamin deficiency, possibly B-complex vitamins, or as a result of aging. The condition may also involve a lack of tone in the blood vessel, surrounding muscle, and connective tissue.

DIAGNOSIS

Examination is performed with a slotted anoscope (which is a short tube inserted into the anal canal) with or without a fiber-optic light, which can show the hemorrhoids or anal lesions more clearly. Sigmoidoscopy or colonoscopy should be performed to rule out other causes of rectal bleeding.

MAINSTREAM MEDICAL TREATMENT

Therapies such as warm sitz baths, anal/rectal cleaning, and hydrocortisone suppositories are often helpful. A high fiber diet and supplementary fiber such as Konsyl or Metamucil are frequently prescribed. (See the entry for constipation for other suggestions on fiber.) The over-the-counter drug Preparation H contains mercury and can be dangerous if used on a prolonged basis because of the tremendous potential for the absorption of mercury from the anal canal.

OUTPATIENT SURGICAL

◆ Internal rubber band ligation, using a rubber ring stretched over a cone and fitted on a firing apparatus. When placed over the hemorrhoid and released, it encircles the tissue and stabilizes it.

◆ Infrared photo coagulation consists of placing a light wand over the base of the hemorrhoid. The instrument superficially cauterizes and seals the blood vessel. This method has a high success rate and is generally the best technique for internal hemorrhoids.

◆ Electrocoagulation is a similar technique that uses electrocautery to cauterize the tissue, but it takes considerably more time and in the author's opinion doesn't work as well as rubber band ligation or photo coagulation.

◆ CO_2 lasers are used in outpatient treatment, for both internal and external hemorrhoid excision and removal. Local anesthesia and occasionally stitches are required. This is typically the most successful technique for external hemorrhoids.

◆ Cryosurgery is not used as frequently now, because it has a long recovery period.

◆ Injection sclerosing therapy is also used less often because it involves an injection of chemicals that can leave ulcers or hard fibrotic scar tissue.

SURGICAL TREATMENT

◆ Blood clots (thrombosis) of external hemorrhoids are treated by surgical removal (excision) and can be performed through laser surgery in the doctor's office or manually with a scalpel. Local anesthesia is required.

◆ Total surgical removal (hemorrhoidectomy) is reserved for prolapsed hemorrhoids that cannot be reduced by internal repositioning or other techniques (fourth-degree hemorrhoids). Very swollen clotted external hemorrhoids may also require complete surgical removal. This is performed under local or general anesthesia in the hospital. However, scarring or stricture of the anal canal can occur and interfere with bowel movements, which may require periodic anal dilation to stretch the strictured area. Postoperative pain may be severe in some patients

TOPICAL PREPARATIONS

◆ Anurex is a suppository chilled in the refrigerator and placed in the anal canal, which reduces inflammation.

◆ Anusol hydrocortisone suppositories are used to reduce inflammation.

◆ Rowasa suppositories contain mesalamine, which is often helpful in the treatment of inflammatory bowel disease and is also helpful in treating hemorrhoids.

DIET

◆ *People with low fiber diets have more hemorrhoids, so a high fiber diet is recommended.* Psyllium or cellulose if tolerated or other fiber supplements are often beneficial.

◆ *Avoid constipation, keep up liquids.* Perhaps keep a chart to be sure you're consuming enough.

NUTRIENTS
+ Vitamin C
+ Vitamins A and E
+ Bioflavonoids such as Pycnogenol may strengthen the vessel wall
+ CoQ10 is a protectant of the engine of our cells (the mitochondria)
+ Trace minerals for chronic inflammation, copper, zinc, and manganese

HERBS
+ Anti-inflammatories such as aloe and slippery elm
+ Ginger, gotu cola, red beet, bilberry, collinsonia taken orally
+ Witch hazel pads (Tucks) are available as astringent wipes and are reported to decrease inflammation
+ Geranium root and plantain as a topical astringent

HOMEOPATHICS
+ If your hemorrhoids are serious, see a well-trained homeopathic physician for either an immediate or long-term remedy. Homeopathics can be a potent cure of hemorrhoids.
+ For homeopathic first aid, see the section on hemorrhoids in Chapter 41.
+ Other first-aid: Metagenics homeopathic (HP5) for preventing flare-ups in people who have the condition
+ Local ointment or suppositories containing Aesculus hippocastanum 3C, and or *Collinsonia canadensis* (homeopathic form).

ACUPUNCTURE
This can often numb the area and decrease pain by unblocking the meridians. Some people with hemorrhoids or other rectal conditions get excellent results with acupressure. A wonderful book that guides the reader through the process with easy-to-find landmarks is K. Serizawa's *Tsubo,* 2nd ed. Japan Publications, 1995. These same points also work well with electro-acustim.

EXERCISE
+ Refrain from heavy lifting and super-vigorous exercise.
+ Moderate exercise is okay, but check with your doctor and let the level of discomfort guide you.
+ If you are able to exercise moderately, this will help to increase tone and improve bowel movements.
+ Kegel exercises can be helpful. If your condition is severe, ask

your doctor to arrange biofeedback (pelvic floor EMG), which can be exceptionally helpful when retraining muscles.

HEPATITIS (Chronic)

For detailed treatment information, please see the section on Liver Disease.

Hepatitis is inflammation of the liver from a variety of infectious agents and other causes.

Here we will focus primarily on hepatitis caused by infection.

CAUSES

♦ Viruses identified as hepatitis A, B, C, D, and E; new strains continue to be identified.

♦ Epstein-Barr virus, which causes hepatitis, also causes infectious mononucleosis.

♦ Cytomegalic virus (also called the fifth disease) can also infect the liver.

♦ Bacterial infections such as tuberculosis and typhoid (caused by salmonella).

SYMPTOMS

Symptoms are similar in all forms, but the potential for liver failure is greater in some forms. Typically, flulike symptoms are accompanied by fever, chills, nausea, and vomiting, aching in joints and over the liver and occasionally jaundice. Some may have intense symptoms.

VIRAL HEPATITIS A

♦ *Transmission:* through food handling, exposure to stool, or contaminated food or water.

♦ *Severity:* Acute and usually mild, rather than chronic; one form can be fatal if not treated.

♦ *Incubation period* is 2 weeks to 48 days, with acute inflammation that eventually goes away and does not become chronic.

♦ *Prevalence:* The potential for epidemics of viral hepatitis A is found most often in the third world or in environments where there are crowded conditions or poor sanitation. In these areas, fifty percent or more of the population test positive for hepatitis antibodies, but often the majority have no symptoms. In the United States, nursing homes, day care facilities, mental institutions, and prisons are high-risk environments.

HEPATITIS B

◆ *Transmission:* most often occurs through needle sharing and intimate sexual contact.

◆ *Severity:* Most often acute; 25 percent of cases become chronic and are at risk for liver failure. Such chronic cases can complain of fatigue but more commonly have no symptoms and are only diagnosed when they are having their blood tested or are donating blood and are rejected.

◆ *Incubation period:* 28 to 160 days

◆ *Prevalence:* Worldwide. More carriers have been exposed to viral hepatitis B than any other type of hepatitis, and 5 percent of the world's population are carriers.

◆ More male than female, more tropical, more urban.

◆ In southeast and central Asia, exposure is as high as 80 percent, almost half acquired in the perinatal period around birth.

◆ *Specifics on transmission:* In the United States, the prevalence is 12 percent. Hepatitis B can be contracted from blood transfusions, contaminated needles, needle sticks, and sexual contact. Even tattoo wells have been implicated and manicure instruments can transmit the virus. The bodily fluids in which hepatitis B is transmitted are saliva, blood, tears, and semen.

◆ *Prevention:* The same type of precautions against HIV are also appropriate for hepatitis B.

HEPATITIS C

◆ *Transmission:* Primarily thought to be through blood transmission such as transfusions.

◆ *Severity:* 50 percent of the cases are acute; 50 percent become chronic with the potential for liver failure.

◆ *Incubation period:* From blood can be 5 to 26 days; the intermediate form has 6- to 12-week incubation period.

◆ *Prevalence:* Found worldwide.

◆ *Specifics on transmission:* Primarily through blood products, especially through multiple transfusions or banking blood/platelet factor transfusions. When you concentrate the blood, the risk increases. Periodically, hepatitis C is transmitted in waterborne epidemics in India and other tropical areas. Sexual transmission and infection from tatoo infections are less likely, but still possible.

◆ *Symptoms:* Same as hepatitis B. Chronic hepatitis can cause an enlarged liver, which can lead to chronic fatigue syndrome, cirrhosis, and liver failure, diagnosed by elevated enzymes in the blood picked up by traditional liver testing (GGT or ALT, AST).

HEPATITIS D

+ *Severity:* The D virus can cause deterioration of the liver.
+ *Prevalence:* Hepatitis D is only associated with hepatitis B infections. It is described as a co-virus or super-infection, and usually found in the Mediterranean region or the Middle East, where as many as 40 percent of hepatitis B virus carriers have been exposed to hepatitis D.
+ *Incubation period:* 20 to 50 days.
+ *Transmission:* It can occur from needles, sexual contact, or transfusions. It is sometimes epidemic in isolated communities in South America.

HEPATITIS E

+ *Prevalence:* Viral hepatitis E is mainly found in third world countries, such as Mexico, India, and Pakistan. It occurs primarily in middle aged or pregnant women. Hepatitis E is largely unknown in North America, except for an outbreak in Mexico in 1986.
+ *Incubation period:* 40-day incubation period.
+ *Transmission:* It can be waterborne, foodborne, or transmitted through feces.

MAINSTREAM AND ALTERNATIVE TREATMENT

See the section in this appendix on Liver Disease for specific information.

HERBS

+ For healing and strengthening: silymarin (milk thistle), St. John's wort, leptotaenia (lomatium), schizandra
+ Systemic Formulas L-Liver; Systemic Formula #5; Systemic VIVI—Lomatium Formula
+ See Chapter 37 on herbal remedies—the section on liver support.

INDIGESTION (Chronic)

See Dyspepsia.

INFLAMMATORY BOWEL DISEASE (IBD) AND CROHN'S DISEASE

IBD is a chronic inflammatory condition of the large or small intestines divided into two types:

+ Ulcerative colitis—affects the colon, but just the lining

- Crohn's disease, an inflammatory condition that can affect all layers of the intestine or even the entire length of the digestive tract from the mouth to the anus

The causes of IBD are still generally unknown. There may be a number of different causes for these conditions. Consequently, treatment that works for one person may not work for the next. These are extremely complex, challenging illnesses. Causal factors suggested by researchers include:

- Possible abnormal overgrowth of bacteria in the GI tract or reaction to viral infections such as measles virus in the wall of the GI tract (in the lining cells).
- Possible contributing disorders such as tuberculosis or pleomorphic bacteria that have no cell walls and therefore are extremely difficult to detect.
- Disordered immune processes (or autoimmune condition). Both ulcerative colitis and Crohn's are considered immune disorders.
- Genetics appears to be a major factor, as these illnesses tend to run in families. This is especially true of Crohn's. For example, it occurs frequently among the Ashkenazi Jewish people and also people from the British Isles, particularly Ireland.
- Stress and inflammation plays a role in this disorder.
- Other factors include altered GI flora, delayed food allergy (such as IgG-related), and diminished blood flow to colon.
- Decreased blood supply (ischemia) such as seen in the elderly. Those on medications that inhibit circulation are more likely to contract this condition.
- Anti-inflammatory drugs, particularly NSAIDs, are implicated in these two disorders because these medications can increase gut permeability.
- Increased oxidative stress and decreased antioxidants may be factors, since this implies lowered cellular defenses.

There are links between immune disorders, IBD, and conditions such as rheumatoid arthritis. This means that when the immune system becomes overly active in our defense, our immune response can actually be toxic to us and cause leaky gut syndrome and overstimulation of the immune system with illnesses such as arthritis, dermatitis, inflammation of the colon (colitis) or lower portion of the small intestine (ileitis), and inflammations of the iris (iritis). Damage due to immune overresponse is similar in these GI conditions and in rheumatoid arthritis.

THE CAUSES OF CROHN'S DISEASE

♦ *Heredity* is clearly associated with Crohn's disease, and it is observed to run in families. Relatives with no symptoms may still have small patches of inflammation seen in a colonoscopic examination and increased gut permeability. However, within a family, some members will develop inflammation and symptoms and others do not.

♦ *Bacterial overgrowth* after antibiotic therapy can promote symptoms of inflammation and bring on attacks of Crohn's disease.

♦ *A change in intestinal permeability* can also trigger symptoms.

♦ *Food allergies* have been directly implicated. Elemental diets (synthetic liquid diets) consisting entirely of powdered soy or rice-based drinks with added nutrients are designed to minimize allergies. This diet tends to be as effective in Crohn's as steroids and can put the patient in remission.

♦ *Autoimmune disorders* that have been associated with Crohn's disease: food allergies, rheumatoid arthritis, eczema, asthma, and hives.

♦ *Viruses, bacteria such as yersinia, and other forms of bacterial overgrowth* can break down bile acids and produce secondary bile salts, which can trigger inflammation.

SYMPTOMS OF CROHN'S DISEASE

♦ Intestinal scarring from chronic inflammation can cause stricturing and narrowing of the gut, resulting in obstruction and requiring surgery.

♦ Diarrhea, abdominal pain, weight loss, rectal bleeding, and/or bloody stools.

♦ Limited growth, excessive weight loss, or in rare cases even weight gain. An overgrowth of bacteria or candida can drive appetite for sweets and starches causing excessive weight gain and triggering symptoms.

♦ Fever of unknown origin.

♦ Crohn's typically manifests in young people in their preteens or teens. The other age group most likely to develop Crohn's is people in their seventies.

♦ In the intestinal tract, active Crohn's is seen as patchy intestinal inflammation.

♦ Symptoms can occur throughout the entire GI system, such as fistulas (draining sores into the rectal, bladder and vaginal tracts or skin).

Symptoms in other parts of the body, seen in Crohn's but also in ulcerative colitis, include

♦ Skin ulcerations and/or swollen, sore red nodules under the skin.

♦ Iritis (inflammation of the iris).

♦ Mouth ulcers: superficial ulcers in the interior of the mouth, on the gums, and on the tongue.

♦ Polyarthritis (aching and swelling of small joints throughout the body)—for example, in the hands or feet, in the elbows or the collarbone, and in the knees.

ULCERATIVE COLITIS

Inheritance is not as clear as in Crohn's, although some genetic factors have been discovered. Genetic models of the inheritance patterns suggest that ulcerative colitis is probably caused by one major gene that has yet to be identified. Symptoms are usually limited to the colon: primarily diarrhea, abdominal pain, discomfort, and bleeding. Weight loss and obstructive symptoms are rare.

Seasonal flare-ups of both Crohn's and ulcerative colitis often occur in the spring and fall. One explanation favored by the author is that the balance between repair factors and inflammation is tipped because intestinal DNA replication is diminished in those seasons.

LAB TESTS FOR CROHN'S AND IBD

Even though these are two distinct conditions, both conventional and functional lab testing is the same for colitis and Crohn's.

Conventional Lab Testing

♦ Stool testing for white cells as an indication of infection
♦ Elevated sedimentation rate (reflects the level of antibodies and indirectly the level of inflammation)
♦ Colonoscopy of the entire colon or enteroscopy of the small intestine
♦ Specialized X-ray of the small intestine
♦ Contrast barium enemas of the colon and the ileum (lower small intestine)

Functional Lab Testing

♦ Antibody testing for bacteria, viruses, or other pathogens
♦ Comprehensive digestive stool analysis—Great Smokies Diagnostic Lab

- Lactulose-mannitol urine test for intestinal permeability. This test is very important in Crohn's and is also relevant in ulcerative colitis.
- IgG blood tests for delayed food allergy
- Organic acids test to check for markers of elusive bacteria
- Testing for vitamin profiles or antioxidant status to indicate any significant nutrient deficiencies that might be affecting general immunity
- Blood testing for trace minerals: low copper, zinc, manganese

MAINSTREAM TREATMENT FOR CROHN'S DISEASE AND IBD
- Steroids (prednisone) are prescribed or used in combination with 5-ASA medications—in the class mesalamine, drugs such as Pentasa or Asacol or sulfasalazine (Azulfidine).
- More recent drugs include chloroquine (Plaquenil), an antimalarial drug that calms the immune system.
- Major immunosuppressants—azathioprine (Imuran) or the parent drug 6-MP.
- Ciprofloxin is an antibacterial that tones down the immune system.

SURGICAL TREATMENT
- Resection (removal) of the entire colon in ulcerative colitis is considered to be a cure for life. This conventional wisdom isn't always true for all people, as the author has seen a number of patients who continued to have lesions elsewhere in the body.
- Resection may be necessary for the scarred section of the bowel in Crohn's that hasn't responded to medical therapy and has either led to obstruction or to recurrent bleeding.

Ulcerative colitis may become so severe that a removal of the entire colon may be necessary, or in the case of Crohn's, removal of a section of the small intestine (referred to as surgical resection). However, we try to minimize this removal, particularly since in the case of Crohn's, removal often doesn't cure the disease. In most cases, the disease process is driven by an overreactive autoimmune response, and when the intestinal tissue is removed, the process simply occurs in other tissue.

RECENT CONTROVERSIAL TREATMENT
- Crohn's: Some people respond to anti-TB therapy (atypical tuberculosis in some patients is suspected as a cause).
- T-cell apheresis reduces the load of T cells through a process like dialysis, which can help in severe conditions, performed at Baptist Memorial Hospital in Memphis, Tennessee.

- Patients with Crohn's who also had bone marrow transplants or AIDS (situations which reduce T-cells) have had a remission of Crohn's because of the decreased number of T cells in the body. This tragic correlation points to the relationship between immune system activity and these severe intestinal inflammations.

- Interleukin and antisense therapy, which turn off the body's signals that promote inflammation.

- TNF-alpha antibody (Infliximab)—turns off tumor necrosis antibodies for Crohn's fistulas, but has been to shown to progress to non-Hodgkin's lymphoma in a few cases because it suppresses the immune system's ability to fight cancer. Therefore indicated for short-term use only or for periodic use.

- Newer 5-ASA medications such as Basalazide, which is probably better absorbed in the colon, squelches free radicals, and turns on manganese superoxide dismutase, a protective enzyme in the mitochondria (the energy center of the cell).

- In Europe, copper superoxide dismutase made from recombinant DNA has been used with success experimentally in treating Crohn's and rheumatoid arthritis.

DIETARY THERAPY

- Enteral and parenteral nutrition are used in treating Crohn's in cases of severe weight loss, chronic diarrhea, or intestinal obstruction. Providing supplemental nutrients can be helpful in many conditions, ranging from mild to severe, and as an adjunct to drug therapy.

- Disaccharide elimination diets. See Elaine Gottschall in *Breaking the Viscous Cycle* (Kirkton Press, 1994).

- Food elimination diets. Research has found that many people with inflammatory bowel disease have major food allergies, including problems with wheat, milk, or citrus. If the allergy is a causal factor, removing the trigger food can make a significant difference.

- *Major nutrients*—the amino acid L-glutamine to decrease gut permeability; omega-3 fish oils to restore vitamin A levels for antibody production; Seacure peptides for repair factors.

- Friendly flora is an underappreciated essential in GI function. Support flora with FOS (fructo-oligosaccharide) in those who can tolerate carbohydrates. The major strains are lactobacillus and bifidobacteria. Also consider mutaflora, a form of beneficial *E. coli* from Germany.

- *Saccharomyces boulardii* is a beneficial yeast especially useful during and after antibiotic therapy.

◆ Many of these nutrients are found in UltraClear Sustain, a powdered nutritional supplement from Metagenics, available by prescription.

◆ Inulin, an active constituent of the Jerusalem artichoke, increases short-chain fatty acids (butyrates); useful for those who cannot tolerate fiber.

◆ Glycoamines found in Mannitec, a glucose and amino acid combination.

HERBS

◆ A useful herbal formula for mild to moderate conditions according to many naturopaths is Robert's Formula. Bastyr also has their own herbal formula.

◆ Aloe vera (liquid); capsules are also helpful, but have a laxative effect, so do not take if diarrhea is present; typically taken at bedtime

◆ Slippery elm or ground flaxseed

◆ Cat's claw as a natural infection fighter; garlic capsules can be helpful, but beware of irritation

◆ Alfalfa, peppermint, or valerian may relieve spasms

COMPLEMENTARY THERAPIES

◆ *Acupuncture*

◆ *EPD allergy treatment*

◆ *NAET therapy.* This is a specialized approach most often used by acupuncturists, which involves using acupuncture and acupressure.

◆ *Gentle exercise.* Increase blood flow to the digestive tract through walking, low-impact aerobic, tai chi, Qigong, and yoga. Be careful not to overdo—aggressive exercise could stimulate bloody diarrhea.

◆ *Mind-body therapies.* Stress reduction/relaxation/self-hypnosis to modify the immune process, host defense, and give adrenal relief.

◆ *Biomagnetic therapy* is a noninvasive treatment just coming into the fore that will be used for treating IBD in the future.

IRRITABLE BOWEL SYNDROME (IBS)

A disorder in the way the intestines function. This condition can occur in the small intestine or the colon, or both. It can be characterized by abdominal discomfort or pain, bloating, mucus in the stools, and irregular bowel habits. IBS is typically a gut motility problem, either constipation or diarrhea, or an alternation between these two extremes. It may also involve low-grade inflammation that is not detected in evaluations, but plagues the patient (termed subclinical inflammation). Pain is sometimes associated with this condition, but is less frequently seen.

CAUSES

At present, the cause is not well understood. IBS may actually describe a number of different conditions or diseases and is something of a catch-all term. Studies have been unable to demonstrate any single physical abnormality that reliably identifies IBS. Current thinking suggests that extended antibiotic use or infection by parasites, bacteria, or viruses may be major factors. It may involve:

- Immediate allergies (IgE), delayed food allergies (IgG), or food sensitivities. Research has detected increased numbers of mast cells, associated with allergic responses (see Chapter 8.)
- Infection, including undetected parasites or viruses
- Increase in immune activity, evidenced by an increase in white blood cells (lymphocytes), which would imply the presence of low-grade inflammation (found in research studies).
- Hormonal imbalance
- Genetic factors
- Psychological trauma or depression
- Imbalance of the autonomic nervous system, which controls many aspects of gut function including motility, so it can cause both diarrhea and constipation

IBS is a chronic disorder that occurs in at least 15 percent of the general population—and twice as many females are affected as males. Among people with digestive problems who are seen by a gastroenterologist, typically 40 percent have IBS. It tends to be a chronic problem, with symptoms that come and go over a period of months, years, or even over a lifetime. The symptoms of IBS often present for the first time early in life; for half of those affected, problems begin before the age of 30.

DIAGNOSIS

Since so many different kinds of conditions are grouped under IBS, a thorough history and chronology of the condition can be quite important. With so many possible causes and diagnoses, it is essential to identify the history of trigger events, such as prior antibiotic therapy, traveler's diarrhea, or food intolerance.

TESTING

Traditional lab testing is generally not helpful in the diagnosis of IBS except to exclude diseases such as cancer of the colon or small intestine, ulcerative colitis, or Crohn's disease. Testing for blood in the stool (hemoccult testing) should be done, as well as a sigmoidoscopy (with biopsy) to exclude conditions such as inflammatory bowel disease or amoebic colitis.

Here are some functional lab tests that may be helpful:

◆ Antibody testing to detect parasites, harmful bacteria, viruses, or yeast
◆ Stool test for parasites
◆ Food allergy testing in blood for IgE and IgG allergies
◆ Intestinal permeability test (lactulose/mannitol test)
◆ Comprehensive digestive stool analysis to assess digestion and identify yeast or bacterial imbalance
◆ Liver detoxification challenge
◆ Oxidative stress evaluation to determine levels of toxic free radicals in the body
◆ Breath testing to identify bacterial overgrowth; this test can also be used to determine lactose intolerance
◆ Testing for the ionized calcium/magnesium ratio to find mineral imbalance (useful in cases of constipation-predominant IBS)
◆ EXA testing can measure minerals within the cell (intracellular electrolytes)

TREATMENT

The overall strategy is the 4 R program.

◆ Remove infective microbes—bacteria, parasites, yeast, or viruses
◆ Remove foods from the diet that may trigger inflammation
◆ Rest the digestive tract to allow the healing of inflammation
◆ Replace digestants and restore friendly flora
◆ Repair GI damage with vital nutrients

DIARRHEA-PREDOMINANT IBS

Two patterns are evident in this condition:

◆ *Lactose intolerance*, which requires the avoidance of lactose-containing foods or in some cases, supplementing with lactase.

◆ *Food hypersensitivity or delayed food allergy,* which requires the discovery and removal of the offending allergenic foods and nutritional support for healing the mucosa. Elimination diets or rotation diets can be helpful once the food allergies have been discovered.

EPD allergy therapy (enzyme-potentiated desensitization) shows promise in desensitizing patients with food or other allergies (see

Chapter 38). Digestible powdered-food supplements of rice protein concentrate have proven to be an excellent element in the hypoallergenic diet. Other nutrients important in healing the GI mucosa include vitamin A, B_5 (pantothenic acid), B_6, C, the mineral zinc, and the amino acid L-glutamine. Choice of dietary fiber may require assessment, or trial and error, particularly if inflammation appears to be present. Other considerations are the elimination of dietary irritants and stimulants, possibly including some spices, alcohol, and tobacco. It is also important to consider the connection between stress and increased tone of the sympathetic nervous system, which can speed up motility, causing diarrhea, cramping, or spasms. If inflammation is present, a blended food diet can be useful, using the blender or a mini-food processor.

CONSTIPATION-PREDOMINANT IBS

This type of IBS syndrome may be due to the inadequacy of fiber or fluids, as well as regular exercise. Dysbiosis, due to parasites or bacteria accompanied by constipation, may also be a factor.

♦ Fiber may be added to the diet in small amounts (5 grams per week) and gradually increased to 25 to 30 grams per day. Insoluble and nonallergenic fiber can enhance the growth of friendly flora. Do not include psyllium or wheat fibers, but consider the use of cellulose fiber, ground flaxseeds, or the use of aloe vera in capsules.

♦ High-quality bentonite clay may be used as long as it is not continued for extended periods of time. Be sure to drink lots of fluid with bentonite or it can cause impaction. Sonne #7 is a quality product.

♦ Chronic lack of magnesium in the diet may also be a factor. Supplement the diet with foods high in magnesium when possible, as well as magnesium (citrate, chloride, maleate, or glycinate). If there is alternating diarrhea with constipation, then magnesium glycinate is preferable.

♦ Mono-meals (the use of a single food at a meal) may also be helpful.

IBS WITH PAIN or GAS AND BLOATING

Gas and bloating can result whenever there is incomplete digestion.

♦ There may not be sufficient hydrochloric acid or digestive enzymes; supplement with betaine hydrochloride and quality enzymes such as the Wobenzyme (see Resources).

♦ Gas and bloating can also result from the overgrowth of opportunistic flora (dysbiosis) and fermentation of starches.

♦ Lactose intolerance or food allergies may be a cause.

♦ Supplement with acidophilus and bifidus if dysbiosis is a factor. FOS products may also be taken to support the friendly bacteria. However, since FOS is a natural sweetener, it may cause increased gas, so start with small doses.

♦ Provide sufficient short-chain fatty acids, found in flaxseed oil and in whole and ground flaxseeds, foods, and supplements with inulin such as UltraClear Sustain and foods such as Jerusalem artichoke. Research has found that olive oil appears to be the most stable of the cooking oils (try Bertolli's Lite).

Abdominal pain may be caused by excessive gas production, impacted stool, or muscle spasms. Antispasmodic medications or calmatives such as peppermint, spearmint, and hawthorn berry may be helpful, and potentially the use of 5HT3 medications.

COMPLEMENTARY THERAPIES

♦ *Diet.* In some forms of IBS, allergies, sensitivities, or tolerance may be an issue. Consider an elimination diet to identify trigger foods or general conditions such as carbohydrate intolerance. (See Chapters 8 and 20 on allergies and Chapter 31 on the Listen-to-Your-Body Diet.)

♦ *Nutrients.* Anti-inflammatory nutrients can be beneficial, such as vitamin A, L-glutamine, and Seacure. If a viral condition underlies the problem, consider Monolaurin capsules from Ecological Formulas.

♦ *Herbs.* Soothing herbs such as aloe vera (liquid, gel, or caps), flaxseed meal, slippery elm, or marshmallow; if infection is present, a wide range of anti-infectives can be beneficial. See the chart on herbs in Chapter 21 on clearing bad bugs; herbs that address spasm (antispasmodics) include alfalfa, peppermint, valerian, and hawthorn.

♦ *Acupuncture* can strengthen immune response and support the body in fighting infection; if there is undetected inflammation present (subclinical inflammation), acupuncture can be helpful in calming it.

♦ *Homeopathy* can be useful in situations with complex, difficult-to-diagnose symptoms and has an excellent track record historically with GI conditions. See a highly skilled practitioner.

♦ *Mind-body therapies.* If there is a history of sexual or physical abuse, psychotherapy and support groups can be extremely helpful. Relaxation techniques, stress management, hypnotherapy, and biofeedback have also been found beneficial.

LACTOSE INTOLERANCE

Inability to digest milk is often due to a *missing enzyme—lactase—* needed to break down the natural sugar in milk called lactose. This condition is different from a food allergy. When there is an allergy to dairy products, the body produces *antibodies against milk protein,* which triggers the activity of the immune system with reactive body chemicals such as histamines. Symptoms include gas and bloating and/or diarrhea.

INCIDENCE

♦ Lactose intolerance is the most common disorder of carbohydrate digestion in humans in the world. Most adults worldwide are unable to digest milk, with the exception of people from Northern Europe.

♦ Age is an important determinant. Children with a genetic predisposition to lactose intolerance show symptoms around the age of five to seven.

♦ Inherited lactase deficiency that manifests at birth is a rare occurrence.

♦ After diarrhea or GI viral infection (enteritis), lactase is often lacking in the regenerated microvilli and appears to be depressed for a longer period than any other metabolic process.

DIAGNOSIS

♦ Home testing for lactose intolerance. In the morning on an empty stomach, drink one or two glasses of milk. If there is an intolerance, diarrhea or gas will be evident.

♦ Breath test consists of measuring hydrogen excretion after drinking milk. This reflects fermentation by colonic bacteria from nonabsorbed lactose. Since milk is normally broken down and absorbed in the small intestine, if undigested milk reaches the colon and is fermented, it implies malabsorption of lactose (milk sugar). When this happens, the milk sugar ferments inappropriately in the colon. Then the colonic bacteria ferments it and releases hydrogen gas. This explains how lactose intolerance can cause gas and bloating.

♦ Lactose tolerance test consists of drinking 15 grams of milk and then measuring blood lactose, which shows how much has been absorbed into the system. In someone who is lactose intolerant, there is very little absorption of this milk sugar, and this will be reflected in the testing levels.

♦ A small bowel biopsy for intolerance can be done in conjunction with other diagnostic testing. The test checks for the presence of the enzyme that digests milk—lactase (found in the brush border of the microvilli).

♦ Blood tests for IgG or IgE antibodies against lactase are not commonly done.

TREATMENT

♦ Lactose-free diet

♦ Lactase enzyme replacement—taking a supplement containing lactase before milk or dairy-containing foods are ingested, such as a lactase enzyme supplement from the health food store or Lactaid from the drugstore.

♦ Cheeses that are almost completely lactose free include Swiss, sharp cheddar, Edam, and Jarlsberg.

♦ Note that if you are allergic to milk protein, you will still have some reactivity to milk or dairy products, even when lactase is supplemented. Symptoms of an allergy to milk protein are highly individual and can range from GI symptoms to respiratory problems (frequent colds), achy muscles, or any of a number of other problems. This allergy can be checked in blood or saliva.

♦ Herbs: For symptomatic relief, ginger, peppermint, gentian, and possibly aloe vera gel.

LIVER DISEASE

Liver disease can range from mild inflammation, jaundice, or minimal scar tissue to conditions as serious as scarring or nodules that can lead to cirrhosis and liver failure. When the flow of blood through the liver is impeded by scarring, portal hypertension occurs. As a result, collateral blood vessels may develop, enlarged veins that develop at the lower end of the esophagus (called varices), around the navel, or rectum (as hemorrhoids). Hemorrhaging can develop due to high blood pressure within the liver (portal hypertension). As the liver becomes less functional, the liver's ability to perform routine duties is impaired:

♦ Protein synthesis cannot be maintained.

♦ Toxins are passed on to the rest of the body and the brain, causing brain fog and confusion.

♦ Fluid seeps out of the arteries and veins into the body cavity, causing generalized edema. When serum albumin declines, edema or ascites occurs.

◆ Decreased circulation can cause a buildup of bile, bilirubin (a breakdown product of red blood cells), and other biochemicals in the liver.

Patients with liver disease should be seen by a gastroenterologist or hepatologist. Severe liver disease can result in confusion, extreme jaundice, and eventually liver failure. In severe cases, hepatic coma or encephalopathy can occur.

PRIMARY CAUSES
◆ *Viral hepatitis*—currently five viruses have been identified, and there may be additional strains
◆ *Chronic alcohol overconsumption*
◆ *Obesity* with fatty liver
◆ *Pregnancy* can sometimes cause fatty liver
◆ *Medication toxicity*—the most frequently occurring is unintentional overdosing with acetaminophen (Tylenol)
◆ *Industrial or environmental toxins*—causing damage through acute or chronic exposure
◆ *Accidental poisoning* from substances such as mushroom ingestion
◆ *Hemochromatosis*—excess iron concentrated in the liver
◆ *Wilson's disease*—excess copper concentrated in the liver
◆ *Crigler-Najjar syndrome and Gilbert's disease*—hereditary conditions that cause jaundice
◆ *Blood clot* (thrombosis) in either of the main veins going into the liver—veno-occlusive disease, clotting in the splenic vein, or Budd-Chiari syndrome, clotting in the hepatic vein.

MAINSTREAM TESTING
◆ *AST-ALT*—measures liver enzymes that indicate liver inflammation (transaminases)
◆ *Bilirubin*—a breakdown product of red blood cells that can cause jaundice if not cleared
◆ *Total protein albumin*—a decrease in albumin shows protein synthesis is diminished
◆ *Immune testing for antibodies* as follows:
  —*Hepatitis A, C, D, and E*—testing for an antibody and antigen
  —*Hepatitis B testing* for the B core antibody and antigen and B surface antigen
  —*DNA polymerase* (a marker for active hepatitis B)
  —*Antibodies for IgG* (reflects chronic conditions, past exposure) *and IgM* (reflects acute current conditions)

◆ *Blood tests to measure for iron overload* (serum iron) and *copper overload* (ceruloplasmin)

◆ *Alpha-antitrypsin*—identifies deficiencies associated with early emphysema, which also results in liver disease

◆ *Liver biopsy* is the best way to tell if chronic liver disease is present. This is done as an outpatient with a very fine needle under ultrasound guidance. When the biopsy is examined under the microscope, scar tissue (cirrhosis) and viral particles can be seen if inflammation is present.

◆ *Imaging using the MRI or CT scan* can show the presence of scar tissue, an enlarged liver, or one that is shrunken and atrophied. Patients with liver disease this serious should be managed by a hepatologist or a gastroenterologist rather than a general practitioner.

FUNCTIONAL TESTING

◆ *Liver detoxification profile* from Great Smokies Diagnostic Lab

◆ *Comprehensive diagnostic stool analysis* (CDSA) to check for dysbiosis and bacterial translocation (Great Smokies Lab)

◆ *Intestinal permeability evaluation,* because increased permeability places an exceptional load on the liver and also reflects elevated cytokines, a marker for inflammation (Great Smokies Lab)

ENVIRONMENT

◆ Minimize all over-the-counter drugs, especially Tylenol.

◆ Minimize exposure to gasoline, fumes, solvents or other chemicals that might burden the liver. Avoid alcohol in any form.
(See Chapter 23 for in-depth information on minimizing toxins.)

TREATMENT

◆ *Hospitalization and liver washout* are required when there is overwhelming hepatitis (fulminant form). The liver may need artificial cultured liver cells, in a procedure comparable to dialysis.

◆ *Specialized diet*

◆ *Actigall or Urso* is derived from bear bile learned from Chinese medicine. Used as an immuno-modulator, this substance rids the liver of secondary bile salts, which tend to be toxic.

◆ *Prednisone* may prep patient for treatment with alpha-interferon therapy (antiviral medication)

◆ *Alpha-interferon*, by injection, is used to stimulate the immune system in cases of hepatitis B and C. Used as aggressive therapy in chronic condition to prevent cirrhosis. Retreatment may be required.

♦ *Alpha-interferon* plus ribavirin is used as combination therapy for retreatment. Ribavirin inhibits the virus from replicating and improves response rate in more than half of patients.

♦ *Amantadine, an anti-influenza drug*, may be useful in treatment of viral hepatitis.

♦ Little is known about therapy for hepatitis D and E.

NUTRITION

♦ Monitor fat-soluble vitamins in chronic liver disease and use water-soluble vitamin E. Vitamins A, E, and any other fat-soluble vitamins can be toxic to the liver in high amounts.

♦ All antioxidants and trace minerals tend to be depleted because of inflammation. *Do not supplement copper or iron, since poor circulation can elevate these minerals.*

HERBS

♦ Silymarin (milk thistle), according to Italian and Chinese data, effective for most forms of hepatitis. However, introduce silymarin gradually. With one form of liver disease, there is reactivity even to silymarin.

♦ Other herbs for healing and strengthening: schizandra, a herb from Chinese medicine that has anti-viral and immune-stimulating effects; St. John's wort; leptotaenia (lomatium).

♦ Systemic Formula L-Liver®; Systemic Formula #5®; Systemic VIVI—Lomatium Formula®.

♦ See Chapter 37 on herbs, the section on liver support.

COMPLEMENTARY THERAPIES

♦ *Minimizing the load on the liver.*

—*Medications*: Under the supervision of an integrative physician, simplify your regimen of medications. The goal is to minimize the amount of drugs and chemicals your liver is required to break down.

—*Toxins:* Also minimize the amount of chemicals you are exposed to at work and at home that may be overworking the liver. (See Chapter 9 on sources of toxins and Chapter 23 on avoiding toxins.)

♦ *Detoxify the liver:* See Chapter 26 on detoxifying and repairing the liver. If you have cirrhosis or liver disease, this process must be done under the supervision of a doctor. Integrative physicians tend to have the dual training relevant to a nutritional approach to liver treatment, performed in a medical context.

◆ *Chelation therapy*: For copper overload, penicillamine is given as an oral supplement to remove some of the metal from the body. For those with iron overload, a form of chelation therapy is used when patients can't have blood drawn to reduce iron levels.

◆ *Treatment for alcoholism*: There are two programs that have a history of high success rates in treating alcoholism

—The multivitamin approach developed by Joan Mathews Larson in Minneapolis, described in her book *Seven Weeks to Sobriety* (Fawcett Columbine, 1997)

—Acupuncture detoxification has been pioneered by Dr. Michael Smith in New York. Practitioners across the country are trained in this method. Ask acupuncturists in your area about the availability of this technique.

◆ *New treatments*: MME treatment (based on technology comparable to the MRI) is currently available at four centers. The device is under research protocol seeking FDA approval; it has a history of being used in mainstream environments, with applications in tissue regeneration. (See Chapter 39.)

◆ *Homeopathy*. Useful in mild, persistent hepatitis. Work with an experienced practitioner.

◆ *Energetic therapies*. Qigong or tai chi, and yoga. Use gentle massage or reiki, but not vigorous massage. If the spleen is enlarged, be sure to check with your doctor before beginning exercise or even vigorous massage, because rupture is possible.

◆ *Mind-body therapies*. Because hepatitis is immune modulated, imagery and stress reduction are useful.

MALABSORPTION

Poor or altered absorption of nutrients due to:

◆ Intestinal infections, overgrowth of bacteria or parasites (severe dysbiosis)
◆ Celiac disease—genetic intolerance of the gluten (protein) in wheat
◆ Severe allergies
◆ Insufficiency of pancreatic enzymes due to conditions such as infection, cystic fibrosis, alcoholism, or pancreatic cancer
◆ The strength of our immunity and our body's ability to repair gut lining tissue

Patients may have one or more of the following symptoms: weight loss, loose stools, diarrhea, flatulence, stools that float (possible from poor digestion of fats and starches), and cramping.

MAINSTREAM TESTING

◆ *The hydrogen breath test* is one of the best. Bacterial overgrowth can be diagnosed.

◆ *Testing for lactose tolerance and celiac disease* is important.

◆ *Pancreatic tests*—Pancreatic stimulation to measure the amount of bicarbonate secreted after stimulating the pancreas with the hormone secretin.

◆ *The d-xylose test* measures malabsorption by indicating whether simple sugar molecules are completely absorbed in the small intestine. This is also a good test for bacteria overgrowth.

◆ *Lactulose-mannitol test* can be used to detect situations in which very few molecules are being absorbed, in addition to measuring leaky gut (the passage of large molecules through the gut wall)

◆ *Testing for the level of bacteria through urine, serum, and breath testing.*

◆ *Bacteria can also be detected by enteroscope* (small bowel endoscope) or other scope to measure the level of overgrowth.

◆ *Biopsy of the small bowel*, through upper endoscopy or by a tethered capsule. This is one of the best ways to determine the cause of malabsorption.

◆ *X-rays of the small bowel,* to indicate the pattern of the mucosa, which reflects whether there is damage to the lining and the villi.

◆ *NG enteroclysis*—a nasogastric tube is used to X-ray the duodenum and jejunum, which contains diluted barium to provide detailed images of the small intestine.

◆ *The small bowel enteroscope* is a new form of scope that can be used to view the small intestine tissue and biopsy it, and in some cases even treat excessive bleeding.

◆ *CT scan* can pick up a diverticulum, an abscess, or even a fistulous tract as is sometimes seen in Crohn's disease, causing bacterial increase (dysbiosis) and therefore malabsorption.

STOOL SAMPLES

◆ *Quantitative, 72-hour fecal fat* (three-day) collection in which a standardized amount of fat is included in the diet and then measured in the stool to show whether the fat is being absorbed.

◆ *CDSA (comprehensive diagnostic stool analysis)* provides multiple information including: profile of absorption of various types of fats, fiber, acidity, friendly flora and pathogenic bacteria, parasites, and yeast. (See Chapter 17 on testing and 21 on clearing bad bugs.)

♦ *Biological terrain assessment (BTA)* involves the analysis of acidity (pH) in blood, urine, and saliva. This test also measures electrical resistance in body fluids which reflects oxidative stress and reflects malabsorption of minerals.

DIET

In this area of treatment mainstream and complementary therapies are in agreement. Diet is determined by the cause of the disorder, and the diet must be individualized in each case. For example, with celiac disease, the primary approach is to avoid gluten. In specific food allergies, it is essential to avoid the offending food and usually also do an elimination or rotation diet (See Chapters 8 and 20 on allergies.) Raw foods and/or juices can be helpful if tolerated because they contain their own enzymes. The Vita-mix is useful for food processing because it retains some of the fiber and pulp in the juice.

NUTRITIONAL THERAPY

♦ *Remove the cause* of the malabsorption such as gluten intolerance or food sensitivities.

♦ *Replace the missing factors*, such as enzymes, hydrochloric acid, or bicarbonate.

♦ *Restore probiotics* with lactobacillus and/or bifidobacteria, and support with inulin and FOS.

♦ *Repair*—provide L-glutamine, glycine, and other essential nutrients to rebuild the GI lining; Seacure to provide healing peptides; trace minerals such as zinc, copper, and manganese; anti-inflammatories such as flaxseed oil (omega-3 acids); antioxidants to repair tissue and protect against oxidative stress.

COMPLEMENTARY THERAPIES

♦ *Herbs.* Include dandelion, aloe, ginger, gentian.

♦ *Acupuncture.* To balance the meridians and improve tone in the GI tract.

♦ *Gentle exercise.* Any movement that simulates peristalsis such as Qigong, yoga, walks, including soothing movement therapies.

♦ *Massage therapy.* To enhance energy from the fatigue of malabsorption.

♦ *Magnetic therapy.* Magnetic sleep systems are believed to improve enzymatic action in the body. The back flex can be worn in the day, over the abdomen to enhance circulation.

SHORT BOWEL SYNDROME

A complex condition typically caused by malabsorption that usually accompanies removal of a significant amount of small intestine. Short bowel syndrome can result from surgery due to Crohn's, cancer, or the clotting of an artery in the digestive tract. This condition often requires intravenous nutrition (hyperalimentation) prepared by a specialist.

A new resource for patients is a center near Boston which uses nutrition to improve regrowth of gut tissue. By supplementing glutamine and growth hormone, they are able to improve patterns of absorption and regrow some tissue while improving absorption in existing tissue. They can be reached at the Nutrition Restart Center, Hopkinton, MA 01748; 800-867-6761.

PANCREATIC CANCER

Pancreatic cancer is now the fifth leading cause of cancer in the United States for both men and women and appears to be increasing in number, as the population grows older. People who have had pancreatitis are more prone to pancreatic cancer. Risk factors include cigarette smoking, alcohol consumption (particularly beer), gallstones, a diet high in animal fats, and diabetes.

SYMPTOMS

Abdominal pain, vague, dull, in the middle of the abdomen, occasionally going through to the back. Weight loss with poor appetite, occasionally with an aversion to meats and a metallic taste in the mouth. Other major symptoms include diarrhea, weakness, vomiting, jaundice, abdominal mass, migratory thrombophlebitis (recurring blood clots in the leg and pelvic veins), and GI bleeding.

DIAGNOSIS

♦ *Lab testing.* Ca 19–9 is the name of a cancer antigen that can be detected through a test based on blood type. Approximately 85% of all pancreatic cancers will have this marker, which is a carbohydrate produced by the cancer cell.

♦ *CAT and MRI scanning.* For CAT scan, the tumor must be at least 2 cm to be visualized.

♦ *Ultrasound* is not as accurate as the scans.

♦ *ERCP* may be performed and samples taken of pancreatic fluid for the examination of cancer cells or markers that may indicate obstruction of the pancreatic duct.

♦ *Biopsy under imaging.* Needle biopsy under CAT or MRI guidance is often needed to provide diagnosis.

TREATMENT

♦ Surgical removal of the pancreas (resection) is possible only in about 50% of cases, those which present with jaundice. Surgical removal is often not possible because detection occurs too late and the pancreas is located so close to other vital organs.

♦ Chemotherapy, especially with gemcitabine.

COMPLEMENTARY TREATMENT

♦ Nutritional adjunctive therapy is receiving good reports; this approach uses antioxidants and organic fruits and vegetables and appears to prolong life and increase quality of life when combined with chemotherapy (NOAT—Nutritional Oncology Adjunctive Treatment, Philadelphia, Pennsylvania). There are various other alternative treatments that include diet therapy, such as the Gerson diet and the work of Dr. Nicholas Gonzales in New York (see Cancer of the Colon for additional information).

♦ Essiac Tea contains five herbs, including burdock root, which has been shown to have anticancer properties. To be used only in combination with adjunctive chemotherapy and nutritional therapy because it doesn't work as a stand-alone cancer therapy.

♦ Detoxification

♦ Acupuncture for pain control and nausea

♦ Subtle energy therapy such as Reiki

♦ Massage therapy, which improves lymphatic drainage and detoxification

♦ Qigong, gentle exercise known for its beneficial effects on lymphatic drainage

♦ Guided imagery

PANCREATITIS

Inflammation of the pancreas is usually results from the blockage of the ducts of the pancreas, causing the enzyme-rich juices of the pancreas to build up inside this organ, breaking down its own tissue, self-digesting (auto-digesting) because the function of the enzymes includes the digestion of protein.

INCIDENCE AND CAUSES

◆ *Gallstones* are the cause of pancreatitis in about 50 percent of patients in industrial nations.

◆ *Alcoholism* is also associated with pancreatitis in men as a causal factor. If gallstones aren't detected by an ultrasound, they are still suspected if there is pain and no evidence of alcoholism. In that case, biliary drainage to clear minute gallstones and biliary sludge can be helpful and is performed through upper endoscopy.

◆ *Malnutrition due to protein deprivation* is a primary cause in underdeveloped countries.

◆ *Familial pancreatitis* occurs as an inherited condition

◆ *Abnormal structure of the ducts.* The pancreatic duct may not be fully developed, or there may be an accessory duct that takes over for the missing duct. When the structure of the duct is malformed, it is called *Pancreas divisum*, and frequent pancreatitis can be associated.

◆ *Scarring of the pancreatic outlet* can occur, called stenosis. Obstruction can result from the scarring due to chronic inflammation. It can be treated by opening the sphincter of the duct, using a specially developed endoscope in a procedure called ERCP (endoscopic retrograde cholangiopancreatography). Pressure measurements can also be taken during this procedure and a special technique can be used to open the scarred duct.

Additional factors in pancreatitis include:

◆ *People with diabetes* are more prone to gallstones, due to chronic inflammation and the presence of proteins within their body that have aged too rapidly due to high blood sugar.

◆ *Drugs* that have been associated as causes include 5-ASAs, tetracyclines, sulfa drugs, Imuran, valproic acid (for seizures), and diuretics, such as thiazides.

◆ *Estrogens.* The body's own natural estrogens are known to cause this condition in rare cases.

◆ *Bacterial infections and viruses,* such as Reye's syndrome and mumps, can cause pancreatitis. Others include AIDS, cytomegalovirus, Coxsackie B, campylobacter, and mycoplasma.

◆ *Elevated calcium levels* in conditions such as hyperparathyroidism.

◆ *Extremely high triglycerides* (blood lipids/fats).

◆ *Trauma* such as an accident that damages the pancreas.

SIGNS AND SYMPTOMS

◆ Abdominal pain that is severe, steady, dull, or boring, generally in the middle of the abdomen, and under the ribs

- Abdominal distention
- Fever or vomiting
- Mild jaundice due to biliary obstruction
- Fluid in the lining covering the lungs
- Shock or in severe cases, coma

DIAGNOSIS

- Blood tests for the presence of enzymes leaking from the pancreas into the bloodstream—particularly amylases (which digest starches) or lipases (which digest fats)
- Ultrasound of the pancreas, which will show swelling
- Abdominal CT scan will show dilation of the duct, hemorrhage, or necrotic areas where cysts and abscesses are occurring.
- Chest X-ray may show fluid in the lining of the lungs (pleural effusion), which indicates the spread of the inflammation from the abdomen into the lung space.
- ERCP. This is an endoscopic dye test used in conjunction with an X-ray. This procedure could cause mild inflammation, but it can also be therapeutic because it can be used to remove gallstones if they are found to be present.

TREATMENT

- There is no known drug treatment for this condition, although in Europe it is treated with marked reduction of mortality using intravenous selenium.
- Hydration using NG tube feeding or intravenous rehydration to replace fluids and rest the gut.
- Pain control such as Demerol.
- Terbutaline, used in asthma treatment and given by injection early on in pancreatitis, has been successful in unpublished research by a Penn State surgical team.
- Surgery may be necessary to remove the abscess or improve drainage.

PREVENTION

- Abstinence from alcohol: Since alcoholism is linked with gallstone formation and pancreatitis, people who overconsume alcohol will want to seek treatment. Alternative therapies with an excellent success rate include acupuncture detoxification and nutritional therapy. See Joan Mathews Larson's program in *Seven Weeks to Sobriety* (Fawcett Columbine, 1997). Both approaches have success rates ranging from 50 percent to 90 percent, even in long-term conditions.

- ◆ Avoidance of fatty foods
- ◆ Supplement with pancreatic enzymes to rest the pancreas
- ◆ Urso or Actigall (ursodeoxycholic acid) to prevent gallstones
- ◆ Statin drugs are used to treat elevated triglycerides

COMPLEMENTARY TREATMENT

- ◆ *Prevention* of gallbladder disease by preventing gallstones. Use silymarin and Urso and observe a low fat diet.
- ◆ *Herbs.* Grape seed extract, bromelain, aloe vera in liquid or capsules, dandelion, licorice (in capsules, extract, or tea)
- ◆ Turmeric root is an anti-inflammatory; silymarin can be used to heal the liver and minimize sludge in the system
- ◆ *Chinese herbal medicine* has been found to reduce mortality from 9 percent to 3 percent in severe pancreatitis. See a knowledgeable doctor of Oriental medicine.
- ◆ *Acupuncture.* For pain relief and prevention of gallbladder disease
- ◆ *Homeopathy* may be helpful for chronic, recurrent gallbladder disease
- ◆ *Mind-body therapies* for pain control; see *Full Catastrophe Living* by Jon Kabat-Zinn (Delta-Dell Books, 1990).

PARASITES/PARASITIC INFECTION

See Chapter 21, "Clear Bad Bugs."

PRURITUS ANI

Pruritus ani is defined as an itchy anus. Some of the potential causes are:

- ◆ Food allergies
- ◆ Poor hygiene
- ◆ Pinworms, candida, parasites, and possibly other GI infections (for example, with cyclospora parasitic infections, in one study 20 percent of patients reported pruritus ani)

DIAGNOSIS

- ◆ Diagnosis depends upon direct inspection with an anoscope
- ◆ Inflammation and redness are visible around the anus
- ◆ Antibody panel for parasites (Immunosciences Lab)
- ◆ Stool sample for yeast, pinworms, and parasites (O & P—ova and parasites)

◆ Allergy testing for IgE and IgG-related allergies—ImmunoLabs in Fort Lauderdale and Great Smokies Diagnostic Lab

DIET

Do a first stage elimination diet, avoiding coffee, citrus, spicy foods, and wheat. If there is no improvement within a month, you can put these foods back in your diet one by one. Use this opportunity to monitor for other allergy symptoms as well (see Chapter 20). Use the same herbals as those for hemorrhoids.

TOPICAL TREATMENT

◆ Sitz baths or showering
◆ Maintain hygiene through the use of witch hazel pads (Tucks)
◆ Suppositories by prescription (Rowasa), hydrocortisone (Anusol-HC)

REFLUX AND HEARTBURN—GERD (gastroesophageal reflux disease)

Acid reflux is a condition in which stomach acid is regurgitated up into the esophagus, causing damage to the lining of the esophagus. This condition is also known as gastroesophageal reflux disease (GERD). A survey of normal hospital employees found that 7 percent experience heartburn daily and 15 percent experience it monthly. A European study found that pregnant women are the most likely to have daily heartburn—48 percent to 78 percent of those surveyed.

SYMPTOMS

Although reflux causes heartburn, by definition it also involves damage to the esophageal lining. Heartburn can be so intense, it can cause angina-like chest pain. A wide range of symptoms are seen in patients with reflux. Common concerns include:

◆ Chest discomfort or pain over the breastbone
◆ Wheezing
◆ Asthma at night (nocturnal)
◆ Hiccups
◆ In the esophagus, stricture or bleeding ulcers
◆ Hoarse voice
◆ Damage to vocal cords

Take heartburn and reflux seriously. Reflux is important, because it can evolve into esophageal cancer. Everyone will have occasional symptoms of heartburn over the course of their life. Heartburn and reflux are one of the most common GI ailments seen in a general medical practice. About half the people who see a doctor with chest pain are found to have heartburn and reflux. However, since it's better to be safe than sorry, whenever there is a question, definitely get your heart checked as soon as possible.

CAUSES

1. *Incomplete closing at the junction between the esophagus and stomach* of the lower esophageal sphincter (LES), which may weaken due to a number of causes: age, pregnancy, or hormones. A drop in pressure can be caused by certain foods, including peppermint, alcohol, and fatty foods, affecting the function of the sphincter.

2. *Hiatal hernia.* About half the people with heartburn and reflux have a hiatal hernia, a defect in the diaphragm muscle that allows part of the stomach to rise into the chest cavity. This makes it more difficult for the sphincter between the esophagus and the stomach to close properly. The incomplete closing of the sphincter can be due to the loss of muscle tone in the lower sphincter or to changes in pressure. Those with larger hiatal hernias are more likely to have significant reflux.

3. *Incomplete esophageal clearing.* We all regurgitate a little, but in people with serious reflux, the esophagus does not fully clear the regurgitated stomach acid. Anything that affects saliva secretion can make reflux worse. Insufficient saliva can be an important factor, since saliva helps clear acid from the esophagus. Insufficient saliva secretion may be due to:

- ◆ Dehydration due to low intake of fluids
- ◆ Drying medications including antihistamines and tricyclic antidepressants
- ◆ Diseases such as Sjögrens syndrome, where there is a defect of saliva

4. *Slowed movement of food in the esophagus* (insufficient esophageal motility) due to aging, medications, or diseases that affect the muscles and interfere with muscle contractions (such as multiple sclerosis, scleroderma, and Parkinson's).

5. *Delayed or slowed emptying of the stomach.* If your stomach is full all the time or if there is delay in emptying, there can be more reflux. Reflux can be aggravated by conditions such as diabetes or medications that delay gastric emptying (these medications include calcium

channel blockers and anticholinergics). One-fourth of patients with reflux have delayed gastric emptying.

PREVENTIVE FACTORS

♦ *Improve the quantity of mucus production.* Interventions that increase the flow of saliva, such as chewing gum, deglycyrrhizinated licorice (DGL), or aloe vera juice or gel.

♦ *Sufficient blood supply to the esophagus.* Try ginkgo biloba or niacin (which both mildly dilate blood vessels). Also try yoga, which can moderately stimulate blood flow.

♦ *Get assistance to quit smoking* because it decreases the mucus barrier, reducing the protection to the lining of the esophagus. Smoking also decreases muscle tone of junction, and decreases the secretion of bicarbonate from the duodenum, which neutralizes stomach acid.

♦ *Cut your intake of foods that decrease sphincter pressure or irritate the esophagus:* mint (which is a smooth muscle relaxant), irritants such as spicy foods, alcohol, coffee, and some oils.

DISEASES ASSOCIATED WITH REFLUX

♦ Diabetes can affect motility.

♦ Obesity places pressure on the abdomen and creates the potential for hiatal hernia, and changes emptying time.

♦ Pregnancy—the pressure of the fetus at the base of the esophagus and the increased production of hormones that cause muscle relaxation.

♦ Neuromuscular disorders that affect coordination throughout the body, including the esophagus, and interfere with swallowing and sphincter pressure, such as Parkinson's, multiple sclerosis, muscular dystrophy, and Alzheimer's.

DIAGNOSIS

♦ Physical exam is often not helpful, although occasionally the doctor can hear gurgling of the stomach in the chest, which is the symptom of a large hiatal hernia.

♦ An upper barium X-ray is often too sensitive, and may pick up variations that do not cause problems.

♦ A double-contrast X-ray is the more helpful because it is able to define the esophageal mucosa and lining better than single-contrast X-rays.

♦ Upper endoscopy is performed to look for damage from reflux, to define hiatal hernias, and to biopsy lesions.

◆ Measuring esophageal pressure is done by evaluating esophageal motility. This technique uses pressure sensors contained in a small tube that is swallowed and then pulled up and down through the various sphincters. Esophageal pressure determinations are not commonly done, but can be very helpful in difficult cases.

◆ Ambulatory pH testing consists of swallowing a small tube with a probe to measure acidity. The patient walks around with a small data recorder that measures acidity (pH), and when it drops below a certain level, acid is suspected of regurgitating up into the esophagus. The recorder can also mark symptoms periodically at the patient's request, which can be evaluated with the pH record at a later time.

◆ A nuclear medicine scan uses radioactively labeled material or food. When reflux occurs, the material regurgitated from the stomach into the esophagus can be scanned with a nuclear medicine device to measure the amount of reflux.

◆ Severe complications can be handled in outpatient endoscopy, which can treat the strictures with dilation or a balloon to stretch them.

◆ Fundoplication is a new technique that is done with the laparoscope. The lower esophageal sphincter can be tightened by laparoscopic fundoplication.

MEDICATIONS

◆ A therapeutic trial of antacids for two weeks is often prescribed by primary care physicians. If this brings about an improvement, the condition may be reflux. The risk is that more serious conditions may be overlooked, such as an erosive condition or Barrett's esophagitis, which is precancerous.

◆ Proton pump inhibitors have generally replaced the histamine blockers for serious reflux conditions. These are medications that block the production of acid by inhibiting the proton pumps of the stomach, specialized cells (chief cells) that produce stomach acid through a molecular pumping action. They include lansoprazole (Prevacid) and omeprazole (Prilosec).

◆ Cisapride(Propulcid) helps empty the stomach and tighten the lower esophageal sphincter (LES).

◆ Histamine blockers are now used less, primarily for short-term therapy—typically two weeks or four treatments. They include cimetidine (Tagamet), ranitidine(Zantac), nizatidine (Axid), or famotidine (Pepcid).

◆ H2 blockers are available as over-the-counter medications at half the prescription dosage—Pepcid AC, Tagamet HG, Zantac 75, or Axid AR. Doctors are now seeing patients who have been self-medicating with these over-the-counter meds, but who actually have more serious conditions such as strictures, erosive or Barrett's esophagitis, episodes with asthma, or false alarm cardiac conditions. The use of these widely available medications may delay more appropriate diagnosis and treatment.

OVER-THE-COUNTER MEDICATIONS

◆ Minimize antacids, which may cause aluminum toxicity.

◆ Minimize bicarbonate, which can change acid balance problems or cause too much alkalinity

◆ Alginic acid (Gaviscon) can be beneficial because it creates a barrier that floats on the stomach acid, so that acid doesn't enter the esophagus. However, it is high in sodium, so minimize sodium in your diet (for delicious salt substitutes, see Chapter 30).

LIFESTYLE CHANGES

◆ Quit smoking. We all now recognize what a battle this addiction can be. Seek medical support, knowing that if you quit, your health risks over time will drop almost to normal.

◆ Consider a weight-loss diet; a good tasty, easy-to-follow diet is *40-30-30 Fat-Burning Nutrition* by Joyce Daoust.

◆ Avoid tight clothing across the abdomen (such as tight belts, girdles).

◆ Eat smaller meals, more frequently.

◆ Don't eat close to going to bed.

◆ Eat slowly and relax after a meal.

DIET CHANGES

◆ *Avoid* fatty foods.

◆ Cut down on fats and simple sugars.

◆ Drink fluids with meals because it helps gastric emptying.

◆ Avoid spicy foods, highly acidic foods.

NUTRIENTS

◆ Magnesium is important for muscle contractions and relaxation. Review your intake and ask your doctor about your optimum level. Generally, there is too much calcium in our diet.

◆ Trace minerals. Low levels of copper, zinc, manganese, and selenium correlates with inflammation.

◆ Bioactive peptides with anti-inflammatory action such as Sea-cure have received positive reports.

HERBS

◆ Avoid mint in candy, herb teas, or any other form.

◆ Aloe vera liquid and gel have anti-inflammatory action; try it whenever you have heartburn; slippery elm is another soothing herb.

◆ MSM (methyl sulfonyl methane) is a therapeutic mineral supplement that is getting good reports.

◆ Noni juice—a tropical tree with herbal properties.

◆ Licorice DGL seems to help mucus, has been found effective in numerous studies.

COMPLEMENTARY THERAPIES

◆ *Acupuncture* seems to be more effective for this condition than acupressure. There are specific points that help gastric emptying that can be treated using a small portable electromagnetic acupuncture device such as the Acu-Stim. These devices are available from Nikken with a prescription from your doctor. (See Resources.)

◆ *Homeopathy* can be useful. See a well-trained homeopathic physician.

◆ *Magnetic sleep systems.* The use of a magnetic mattress or large magnet over the offending area may improve the tone of the sphincter muscle or help the stomach's emptying by retraining of the gastric pacemaker. At present, these reports are anecdotal, from physicians and patients.

◆ *Exercise.* It is good for heartburn to exercise: walking, running, yoga.

◆ *Stress reduction.*

COMPLICATIONS

◆ *Barrett's esophagitis* can be a precancerous condition. Treatment is proton pump inhibitor and periodic surveillance via upper endoscopy with multiple biopsies.

◆ *Dysphagia* (difficult or painful swallowing) is an alarm that most often suggests the presence of cancer. It is important to evaluate the condition through an endoscopic examination and a biopsy.

◆ *Alcohol overconsumption* is associated with reflux because it lowers the pressure in the esophagus and sphincters. It also creates the risk of esophageal varices, varicose veins in the area of the esophagus that can cause symptoms of dysphagia.

STRICTURES and STRUCTURAL CONDITIONS

ESOPHAGEAL STRICTURE

This is a narrowing of the esophagus, a condition that may be present from birth, in tissue structures described as webs or rings within the esophagus. It may be caused by inflammation due to reflux, which can scar the tissue or be caused by tumors.

In general, symptoms include difficulty swallowing or getting food stuck after eating, especially dense or dry foods such as beef or chicken; in some cases pain may be prominent or there may be heartburn. In other cases, the condition may be painless.

DIAGNOSIS

♦ *The upper GI-barium swallow* can be quite useful in diagnosing these conditions. The test can be done in real time, so that the technician can observe the esophagus during the test to evaluate the transit time of food or whether contractions are occurring. The contractions are found in conditions described as corkscrew esophagus, rosary bead esophagus (with spasms caused by acid reflux), stricture (a narrowed area), or when a tumor is present.

♦ *Endoscopy* allows the physician to view the tissue directly with a scope. This procedure can also be therapeutic, because the tissue can be dilated with a balloon-like attachment or other scoping techniques. When the passageway is expanded, the scar tissue is stretched and the correction may need only periodic attention, or may even be permanent. Biopsies can also be performed to assess tumors or inflamed tissue.

♦ *Manometry* involves the measure of pressure in the esophagus to detect excessive increases or decreases. This information can be used, for example, to diagnose low pressure of the esophageal sphincter, a form of stricture that can result when the acid or bile from reflux actually scars the esophagus. A high pressure condition is also possible, called achalasia, in which the muscles are too tight due to increased muscular tension. Esophagomyotomy may be performed in cases that do not respond to other forms of therapy. In this surgery, a strip of muscle is removed from the lower sphincter to prevent the muscle from tightening excessively. Cancerous tumors of the esophagus often have to be removed by surgery, or in some cases can be removed by laser through the endoscope.

OTHER TREATMENT

Medication can be used to relax spastic disorders of the smooth muscles of the esophagus, including sub-lingual long-acting nitrates (amyl nitrate or nitroglycerin) or calcium channel blockers such as nifedipine or diltiazem that affect smooth muscles. Medication is useful in cases that are not true strictures but rather narrowing due to spasm, like corkscrewing. Antidepressants may be helpful, such as trazodone (Desyrel) because it improves communication between the brain and the autonomic/cholinergic nervous system. These conditions are comparable in some ways to an irritable bowel syndrome of the upper esophagus.

OTHER STRUCTURAL PROBLEMS OF THE GI TRACT

Gastric volvulus occurs when the stomach twists upon itself. This condition is due to a hernia of the diaphragm, causing the stomach to ride up through the diaphragm area and get caught. Sudden severe pain can accompany this condition, with vomiting. This is to be considered a medical emergency. It is diagnosed through a barium swallow and typically corrected through surgery. However, in some cases it is self-correcting when a nasogastric tube is inserted and changes the gastric pressure. At that point, the stomach may return to the proper position naturally.

CHRONIC ULCER DISEASE WITH STRICTURE

Chronic duodenal ulcers can cause the narrowing of the outlet of the stomach, termed duodenal stenosis. The symptoms include nausea, vomiting, inability to eat a full meal, and history of chronic ulcer disease. Often dilation of the pylorus with the scope may correct this condition. Diagnosis is made by both upper GI X-ray series *and* endoscopy to rule out the presence of cancer in any form.

If the ulcer is active, it is important to address it, using proton pump inhibitors, H2 blockers given intravenously, and a nasogastric tube to remove the fluid in the stomach. In some cases, the narrowed area of the pylorus can be dilated using an endoscope with a balloon inserted through the scope, which often corrects this condition. In rare cases, surgery is necessary. Again, it is important to rule out gastric cancer.

INTESTINAL OBSTRUCTION

Obstruction typically occurs in the small intestine following surgery, due to scar tissue from prior operations. It can also be caused by Crohn's disease. Diagnosis is made by X-ray, CT scan, or by endoscopy.

Symptoms can include intermittent or acute abdominal pain or distention. In some cases, just resting the bowel takes care of the problem. In other cases, surgery, nasogastric tubes, and IVs are helpful. The long tube or the nasogastric tube may be used to remove fluid from the small intestine or the stomach. Again, it is important to rule out tumors. It is necessary to correct electrolyte imbalance and replace fluids as needed.

COMPLEMENTARY THERAPIES

Because these conditions are mechanical, they typically require surgical or mechanical intervention rather than alternative therapies. Acupuncture is probably the only alternative to be explored. For example, in the case of achalasia, using an electromagnetic TENS unit on relevant acupuncture points can lower the pressure and in some cases that is sufficient to restore functioning.

STRICTURE OF THE COLON

Strictures of the colon can occur, typically caused by ulcerative colitis or Crohn's disease and evidenced by the inability to have normal bowel movement or resulting in very small bowel movements. Diagnosis is by barium enema or colonoscopy. Therapies include balloon dilatation and biopsy to rule out cancer, or surgery.

CHRONIC INTESTINAL PSEUDO-OBSTRUCTION

This condition occurs when there is ineffective intestinal motility, characterized by symptoms of chronic intestinal obstruction. The colon is dilated and there is no motility. This condition is accompanied by chronic constipation, distention and bloating, slow transit, and an absence of bowel sounds.

The acute form can require surgery. The chronic form may be due to muscular dystrophy, nerve degeneration, visceral neuropathy, Schuster's syndrome (a hereditary condition with chronic constipation, with or without chronic fatigue syndrome), Parkinson's disease, brain or spinal cord tumor, chronically low parathyroid function (hypoparathyroidism), or due to dysfunction on a cellular level. Decompressive colonoscopy can be very helpful to remove as much fluid and air as possible from the colon. In some cases, this procedure is so successful, surgery is unnecessary.

Poor motility has become quite common in our society, due to the increase in GI surgeries and the use of narcotic painkillers and antipsychotic medications, which can slow motility drastically. Patients using these medications should take a lot of fiber and a lot of fluid. Many of these conditions are reversible if you catch them early enough. Avoid the long-term use of laxatives, which may work initially, but cause poor tone of the colon muscle and may make the problem worse. Cholinergic drugs are now being used to treat this condition.

ULCERS/ULCER DISEASE

An ulcer is a lesion in the lining of the stomach or the first part of the small intestine (duodenum). Researchers have found ulcers to be caused by infection due to the bacteria, *Helicobacter pylori (H. pylori)*. Researchers once believed ulcers resulted from hyperacidity and stress.

In humans, *H. pylori* was considered a harmless resident of the stomach and GI tract. Dr. Barry Marshall, an Australian researcher, investigated the bacteria in the early 1980s. When his request for a grant to do further research was rejected, to prove his point he ingested a test tube of *H. pylori* bacteria and days later developed a major case of stomach ulcers. He was evaluated, treated with antibiotics which resolved his symptoms and infection, and the rest is history.

Unfortunately, surveys show that about 40% of doctors are unaware of the discovery of *H. pylori*. Gastric ulcers in the elderly are worrisome because of their association with cancer and should be endoscoped and biopsied for that reason.

SYMPTOMS

- Chronic abdominal pain in the area of the stomach
- Pain that occurs after eating (postprandial) when the stomach is empty, at 11 A.M., 4 P.M., 10 P.M., and 1 to 2 A.M. This is most common for duodenal ulcers, which are relieved by antacids or eating.
- Frequent heartburn that may resemble reflux.
- May be intermittent or even be silent and be apparent only after GI bleeding; this is more characteristic of ulcer disease caused by the use of NSAIDs.
- Nausea and vomiting. Prolonged vomiting is rare, unless a stricture or obstruction is present.
- GI bleeding

CAUSES

Peptic ulcer disease is like being on a teeter-totter—it is a matter of balance between protective factors and ulcerative factors, as well as exposure to infection.

- *Exposure is more frequent in certain environments* such as medical care facilities. Among medical students, positive titers for *H. pylori* (reflecting exposure to the infection) increase by 33 percent over the course of their medical education.
- *Animals can be carriers.* For example, in San Francisco about 40 percent of all cats are said to be carriers. *H. pylori* is also associated in the body with gingivitis.

♦ *Old water systems and piping* have been found to harbor *H. pylori.*

♦ *Factors that compromise the protective mucous barrier:* smoking, alcohol, NSAIDs (nonsteroidal anti-inflammatory drugs), stress (including physical stressors such as surgery, burns, or traumatic injury), decreased blood flow.

♦ *Seasonal variations of ulcer disease.* Repair is less active in the spring and fall because growth factors, cell turnover, and DNA for intestinal repair are the lowest when we are adapting to the change in season.

DIAGNOSIS

♦ Upper endoscopy

♦ X-ray—upper GI barium series (contrast or double contrast which involves air and barium)

♦ A therapeutic trial is often recommended with H2 blockers for two weeks, but some patients may have acid reflux. If a gastric ulcer is present, this treatment will be masking the symptoms and may allow more serious complications to develop. With OTC availability of H2 blockers such as Pepcid AC and Tagamet HB, there will be a greater tendency for this kind of problem.

♦ Testing for *H. pylori* antibodies in blood draw, finger stick, saliva test, or breath test. Unless the test is measuring IgM antibodies in response to a current infection, the test may show the presence of *H. pylori* bacteria but still doesn't necessarily indicate the presence of an active ulcer infection.

MAINSTREAM TREATMENT

For ulcers caused by *H. pylori* infection:

♦ Triple therapy—two antibiotics such as ampicillin and clarithromycin, plus a proton pump inhibiting drug such as omeprazole (Prilosec) or lansoprazole (Prevacid).

♦ Another triple therapy combination is bismuth/metronidazole/tetracycline (Helidac).

♦ Remember to take probiotics with antibiotic therapy, such as acidophilus or live-culture yogurt.

♦ Dual therapy raniditine bismuth citrate (RBC—Tritec) given with an antibiotic such as clarithromycin.

For ulcers not caused by *H. Pylori* infection:

♦ Proton pump inhibitors such as omeprazole or lansoprazole

♦ H2 blockers such as cimetidine (Tagamet), nizatidine (Axid), famotidine (Pepcid), or ranitidine (Zantac) in prescription strength

SURGERY

In cases of extensive bleeding.

DIET

Diet therapy has fallen out of vogue, but earlier was the only therapy available. This typically consists of all soft food, including milk and cream (not great for dairy-intolerant people or those with cholesterol problems). When there is a lot of inflammation, some relief can be gained by blending foods—the small jar attachment to a blender or a mini-food processor can be invaluable in this regard. Fresh juices can also be helpful if tolerated, but care must be taken not to take in too much carbohydrate (carrot juice, for example, is quite sweet).

COMPLEMENTARY THERAPIES

◆ *Nutrients.* Vitamins A and E to promote mucous membrane healing; copper, zinc, manganese tend to be depleted in chronic inflammation; rice bran extract—gamma-oryzanol.

◆ *Juices.* A cabbage juice regimen has anecdotal reports of benefit with ulcer conditions.

◆ *Herbal therapies.* Deglycyrrhizinated licorice, DGL; aloe vera; slippery elm; grape seed extract; citrus seed extract; ginger (tea or capsules).

◆ If *H. pylori* is detected through lab work, consider garlic oil in caps, grape seed extract, gentian, goldenseal (for no longer than three weeks).

◆ Plautonol is a Japanese nutraceutical found to inhibit growth of *H. pylori.*

◆ Sublingual SOD is a supplement that works on superoxide dismutase (SOD) and is a free radical squelcher.

◆ *Acupuncture.* With chronic problems, there are specific points that are useful which can help with pain and nausea and assist gastric emptying.

◆ *Homeopathy.*

◆ *Energy Exercise.* Yoga, tai chi, and Qigong.

◆ *Mind-body therapies.* Meditation and stress reduction.

ULCERATIVE COLITIS

See Inflammatory Bowel Disease.

VIRAL BOWEL DISEASE

See Chapter 22.

RESOURCES

❖

GENERAL RESOURCES ON DIGESTIVE HEALTH— THE TEAM

BOOKS

Baker, Sidney. *Detoxification and Healing*. Keats, 1997.

Bland, Jeffrey. *The 20-Day Rejuvenation Diet Program*. Keats, 1997.

Crook, William, M.D. *The Yeast Connection Handbook*. Publishers Group West, 1999.

D'Adamo, Peter. *Eat Right 4 Your Type*. Putnam, 1996.

Galland, Leo. *Power Healing*, 2nd ed. Random House, 1998.

Gates, D. *The Body Ecology Diet*. Bookpeople, 1998.

Gittleman, Ann Louise. *Guess What Came to Dinner: Parasites and Your Health*. Avery Publishing Group, 1993.

Golan, Ralph. *Optimal Wellness*. Fawcett, 1995.

Gottschall, Elaine. *Breaking the Vicious Cycle*. Kirkton Press, 1994.

Haas, Elson. *Staying Healthy with Nutrition*. Celestial Arts, 1992.

———. *The Staying Healthy Shopper's Guide*. Celestial Arts, 1999.

Jahnke, Roger. *The Healer Within*. HarperCollins, 1999.

Kellas, William, and Andrea Dworkin. *Thriving in a Toxic World*. Professional Preference Publications, 1996.

Lipsky, Elizabeth. *Digestive Wellness*. Keats, 1996.

Lockie, Andrew, and Nicola Geddes. *The Complete Guide to Homeopathy*. Dorling Kindersley, 1995.

Rossman, Martin. *Healing Yourself*. The Academy for Guided Imagery, 1997.

Serizawa, K. *Tsubo*. Japan Publications, 1995.

Timmins, W. *The Foundational Health Program*. Program guide and tapes, 1999.

Werbach, Melvyn. *Nutritional Influences on Illness*. Third Line Press, 1993.

Wright, Jonathan. *Dr. Wright's Guide to Healing with Nutrition,* rev. ed. Keats, 1993.

PATIENT INFORMATION RESOURCES

The Health Resource, 933 Faulkner Street, Conway, AR 72032; 800-949-0090; e-mail: moreinfo@thehealthresource.com

Hermes Health Education Resources and Medical Extract Service, 1200 Arguello Blvd., San Francisco, CA 94122; 415-289-6550; e-mail: perryolesen@ hotmail.com

Institute for Health and Healing Library (formerly Planetree Health Resource Center), 2040 Webster Street, San Francisco, CA 94115; 415-923-3681, ihhlib@sirius.com

National Digestive Diseases Information Clearinghouse, 2 Information Way, Bethesda, MD 20892; 301-654-3810

World Research Foundation, 41 Bell Rock Plaza, Sedona, AZ 86351; 520-284-3300

WEBSITES

Great Smokies Diagnostic Laboratory, www.gsdl.com

HealthComm International, www.healthcomm.com

Health Medicine Forum, information on alternative medicine, www.health medicine.org

Health Medicine Network. Television-style broadcasts, both live and taped, of talks and conferences on complementary medicine. www.health broadcastnetwork.com

Health On-Line, www.healthonline.com

Health World, www.alternativemedicine.net

Medline on the Internet, www.nlm.nih.gov, tends to be a user-friendly system. Click on Medline, then Pub Med, and enter the key word.

GASTROENTEROLOGY REFERENCES

Bayless, Theodore, ed. *Current Therapy in Gastroenterology and Liver Diseases*, 4th ed. Mosby-Year Book, 1994.

Feldman, Mark, Bruce Scharschmidt and Marvin Sleisenger, eds. *Sleisenger and Fordtran's Gastrointestinal and Liver Disease*, 6th ed. W. B. Saunders, 1997.

Kirsner, Joseph, and Roy Shorter, eds. *Inflammatory Bowel Disease*, 4th ed. Williams & Wilkins, 1995.

Spiro, Howard. *Clinical Gastroenterology*, 4th ed. McGraw-Hill, 1993.

NUTRITIONAL REFERENCES FOR PROFESSIONALS

Bland, Jeffrey. *New Perspectives in Nutritional Therapies: Improving Patient Outcomes*. HealthComm International, 1996. *Nutritional Improvement of Health Outcomes: The Inflammatory Disorders*. HealthComm International, 1997.

HealthComm International, Gig Harbor, WA; 800-843-9660. Monthly medical updates on audiotape, publications, regional workshops, and yearly conferences.

Kiminski, Mitchell, Steven Weil, Jeffery Bland, et al. "AIDS wasting syndrome as an entero-metabolic disorder: The gut hypothesis." *Alternative Med Review*, 3:40–53, 1998.

Liska, DeAnn. "The detoxification enzyme systems." *Alternative Med Review* 3:187–198, 1998.

SOURCES OF REFERRALS TO PRACTITIONERS

American Academy of Environmental Medicine, 7701 E. Kellogg, Suite 625, Wichita, KS 67207; 316-684-5500

American Academy of Medical Acupuncture, 5820 Wilshire Blvd, Suite 500, Los Angeles, CA 90036; 213-937-5514

American Association of Naturopathic Physicians, 601 Valley St., Suite 105, Seattle, WA 98109; 206-298-0125. Directory/brochures mailed for $5 or by accessing www.naturopathic.org

American Association of Oriental Medicine, 433 Front St., Catasauqua, PA 18032; 610-266-1433

American Chiropractic Association, 1701 Clarendon Blvd., Arlington, VA 22209; 800-986-4636; www.amerchiro.org

American College for the Advancement of Medicine, PO Box 3427, Laguna Hills, CA 92654 (enclose a self-addressed envelope with two stamps); 800-532-3688.

American EPD Society, 141 Paseo de Peralta, Suite A, Santa Fe, NM 87501; 505-984-0004. For a list of physicians trained in EPD, send a $10 tax-deductible donation and a self-addressed, stamped envelope. Information is also available at www.epdallergy.com

American Holistic Medical Association, 6728 Old McLean Dr., McLean, VA 22107; 703-556-9728; www.holisticmedicine.org

American Holistic Veterinary Medical Association, 2214 Old Emmorton Rd., Bel Air, MD 21015; 410-569-0795

The American Preventive Medical Association 459 Walker Road, Great Falls, VA 22066; 703-759-0662

Bastyr University Referral Line, Kenmore, WA; 425-602-3390; www.bastyr.edu. Referrals to naturopathic physicians

Broda Barnes Foundation, Bridgeport, CN; 203-261-2101

Certified Natural Health Professionals, 400 Oak Hill Drive, Winona Lake, IN 46590; 219-267-4230. Referrals to naturopathic physicians

Environmental Dental Association, 800-388-8124. For book orders, call EDA at 619-586-7626. To receive a list of alternative dentists, send a self-addressed stamped envelope with 55¢ postage. Enclose $3. Mail to EDA, PO Box 2184, Rancho Santa Fe, CA 92067

HealthComm International, PO Box 1729, Gig Harbor, WA 98335; 800-843-9660. Referrals: physicians and practitioners trained in functional medicine. www.healthcomm.com

International Chiropractor Association, 1110 N. Glebe Road, Suite 1000, Arlington, VA 22201; 800-423-4690; www.chiropractic.org

National Center for Homeopathy, 801 N. Fairfax Street, Suite 306, Alexandria, VA 22314; 703-548-7790; www.homeopathic.org

Orthomolecular Health-Medicine, 2698 Pacific, San Francisco, CA 94115; 415-922-6462

COMPOUNDING PHARMACIES

Referrals to compounding pharmacies:

International Academy of Compounding Pharmacists, Houston, TX; 800-927-4227

Professional Compounding Centers of America (PCCA), Houston, TX; 800-331-2498.

Specific pharmacies:

Abbott's Compounding Pharmacy, Berkeley, CA; 800-327-6842

College Pharmacy, Colorado Springs, CO; 719-262-0022

Wellness Pharmacy, Birmingham AL; 800-227-2627

Women's International Pharmacy, Madison, WI; 800-699-8144

How to find a physician who uses low-dose hormone therapy:

Check with organizations that provide practitioner referrals, such as the American College for the Advancement of Medicine (ACAM) at 800-532-3688.

SOURCES FOR NUTRIENTS

These are companies that sell to the public and to physicians. All provide mail-order service and many will send catalogues on request.

Allergy Research Group/Nutricology, San Leandro, CA; 800-545-9960. An outstanding line of nutritional supplements

Gaia Herbs, Brevard, NC 28712; 800-831-7780. Quality herbal tinctures

Klaire Laboratories, from Wellness Pharmacy; 800-227-2627. Probiotics, glandulars, etc.

Nutri-Source, Tyson Nutriceuticals; 800-293-1683. Quality line of amino acids, vitamins, minerals

Pure Encapsulation, Sudburg, MA; 800-753-CAPS

Seacure from Proper Nutrition, Inc., PO Box 13905, Reading, PA 19612; 800-555-8868. Available to the general public, as well as physicians. Next-day shipping is available if desired.

Smart Basics, San Francisco; 800-868-7627; www.smartbasic.com. Mail-order service, discounted prices, providing many specialty products

Vitamin Express, San Francisco; 800-500-0733; www.vitaminexpress.com. Mail-order service, discounted prices, providing both familiar and specialty brands

Vitamin Research Products, Carson City, NV; 800-877-2447. Custom line of vitamin products

The Vitamin Shoppe, North Bergen, NJ; 800-223-1216. Mail-order service, discounted, providing familiar brands

Nutrient and herb companies that sell to physicians and pharmacies only:

Interplexus, Seattle, WA; 800-875-0511. Specialty products, including immune support

MarcoPharma, Denver, CO; 800-999-3001. A variety of German imports, including enzymes

Metagenics, San Clemente, CA; 800-638-4362. Edison, NJ; 800-638-2848. Products formulated by Jeffrey Bland, Ph.D., including UltraClear and Sustain

Thorne Research, Dover, ID; 800-228-1966. Wide range of products and specialty formulas

Tyler Encapsulations, Gresham, OR; 800-869-9750. Specialty products

LABORATORIES

Information to the public and doctors on testing:

BioHealth Diagnostics, San Diego; lab test panels and consultation; 800-570-2000

Great Plains Laboratory, Overland Park, KS; organic acids testing; 913-341-8949

Great Smokies Diagnostic Lab, Ashville, NC; intestinal permeability, digestive, stool analysis, liver function, oxidative stress; 800-522-4762. Contact Client Services for educational materials and general information for both patients and physicians. Publications include "Solving the Digestive Puzzle." Website at www.gsdl.com

Immuno Laboratories, Fort Lauderdale, FL; food allergy testing for IgE & IgG; 800-231-9197

SpectraCell Laboratories, Houston, TX; vitamins, minerals, fatty acids; 800-227-5227

Information for health care professionals only:

Body Bio, Millville, NJ; consultation on fatty acid analysis and blood chemistry; 609-825-8338

Diagnos-Techs, Kent, WA; testing digestive and hormone function; 206-251-0596

Diagnostic Labs, Phoenix, AZ; evaluation of stool for parasites, yeast, and certain bacteria; 602-955-4211

Immunosciences Lab, Beverly Hills, CA; wide range of antibody testing; 310-657-1077; www.immuno-sci-lab.com

Meridian Valley Clinical Laboratory, Kent, WA; full service lab, allergy tests; 253-859-8700

National Medical Services, Willow Grove, PA; reference lab used by hospitals, and major labs across the country, highly specialized testing, including heavy metals; 215-657-4900

Vitamin Diagnostics, Cliffwood Beach, NJ; vitamins, minerals, fatty acids; 732-583-7773

BIO-ELECTRIC MAGNETISM—RESOURCES— TRENT NICHOLS, JR., M.D.

BOOKS

Becker, Robert and Gary Selden. *The Body Electric: Electromagnetism and the Foundation of Life.* Morrow, 1987.

Blank, Martin, ed. *Electromagnetic Fields: Biological Interactions and Mechanisms.* American Chemical Society, 1995.

Lawrence, Ron, and P. Rosch. *Magnet Therapy: The Pain Cure Alternative.* Prima Health, 1998.

Null, Gary. *Healing with Magnets.* Carroll and Graf, 1998.

Rubik, Beverly, Robert Becker, Robert Flower, and others. "Bioelectromagnetics applications in medicine." *Alternative Medicine, Expanding Medical Horizons,* 1993. A report to the NIH on alternative medical systems and practices in the United States.

Advanced Magnetic Research Institutes are currently located at:
5421–11 Street N.E., #109, Calgary, Alberta T2E 6M4; 800-265-1119
27652-B Camino Capistrano, Laguna Niguel, CA 92677; 949-367-0877

Dayspring Medical Center, 217 Dayspring Way, Mocksville, NC 27028; 336-492-2812

Eichelberger Professional Building, 195 Stock St, Suite 200, Hanover, PA 17331; 717-632-0300

CHINESE MEDICINE RESOURCES— EFREM KORNGOLD, O.M.D.

Presently, in the United States, there are about 10,000 certified or licensed practitioners of acupuncture and herbal medicine. There are more than three dozen schools of Chinese medicine, offering three- and four-year programs that graduate hundreds of new practitioners annually. There are also numerous state and national organizations of Chinese medicine professionals, researchers, and educators. The following list identifies books, organizations, institutions, and businesses that provide information, services, and products related to Chinese medicine.

BOOKS

Beinfield, Harriet, and Efrem Korngold. *Between Heaven and Earth: A Guide to Chinese Medicine.* Ballantine, 1991. Available in hardcover and paperback.

Pitchford, Paul. *Healing with Whole Foods.* North Atlantic Books, 1993.

REFERRALS

The Association of Acupuncture and Oriental Medicine (AAOM), 433 Front Street, Catasauqua, PA 18032-2506; 610-266-1433

The National Acupuncture and Oriental Medicine Alliance (NAOMA), P.O. Box 77511, Seattle, WA 98177-0531; 206-524-3511; e-mail: 76143.2061@ compuserve.com

The National Commission for Certification in Acupuncture and Oriental Medicine (NCCAOM), 1424 16th St. NW, Suite 501, Washington, DC 20036; 202-232-1404

INFORMATION ABOUT CHINESE MEDICINE

The Council of Colleges of Acupuncture and Oriental Medicine (CCAOM), 1424 16th St. NW, Suite 501, Washington, DC 20036-2211; 202-265-3370

The Institute for Traditional Medicine and Preventive Health Care, 2017 SE Hawthorne Blvd., Portland, OR 97214; 503-233-4907; website www. europa.com/~itm

The American Foundation of Traditional Chinese Medicine, 505 Beach Street, San Francisco, CA 94133; 415-776-0502

CHINESE HERBAL PRODUCTS AND SUPPLIES

Institute Herb Company (available to the general public and to professionals), 1190 NE 125th St., North Miami, FL 33161; 305-899-8704

Shen Nong Herbs (available to the general public and to professionals), 1600 Shattuck Ave., Store #125, Berkeley, CA 94709; 510-849-0290

K'AN Herb Company (available to health care professionals), 6001 Butler Lane, Scotts Valley, CA 95066; 800-543-5233

The Institute for Traditional Medicine and Preventive Health Care—above (professionals only).

ENVIRONMENTAL MEDICINE RESOURCES— JEFFREY ANDERSON, M.D.

BOOKS

Ashford, N.A., and C.S Miller. *Chemical Exposures: Low Levels and High Stakes.* Van Nostrand Reinhold, 1997. This is the definitive text addressing the whole subject of chemical exposure, both medical and scientific, and the political, social and economic consequences of chemical injury, including chemical sensitivities. Meaningful to both general audiences and professionals.

Audesirk, T. and G. *Biology: Life on Earth,* 4th ed. Prentice Hall, 1996. Broad presentation on the biology of life on our planet, including good general information on the dynamics of the cell.

Colborn, Theo, Dianne Dumanoski, and John Myers. *Our Stolen Future.* Dutton, 1996.

Merck Manual of Medical Information, Home Edition, 1997. A good introduction to medical information from specific diseases to basic physiology and anatomy.

Randolph, Theron, M.D. *Human Ecology and Susceptibility to the Chemical Environment.* Charles C Thomas, 1976. First published in the 1960s by the father of environmental medicine, this is the original definitive text, still in print. Appropriate for general readers and practitioners.

Rogers, Sherry A., M.D. *Tired or Toxic?* Prestige Publishers, 1990. An informative book written for patients linking chronic fatigue and other common complaints with the effects of environmental toxins.

Steingraber, Sandra. *Living Downstream.* Vintage, 1998. The personal perspective of a world-class scientist, oriented toward chemicals and cancer, with a definitive resource list for professionals.

Wallace, Robert A. *Biology: The World of Life.* Benjamin Cummings, 1996.

World Book, Rush-Presbyterian-St. Luke's Medical Center Medical Encyclopedia. World Book, 1998. Clear descriptions of cell anatomy and function and a good compendium of medical diagnosis and treatment.

ORGANIZATIONS

The American Academy of Environmental Medicine. 7701 E. Kellogg, Suite 625, Wichita, KS 67207; 316-684-5500. Sponsors conferences and training for health care professionals and the general public. Publishes/distributes books, monographs and audiotapes on environmental health subjects, for both audiences. Provides referrals to physicians.

The American Environmental Health Foundation. Dallas, TX, 214-361-9515; 800-428-2343. Sponsors scientific symposiums for professionals. Funds scientific research on environmental issues. Extensive resource center and mail-order catalogue for media, educational books, abstracts, and audiotapes), treatment strategies and products; environmentally safe products for the home and personal care.

The Chemical Injury Information Network. White Sulphur Springs, MT, 406-547-2255; website: http://biz-comm.com/CIIN. Education, research, and advocacy related to chemical injury. Extensive referral resources and educational materials including monthly newsletter, research services, and more.

PROFESSIONAL RESOURCES IN ENVIRONMENTAL MEDICINE

BOOKS

Alberts B., D. Bray, J. Lewis, M. Raff, K. Roberts, and J.D. Watson. *Molecular Biology of the Cell*. Garland, 1994.

Board on Environmental Studies and Toxicology, Commission on Life Sciences, National Research Council. *Biological Markers in Immunotoxicology: Multiple Chemical Sensitivities*. National Academy Press, 1992.

Doull, Klaassen, Amdur, Eds. *Casarett and Doull's Toxicology: The Basic Science of Poisons*. Macmillan, 1997.

Rea, William, M.D. *Chemical Sensitivities,* vols 1–4. Lewis Publishers, 1997.

JOURNALS

The Journal of Nutritional and Environmental Medicine. Official journal of the American Academy of Environmental Medicine, the British Society for Allergy, Environmental and Nutritional Medicine, and the Australian College of Nutritional and Environmental Medicine. Carfax Publishers.

Toxicology and Industrial Health. Princeton Scientific Publishing.

GUIDED IMAGERY RESOURCES— MARTIN ROSSMAN, M.D.

BOOKS

Rossman, Martin. *Healing Yourself: A Step-by-Step Program for Better Health Through Imagery,* 2nd ed. The Academy for Guided Imagery, 1997.

CONSULTATIONS

Rossman, Martin, M.D., Mill Valley, CA; 415-383-3197. Available for phone consultations on health conditions and also the use of mind-body approaches to resolve them.

RESOURCES AND TRAINING FOR THE PUBLIC AND PROFESSIONALS

The Academy for Guided Imagery, Mill Valley, CA, 800-726-2070. A free catalogue of imagery related tapes and videos; training for health professionals to use guided imagery including certificate programs and conferences. Referrals through the *Directory of Imagery Practitioners*

The Institute of Transpersonal Psychology, Palo Alto, CA; 415-493-4430. Offers training in the many uses of imagery, including its applications in healing.

HERBS AND BOTANICAL RESOURCES— TIMOTHY KUSS, PH.D.

Seek the advice of a trained herbalist whenever possible. The small expense can turn into a great savings by using the proper herbs for your own unique situation. Look in the yellow pages of your local phone directory under Herbalist or contact the American Botanical Council.

HERB ASSOCIATIONS

American Botanical Council, PO Box 201660, Austin, TX 78720; 800-373-7105 for a catalogue; 512-331-8868; www.herbalgram.org
American Herbalists Guild, PO Box 746555, Arvada, CO 80006; 303-423-8800
Herb Research Foundation, 1007 Pearl St., Ste. 200, Boulder, CO 80302; 303-449-2265; www.herbs.org
International Herb Association, 1202 Allanson Rd., Mundelein, IL 60060; 847-949-4372

RECOMMENDED BOOKS ON HERBS

Castleman, Michael. *The Healing Herbs*. Bantam, 1995.
Duke, James A. *The Green Pharmacy*. Rodale Press, 1998.
Hoffman, David. *The New Holistic Herbal*. Penguin/Element Books, 1991.
Landis, Robyn, with K.P. Khalsa. *Herbal Defense*. Warner Books, 1997.
Mowrey, Daniel B. *The Scientific Validation of Herbal Medicine*. Cormorant Books, 1990.
Murray, Michael T. *The Healing Power of Herbs*. Prima Publishing, 1995.
Werbach, Melvyn. *Botanical Influences on Illness*. Third Line Press, 1994.

PUBLICATIONS ON HERBS

The Herb Quarterly, Long Mountain Press, PO Box 689, San Anselmo, CA 94960; 415-455-9540
HerbalGram, PO Box 201660, Austin, TX 78720; 512-331-8868; www.herbal gram.org

HERBAL STUDY PROGRAMS

Bastyr University, Distance Learning Program, Seattle, WA; 206-517-3549
Blazing Star Herb School, PO Box 6, Shelburne Falls, MA 01370; 413-625-6875

Sage: Home Study Herbology Course, Rosemary Gladstar, PO Box 420, East
    Barre, VT 05649
Western States Chiropractic College, "Botanical Medicine" for health profes-
    sionals, 2900 NE 132nd Ave, Portland, OR 97230; 503-251-5719

HERBAL PRODUCTS

Herbs that have been gathered fresh and well processed can be obtained
    from Nature's Way, Nature's Answer, Eclectic, Gaia, and other compa-
    nies found in health food stores. Exceptional herbal formulas available
    from health professionals include PhytoPharmica and Systemic For-
    mulas.
East Earth Trade Winds, PO Box 493151, Redding, CA 96049; 800-258-
    6878, 916-223-2346; www.snowcrest.net/eetw/.Chinese herbal formulas
Eclectic Institute, 4385 Southeast Lusted Rd., Sandy, OR 97055; 800-332-
    4372; www.eclecticherb.com. Organic herbs
Gaia Herbs, Brevard, NC 28712; 800-831-7780. Quality herbal tinctures
Herbs for Kids, PO Box 837, Bozeman, MT 59717; 800-735-0299, 406-587-
    0180. Pesticide-free and alcohol-free glycerites for children
Infinity Health, Highlands Ranch, CO; 303-346-7212; order line 800-733-
    9293. www.wellnessplace.com/cat/ih. Carries a wide range of combina-
    tion remedies and the most popular single herbs from companies
    including Nature's Answer and Systemic Formulas
PhytoPharmica, PO Box 1745, Green Bay, WI 54305; 800-553-2370, 920-
    469-9099; www.phytopharmica.com; quality standardized herbal ex-
    tracts

RESOURCES FOR MIND-BODY MEDICINE— LEN SAPUTO, M.D.

Bolen, Jean Shinoda. *Close to the Bone.* Simon & Schuster, 1998. Using ill-
    ness as a means of opening the heart and as a door to personal trans-
    formation.
Cousins, Norman. *Anatomy of an Illness.* Bantam, 1995. Using laughter and
    nutrition to heal the body; an account of Cousins's personal experi-
    ence in self-healing.
Kabat-Zinn, Jon. *Full Catastrophe Living: Using the Wisdom of Your Body and
    Mind to Face Stress, Pain, and Illness.* Delta-Dell Books, 1990. Resources
    for healing, including hatha yoga, mindfulness meditation, pain man-
    agement, and stress reduction.
Myss, Caroline. *Why People Don't Heal and How They Can.* Harmony
    Books, 1998. An expanded understanding of the nature of illness and
    the value and relevance of addressing illness on many levels.
Pescosolido, Bernice A, Eric R. Wright, and William Patrick Sullivan.
    "Communities of care: A theoretical perspective on case management

models in mental health." *Advances in Medical Sociology* 6: 37–79, 1995.

Remen, Rachel Naomi. *Kitchen Table Wisdom.* Riverhead Books, 1997. Remarkable true stories, shared wisdom that humanizes the face of illness.

Shuman, Robert. *The Psychology of Chronic Illness.* Basic Books/HarperCollins, 1996. Insight into the nature of chronic illness and healing resources, written by a wise and honest psychologist who has experienced chronic illness.

NATIONAL ASSOCIATIONS FOR DIGESTIVE DISORDERS

American Liver Foundation and the Hepatitis Liver Disease. Hotline and information on gallbladder disease. 1425 Pompton Avenue, Cedar Grove, NJ 07009; 800-223-0179 or 212-668-1000; www.liverfoundation.org

Crohn's and Colitis Foundation of America, 3386 Park Avenue South, New York, NY 10016; 800-932-2423, 212-685-3440

The Digestive Disease National Coalition, 711 2nd Street NE, #200, Washington, DC 20002; 202-544-7497

Gluten Intolerance Group of North America, PO Box 23053, Burien, WA, 206-246-6652

National Digestive Diseases Information Clearing House, Box NDDIC, 900 Rockville Pike, Bethesda, MD 20892; 310-654-3810

RESOURCES FOR PARASITIC INFECTION— OMAR AMIN, PH.D.

BOOKS OF INTEREST

Garcia, L. S., and D.A. Bruckner. *Diagnostic Medical Parasitology.* Washington, DC: American Society of Microbiology, 1997.

Gillespie, S. H., and P. M. Hawkey. *Medical Parasitology: A Practical Approach.* Oxford University Press, 1995.

Weintraub, S. *The Parasite Menace: A Complete Guide to the Prevention, Treatment, and Elimination of Parasitic Infection.* Pleasant Grove, UT: Woodland Publishing, 1998.

WEBSITES

Stanford University: www.bio.net
University of Nebraska: www.museum.unl.edu/asp/
Referral site: www.paru.cas.cz/parasito.htm

PROFESSIONAL RESOURCES

Omar Amin, Ph.D., director, Institute of Parasitic Diseases, PO Box 28372, Tempe, AZ 85285. The laboratory provides analysis for specimens of parasites and yeast. Dr. Amin, a faculty member of Arizona State University, provides training in parasitic detection and laboratory protocols.

BOOKS OF INTEREST TO PRACTITIONERS

Ash, L.R., and T. C. Orihel. *Atlas of Human Parasitology.* Chicago: American Society of Clinical Pathology, 1997.

Mahon, C.R., and G. Manuselis, Jr. *Diagnostic Microbiology.* W. B. Saunders, 1995.

Peters, W., and H.M. Gilles. *A Color Atlas of Tropical Medicine and Parasitology.* Weert, Netherlands: Wolf Medical Publishing, 1989.

TRAINING VIDEO

Amin, O. M. *Parasitic Infections in Humans: Diagnosis and Pathology,* a five-part video set. The Center for the Improvement of Human Functioning, 1997. To order, contact the center in Wichita, KS, at 800-447-7276.

PROFESSIONAL JOURNALS

Journal of Parasitology, Parasitology, Annals of Tropical Medicine and *Parasitology*

PROFESSIONAL ORGANIZATIONS

American Society of Parasitologists, Iowa City, IA; 319-335-1061
American Society of Microbiology, Washington, DC; 202-737-3600
American Society of Tropical Medicine and Hygiene, Northbrook, IL; 847-480-9592

INDEX

❖

A

Achalasia, 312
  treatment, 381
Acid-alkaline diet, 291–92
Acidophilus. *See Lactobacillus acidophilus*
Acupuncture, 400–401, 538, 540, 552,
  571, 584
Adenovirus, 210
Adrenal glands, DHEA support, 326–28
Adrenaline, stress response, 98, 426
Aerobic bacteria, types of, 144
Aerobic exercise, detoxification, 258
Aesculus, 413
Ag-CIDAL, 206
Aging
  and free radical formation, 120
  minimizing with antioxidants, 123
AIDS
  nutritional support, 342
  parasite infections in, 197, 198
Alcohol use
  alcoholism treatment, 571, 577
  and cirrhosis, 522–25
  and free radical formation, 121–22, 124
  health problems from, 266–67
  and pancreatitis, 576, 577
  and reflux, 584
Alexander technique, 434–35
Alginic acid, 583
Alkaline diet, 280–81, 291–92, 528
Alka-Seltzer Gold, 185, 186, 234, 313
Allergies
  EPD treatment, 370–77
  and leaky gut, 17–18, 68
  See also Food allergies
Aloe vera, 319, 355, 529, 538, 584
Alumina, 410
AMAS Test, 512–13
Amino acid supplements
  chelation with, 261
  detoxification, 260
  liver support, 113
Amin, Omar, 145, 195, 196
Amoebic dysentery. *See Entamoeba
  histolytica*

Amylase, 31, 230
Anaerobic bacteria, 144, 198–200, 376–77
  diagnostic testing for, 199–200
Anderson, Jeffry, 80, 95, 125, 247, 252
Anderson, Scott, 26, 34
Angustora Bitters, 234
Antacids, 582, 583
  dangers of, 408–409
Antibiotics
  destruction of microflora, 51, 52, 58, 59,
    197, 346
  for diarrhea, 532
  parasite elimination, 202–203
  for ulcers, 589
  yogurt with course of, 236, 589
Antibodies
  and food allergies, 77
  functions of, 32–33, 38, 40, 143
  testing levels. *See* Antibody testing
Antibody testing, 141–44
  bacterial panel, 144
  microflora immune competence test,
    144
  parasite antibody panel, 144, 150
  SIgA level testing, 171–73
  viral screens, 144
alpha-antichymotrypsin, measurement
  of, 173
Antigens, 32–33, 38
  defenses against, 32–33
  and illness, 32, 38
Antimony, 406
Antioxidants, 61, 258–60
  against free radicals, 122–23, 124
  liver support, 113, 255
  sources of, 124, 207, 259
  and stamina, 122–23
Anus
  fissures, 541
  fistulas, 541–42
  nutritional needs, 321
  pruritus ani, 578–79
  viral diseases of, 212
Appendix infections, and Crohn's disease,
  39–40

Arnica, 413
Arsenicum, 406, 411
Art, benefits of, 475–76
Artemisia annua, 206, 367–68
Aspergillus parasiticus, 362
Astragalus, 207, 363
Attention deficit disorder
  and candida, 196–97
  and leaky gut, 69
Attitude, positive, 276–77
Autism, and candida, 196–97
Autoimmune disorders
  and exposure to toxins, 84
  and leaky gut, 67–68, 377
  and T cell activity, 375–76
  treatment, 372
Ayurvedic medicine, 206, 354, 358, 359,
    415–21
  basic principles, 419–20
  energies in, 416–17

B
Bacteria
  aerobic, 144
  anaerobic, 144, 198–200, 376–77
  antibiotic-resistant bacteria, 90–91
  antimicrobial/antibacterial herbs,
    360–64, 361
  friendly. *See* Microflora
  harmful. *See* Pathogens
Bacterial panel, 144
Baikal skullcap, 363
Baker, Sidney MacDonald, 156, 159
Barium enema, 136
Barium X-ray, 135–36, 585
Barrett's esophagitis, 584
B cells, functions of, 39
Beaumont, William, 96–98
Bentonite clay, 529
Berberine, 364, 517
Beta-carotene, 207
Beta-glucuronidase, 375
  measurement of, 162–63
Betaine hydrochloride, 205, 321
Betalactulose, 528
Bicarbonate
  and digestion, 30
  for food allergy reactions, 184–85, 186
  measurement of, 140, 231–32
  supplemental, 186, 234
Bifidobacteria, 48, 49, 237
Biochemical individuality, 4–5
Biocidin, 206
Bioelectromagnetic therapy, 379–83
  disorders treated with, 380–81
  electro-acupuncture, 381
  microwave resonance therapy, 382
Bioflavonoids, 61, 242, 542
Biological terrain assessment (BTA), 573
Biopsy, parasite testing, 151
Biorhythm, 291
Bismuth, 334
Bitters, gentian, 234, 353, 366

Black elderberry, 365
Black-eyed Susan, 365
Black walnut, 360
Bladderwrack, 546
Bland, Jeffrey, 105, 114, 115, 181
Blastocystis hominis, 147, 148, 195
  signs of infection, 198
Blood tests
  candida diagnosis, 165–66
  parasite testing, 150
Boldo leaf, 357
Borage oil, 245
Bragg's Liquid Aminos, 284
Breath fresheners, herbal, 361
Breathing
  meditation, 446, 449–50
  for relaxation, 274
Bryonia, 410
Buckthorn bark, 355
Butyrate, 249, 319–20, 534, 537–38
  measurement of, 163, 198, 200
Byronia, 405

C
Cabbage juice, 359, 590
Caffeine, 267–68, 286–87
  detox from, 268
  health problems from, 267–68
Calcium polycarbophil, 528
Cancer
  and chemical toxins, 93–94
  and cigarette smoking, 265
  colon cancer, 511–15
  pancreatic cancer, 574–75
Cancer protection, and *L. acidophilus*, 48
Candida, 19–20, 515–19
  anti-yeast herbs, 360, 361, 365–67, 517
  causes of, 20, 126, 516
  diagnostic tests, 164–66, 516
  and liver, 166
  and parasites, 151
  physical damage from, 196
  signs of, 19–20, 515–16
  treatment, 372, 517–19
Canned foods, avoiding, 287
Carbamates, 227
Carbohydrates
  diet for finding balance, 297–300
  minimizing, 246, 294–301
  negative health effects, 296
Carbonated drinks, avoiding, 285–86
Carbo vegetalis, 405, 407
Carcinoma embryonic antigen, 512
Cardamom, 353
Carnitine, 318–19
Cascara sagrada, 355–56
Cat's claw, 206, 356
Celandine, 366
Celiac disease, 519–22
Cellulose, 527
Chamomile, 353
Chamomilla, 405
Chaparral, 364

Chaparro amargosa, 368
Cheese, healthy choices, 288
Chelation, 571
  drugs for, 261
  foods/supplements for, 261
Chelation challenge test, heavy metal
  exposure, 226
Chemicals. *See* Toxins
Chewing, importance of, 26
China, 407
Chinese medicine, 384–401
  acupuncture, 400–401
  body, organization of, 384–85, 388
  communication within body, 399–401
  eating guidelines, 393–97
  good digestion, signs of, 388–89
  immune system in, 397–98
  origin of digestive problems, 390–92
  Qi, 384, 385, 387–88
  stress management, 398–99
  tongue diagnosis, 389–90, 391
Chlordane, 223, 227
Chlorophyll, 280–81, 306–307
Chmotrypsin, 162
Cholecystokinin (CCK), 76–77, 92
Cholesterol level, and *L. acidophilus*,
  47–48
Chorella, 306
Chromium, 264, 518
Chronic fatigue syndrome, 210
Chyme, 30
Chymex Test, 78
Cigarette smoking, benefits of stopping,
  123–24
Cinchona bark, 363
Cirrhosis, 522–25
Cisapride, 582
Clear, 206
Clostridium difficile, 51, 237, 346
  causes of, 59
  testing for, 199–200
Clove, 360
Coca Test, 184
Cocsackie viruses, health effects, 210
Coenzyme Q10, antioxidant, 124, 207
Colcoynithis, 406
Cold sores, 209–10
  treatment, 210
Colic, treatment, 353, 354
Colitis, treatment, 59, 236, 237
Collinsonia, 413
Colon
  colon cancer, 511–15
  and digestive process, 31
  nutritional needs, 319–20
  stricture of, 587
Colonics, for constipation, 530
Colostrum, 238, 239, 247, 535
Comprehensive digestive stool analysis,
  162–63
  candida testing, 165, 516
  elements measured in, 162–63, 235
  enzyme measurement, 231

Congestion, herbs for clearing, 351
Constipation, 125, 525–30
  treatment, 303, 306, 355–56, 357, 372,
    409–10, 527–30, 564
Copper, 124
  deficiency, 312, 313
  overload, 568, 571
Corticosteroids, 346
Cortisol, measurement of, 174–75
Cortisone, 328–29
Cranberry, 366
Crigler-Najjar syndrome, 568
Crohn's disease, 555–61
  and appendix infections, 39, 40
  causes, 57, 557
  diagnosis of, 558–59
  signs of, 557–58
  treatment, 359, 372, 559–61
Cryptosporidium, 142, 146, 194
  signs of infection, 197
CT scan, 137–38
Cuprum arsenicosum, 411
Curcumin, 358
Cyclospora, 146, 147, 195
N-acetyl-cystein, 212, 238, 242, 248
Cytokines, 42
Cytolog, 243

D
Dairy products
  alternative products, 288
  lactose intolerance, 176
  problems with, 288
Dandelion, 357, 363, 524, 546
Depression, DHEA support, 327–28
Detoxification
  aerobic exercise, 258
  amino acid supplements, 260
  antioxidants, 258–60
  Ayurvedic, 420
  chelation, 261
  and liver, 17, 254–56
  sauna therapy, 257–58
DGL (deglycyrrhizinated licorice), 190,
  207, 250, 345–46, 359, 584, 590
DHEA, 325–328
  abnormal, signs of, 174, 325
  function of, 174, 326–28
  measurement of, 174, 325
Diabetes, 311, 314
  and candida, 518
  and diet, 233
Diagnostic tests
  for anaerobic bacteria, 199–200
  antibody testing, 141–44, 171–73
  barium enema, 136
  barium X-ray, 135–36
  comprehensive digestive stool analysis,
    162–63
  cortisol level measure, 174–75
  CT scan, 137–38
  DHEA measure, 174
  endoscopic ultrasound, 137

endoscopy, 136–37
for enzyme levels, 139–40, 231–32
esophageal motility test, 139
food allergy testing, 156–59, 183–85
functional assessment, 140, 153–55
gastric acid testing, 139–40
gluten intolerance test, 175–76
for infection, 174
for inflammation in large intestine, 173
for inflammation in small intestine, 173
intestinal permeability, 164
lactose intolerance test, 176
laparoscopy, 138–39
liver challenge test, 167–68
liver detox profile, 167
metabolic profile, 176–77
microflora measurement, 235
MRI testing, 137–38
oxidative stress testing, 168–69
pancreatic enzyme measurement, 78
parasite detection, 150–51
for toxic exposures, 224–29
and treatment design, 161, 177
Diarrhea, 530–35
treatment, 306, 335–36, 411–12,
532–35, 563–64
Dientamoeba fragilis, 149, 198
Die-off reaction, 204–205
Diet
alkaline diet, 280–81, 291–92
antioxidant-rich, 259
basic foods to include, 281–85, 294
basic guidelines, 271–72
cancer prevention, 515
candida treatment, 517–18
carbohydrates, minimizing, 246,
294–301
and dysbiosis, 57
eating and biorhythm, 291
effects on microflora, 51, 52
fluid needs, 280
and food allergy control, 78–79, 186
food combining, 290–91
and food cravings, 295–96
foods to avoid, 285–89
gluten-free, 521–22
and glycemic index, 281
natural chelators, 261
Diflucan, 517
Digestion
Chinese view, 395–96
herbs for support of, 353–55
and nutrient absorption, 16
and pathogens, 16
process of, 29–32
and stomach acid, 27, 29
Digestive enzyme supplements, 29
betaine hydrochloride, 205, 232
bicarbonate, 186, 234
bitters, 234
choosing supplement, 233–34
pancreatic enzymes, 186, 205

Digestive problems
causes of, 14–15, 130
leaky gut, 16–17
and poor health, 125–26
solutions to, 132
Digestive system
anatomy of, 28
ecosystem of, 14, 55
microflora, 14, 16, 34, 36
Digestive system and immunity
antibodies, 32–33, 38
cellular immunity, 38, 39, 40
complexity of protection, 35–36
gut-associated lymphoid tissue, 38–40
influencing factors, 44–45
and leaky gut, 66–67
lymph tissue, 38
lysosomes, 42
malfunction, causes of, 60
M cells, 40
oral tolerance, 42–44
secretory immunoglobulin A (SIgA),
32–33, 40–42
stomach acid, 38
T cells (killer cells), 38
and toxic exposures, 88–89
Diverticulosis, 535–38
treatment, 537–38
Diverticultis, 535–38
treatment, 356, 359, 537–38
Drug abuse, health problems from, 269
Drug treatment. *See* Medications
Dysbiosis
causes of, 57–60
diagnosis of, 60
effects of, 54
and illness, 57–58
and irritable bowel syndrome, 564
and leaky gut, 68
meaning of, 16, 54, 55
restoring balance, 56, 60–61, 533–34
Dyspepsia, 538–41
Dysphagia, 584

E
Echinacea, 206, 360–61
EDP therapy
for allergies, 374–75, 542
course of treatment, 373–74
for digestive disorders, 372, 376–77
mechanism of action, 375–76
success of, 372–73, 377
Eggs, in diet, 282–83
Electro-acupuncture, 381
Elimination diets
for food allergies, 156–57, 188–89
withdrawal phase, 188–89
Endoscopic ultrasound, 137
Endoscopy, 136–37, 585
Enemas, for constipation, 530
Energy
and antioxidants, 122–23
from foods, 268

Entamoeba coli, 47, 50, 52, 195, 362
Entamoeba hartmanii, 195, 198
Entamoeba histolytica, 147, 149, 150, 195,
    361, 362
  signs of infection, 197
Enteral nutrition, 337
Environmental factors
  environmental toxins. *See* Toxins
  and health, 7
Enzymes
  functions of, 27, 29, 230–31
  measurement of, 231
  of mouth, 230
  of pancreas, 30–31, 230–31
  of stomach, 27, 29, 230–31
  See also Digestive enzyme supplements
EPD treatment, 370–77
Epithelial growth factors, 207, 249
Epstein-Barr virus, 212
Esophageal motility test, 139
Esophagus
  esophageal stricture, 585–88
  nutritional needs, 332–33
Essential fatty acids, 61, 207, 318
  omega-3 fatty acids, 244, 318
  omega-6 fatty acids, 244–45, 318
  supplements, 244–46
Evening primrose oil, 245
Exercise
  Alexander technique, 434–35
  basic guidelines, 272–73
  benefits of, 425–26
  Feldenkrais method, 435–36
  and free radical formation, 122
  gentle practices, 423–24
  isometrics, 436
  Pilates, 436–37
  Qigong, 428–31
  walking, 426–28
  weight training, 432–34
  yoga, 431–32

F
Faass, Nancy, 469, 503
Fats in diet
  fats to avoid, 286
  healthful types, 284, 294
Fecal fat analysis, 231
Feldenkrais method, 435–36
Fennel, 354
Ferguson, Tom, 464, 468, 491
Fermented foods, in diet, 284
Fiber
  and digestive health, 58, 321–22, 347,
    528
  supplement, 242, 527
Fibromyalgia, 210
Fight-or-flight, stress response, 98–99
Fissures, anal, 541
Fistulas, 541–42
Flagyl, 203
Flaxseed, 306–307, 356, 527
Flaxseed oil, 245, 284, 303–304, 306, 323

Flora. *See* Dysbiosis; Microflora
Fluoride, toxic effects, 82, 221–22
Folic acid, 311, 316
Food additives, sensitivity to, 74, 77
Food allergies, 542–43
  antibody protection, 77
  and food additives/pesticides, 77
  and leaky gut, 17–18, 74–75, 189–90
  mental effects, 75–76
  peptides as trigger, 76–77
  signs of, 158
  sublingual antidote treatment, 187–88
  treatment, 78–79, 184–88, 372, 374,
    542–43
  types of, 72–74
Food allergy testing, 156–59
  elimination diet, 156–57, 188–89
  food challenge test, 183–84
  IgG ELISA test, 157
  pulse test, 184
  research on, 157–59
  skin testing, 187
Food combining
  control of food allergies, 78–79
  guidelines, 290–91
Food cravings, 295–96
  mechanism in, 75
  sugar, 264–65, 295
Food poisoning, bacteria in, 195
Formula, 2, 260
Forsythia, 365
FOS (fructo-oligo-saccharides), 238, 319
Free radicals, 18–19
  antioxidant protection, 122–23, 124
  causes of, 120–22
  dangers of, 19, 119
  formation of, 115–16, 118–19
  lifestyle and reduction of, 123–24
  and liver, 119–20
  oxidative stress testing, 168–69
Fried foods, avoiding, 288
Fruit juice, 286
Fruits, nutritional benefits, 283
Functional testing, 5–6, 140, 153–55
  candida testing, 164–66
  comprehensive digestive stool analysis,
    162–63
  intestinal permeability, 163–64
  purpose of, 154–55, 171
  See also Diagnostic tests
Furlong, John, 160, 169

G
Gallstones, 543–46
  treatment, 357, 545–46
Gamma globulin, oral, 533
Ganoderma, 517
Garden, toxins, in, 220–21
Gardening, benefits of, 474–75
Garlic, 361, 517
Gas, treatment, 353–54, 358, 361,
    407–408, 564–65
Gastric volvulus, 586

Gastritis, 333–34, 546–49
  treatment, 548–49
Gastrointestinal reflux disease, 579–84
  causes of, 580–81
  diagnosis of, 581–82
  treatment, 582–84
Gelsemium, 411–12
Genetics, and health, 7
Gentian, 234, 353, 366
Giardia lamblia, 145–46, 148, 150, 193,
  362
  diagnostic difficulty, 197
  signs of infection, 197
Gilbert's syndrome, 339, 568
Ginger, 354, 359, 362
Ginkgo biloba, 207, 250
GLA (gamma linolic acid), 244
Glandular supplements, pancreas support,
  232
Gliadin, measurement of, 175–76
Glutathione, 207, 255, 321, 534
Gluten intolerance
  celiac disease, 519–22
  gluten intolerance test, 175–76
  signs of, 175
Glycemic index, 281
Goldenrod, 366
Goldenseal, 364
Goldthread, 364
Grains, nutritional benefits, 281–82, 312
Grapefruit juice, drug interactions,
  340–41
Grapefruit seed extract, 206, 207, 362, 517
Graphites, 410
Growth factors, for leaky gut, 190
Guided imagery, 103, 452–82
  effects of, 456–60
  with hypnosis, 454–55, 459
  types of, 453–54
Gums, bleeding, 310–11
Gut-associated lymphoid tissue, 38–40
Gut reactions, 34

H

H2 blockers, 345, 583, 589
Haas, Elson, 262, 270, 271
Hair analysis, heavy metal exposure, 226
Healer within concept, 495–502
  self-healing, 500–502
Health, influencing factors, 7–8
Health evaluation profile, 9–13
Heartburn, 579–84
  treatment, 312, 354, 377, 582–84
Heavy metal exposure, 80, 225–26
  detoxification from, 256–61
  testing for, 226
Heidelberg capsule, 231
Heimlich, Jane, 402, 414
Helicobacter pylori, 201, 202, 334
  ulcers, 588–90
Helminths, types of, 144
Hemoccult blood testing, 512
Hemochromatosis, 568

Hemorrhoids, 549–53
  treatment, 412–14, 550–53
Hepatitis, 212, 339, 522, 553–55
  treatment, 555
  types of, 553–55
Herbal therapy
  anti-bacterial herbs, 363–64
  anti-microbial herbs, 360–63
  antioxidant herbs, 124
  anti-viral herbs, 364–65
  digestive support, 353–55
  intestinal healing, 355–57
  leaky gut, 250
  liver support, 113, 357–58
  parasite elimination, 203–204, 206,
    360–62, 367–69
  with sauna therapy, 258
  therapy routine, 203–204, 350–53
  ulcers, 359
Herpes virus, 209–10, 211
Histamine blockers, 582
Home, toxins in, 220–21
Homeopathic remedies, 402–14
  for constipation, 409–10
  for diarrhea, 411–12
  for gas, 407–408
  hemorrhoids, 412–14
  for indigestion, 404–406
  mechanism in, 403–404
  for nausea/vomiting, 406–407
Homeostatic soil organisms, 237
Homocysteine, 320–21
Honeysuckle, 363
Hormones
  cortisone, 328–29
  DHEA, 325–28
  progesterone, 329–31
H. pylori, 201, 202, 334
Hydrochrolic acid (HCl), 39
  functions of, 27, 29, 230
  measurement of, 139–40, 231–32
  supplementation of, 205, 232
Hyperpermeability, 17
  See also Leaky gut
Hypnotherapy, 454–55, 459

I

IgG ELISA test, 157
Ignatia, 405
Illness, as time for change, 471–72, 478
Immune system
  and allergies, 17–18
  autoimmune disorders, 18
  basic support, 278–79
  cellular/humoral immunity
    interactions, 37
  Chinese medicine, 397–98
  and free radicals, 18–19
  supplements for support of, 207, 238,
    247, 326–27, 342, 360–61
  See also Digestive system and immunity
Immunoglobulin A (IgA), 41–42, 43, 44,
  74

Immunoglobulin E (IgE), 73
Immunoglobulin G (IgG), 43, 73, 157
Immunoglobulin M (IgM), 42, 43, 142
Indigestion
    dyspepsia, 538–41
    treatment, 404–406
Infection
    diagnostic test for, 174
    See also Inflammation
Inflammation
    signs of, 243
    treatment, 243–45, 303–307, 328–29,
        353, 355–57
Inflammatory bowel disease, 555–61
    causes, 556–57
    diagnosis of, 558–59
    treatment, 559–61
    types of, 555–56
    See also Crohn's disease
Inositol hexaphosphate, 207
Insulin, 30
    and candida, 518
Interferon, 569–70
Intestinal obstruction, 586–87
Intestinal permeability
    testing for, 164
    treatment, 164, 242
Intradermal testing, for food allergies, 187
Ipecac, 406
Irritable bowel syndrome, 19, 561–65
    causes, 82, 90, 562
    treatment, 238, 336–38, 372, 563–65
Isometrics, 436

J
Jahnke, Roger, 422, 437, 495
Junk food, avoiding, 289

K
Kabat-Zinn, Jon, 443, 451
Kamala, 368
Kapha, 416–17
Ketones, measurement of, 297
Korngold, Efrem, 384, 401
Kunin, Richard, 198, 209, 212, 293, 309
Kuss, Timothy, 192, 203, 349, 369

L
Lactobacillus acidophilus, benefits of, 46,
    47, 48, 235–38, 240
Lactobacillus bulgaricus, 48
Lactobacillus DDS, 237
Lactobacillus plantarum, benefits of, 238
Lactoferrin, 237, 238, 247
Lactose intolerance, 566–67
    diagnosis of, 176, 566–67
    management of, 47, 567
    signs of, 176, 563
Lad, Vasant, 415, 421
Laparoscopy, 138–39
Large intestine
    and digestive process, 31
    testing for inflammation, 173
Laughter, and healing, 473

Leaky gut, 16–17
    causes, 17, 61, 63–64, 127, 129
    chemical toxins as cause, 94
    and food allergies, 17–18, 74–75,
        189–90
    genetic factors, 69
    immune response to, 66–67
    physical effects of, 62–63, 67–69,
        130–31
    sequence of events in, 65–67
    treatment, 132, 189–91, 247–50, 306
Legumes, 282
Leptotaenia, 365
Lerner, Michael, 441, 442
Leukotriene, 375
L-glutamine, 61, 207, 247–48, 264, 303,
    304–305, 306, 318, 534
Lice, toxic therapy, 222
Licorice root, 250, 359, 362–63, 366
    See also DGL (deglycyrrhizinated
        licorice)
Lifespan Institute, 13
Lifestyle
    beneficial changes, 262–70
    and health, 7–8
Lipase, 30, 230
Lipoic acid, 207, 212
Liver
    and candida, 166
    detoxification function, 17, 33, 105–10,
        166–67
    detoxification procedure, 254–56
    factors affecting function, 93, 113–14,
        254–55
    and free radicals, 119–20
    herbal support, 113, 357–58
    leaky gut, effects on, 67
    liver function testing, 110–11, 167–68,
        568–69
    nutritional support, 111–13, 255–56,
        320–21, 338–41
    overload, effects of, 112, 129, 254–55
Liver disease, 567–71
    cirrhosis, 522–25
    diagnosis of, 568–69
    hepatitis, 553–55
    treatment, 569–71
    types of, 212, 568
Luncheon meats, avoiding, 287
Lycopodiun, 407
Lymphocytes, 38
Lymph system, exercise effects on, 426
Lymph tissue, gut-associated lymphoid
    tissue, 38–40
Lynn, Paul, 302, 308, 324
Lysosomes, 42
Lysozyme A, measurement of, 173

M
McLean, Rebecca, 482, 490
Magnesium, 207, 243, 340, 528, 529, 583
Magnets. *See* Bioelectromagnetic therapy
Malnutrition, and leaky gut, 68

Manganese, 124
  deficiency, 336
Manometry, 585
Marshmallow root, 356
Massage, 538
  self-massage, 274
M cells, 40
Meadowsweet, 359
Measles, in GI tract, 211
Meat, in diet, 282
Medications
  combined with nutritional support,
    332–42
  effects on microflora, 59
  health problems from, 269 compared to
    natural therapies, 344–48
Meditation, 275, 443–51
  basic guidelines, 447–49
  sitting meditation, 445–47, 449–51
Medline, 198
Megadophilus, 239
Memory cells, functions of, 39
Mental disorders
  and candida, 196–97
  and exposure to toxins, 85, 90
  and leaky gut, 69, 130
  and liver function, 340
  and parasite infection, 151
Mercury amalgams, toxic effects, 82,
    90–91, 222–23
Metabolic profile, 176–77
Methionine, 321
Metronidazole, 202
Microflora, 14, 16, 34, 36
  balance, affecting factors, 51–52
  beneficial effects of, 46–48
  destruction by toxins, 89–90
  imbalance, signs of, 52
  measurement of, 235
  origin of, 49–50
  primary strains of, 48, 50
  supplementation of, 235–39
Microflora immune competence test, 144
Microsporidia, signs of infection, 198
Microwave resonance therapy, 382
Milk thistle, 212, 250, 357, 524, 570
Mind/body methods
  guided imagery, 452–82
  healer within concept, 495–502
  meditation, 443–51
  proactive patient, 503–507
  self-care, 463–68
  support system, 469–90
Minerals, 255
  liver support, 113
  malabsorption of, 27, 29
  parasite elimination, 206
  with sauna therapy, 258
Monolaurin, 211, 212
Motility, pseudo-obstruction, 587
Motion sickness, 381
Mountain mahogany, 357–58

Mouth
  digestive enzymes of, 230
  nutritional needs, 310–12
  and nutritional status, 310–11
  viral diseases of, 209–10
MRI testing, 137–38
MSM (methyl-sulfonyl-methane), 124,
    529, 542, 584
  for inflammation, 243, 307
  for leaky gut, 190, 249
  for parasite elimination, 206
Music, benefits of, 475

N
N-acetyl-glucosamine, 249, 319
Nat Cell Thymus, 247
Natrum mur, 410
Nausea, treatment, 406–407
Neem leaf, 354, 359
Neurotransmitters
  and food allergies, 75–76
  peptides as, 76
Niacin, 316
  with sauna therapy, 257
Nichols, Trent, 135, 197, 332, 379, 383,
    509
Nicotine
  health problems form, 265
  smoking cessation, 266
Nitric acid, 413
Nitric oxide, measurement of, 174
Nizoral, 517
Nonsteroidal anti-inflammatory drugs
    (NSAIDs), 345, 390
Nutrient absorption
  and digestion, 16
  improvement of, 573–74
  malabsorption, 66, 68, 88, 571–74
Nutritional medicine, 6
Nutrition. *See* Diet
Nuts, in diet, 283
Nux vomica, 405, 406, 409, 413
Nystatin, 517
N-Zymes 10, 233

O
Occupation, toxic exposures, 84, 224
Oils
  beneficial types of, 284
  and digestive health, 322
Okra, 359
Olive leaf extract, 206, 250, 363
Omega-3 fatty acids, 244, 318, 528–29
Omega-6 fatty acids, 244–45, 318, 534
Online resources, 491–94
  support system, 476–77, 493–94
Oral tolerance, and immunity, 42–44
Oregano oil, 366, 517
Organic acids testing, 200, 201
Organic foods, benefits of, 219
Organochlorines, 227–28
Organophosphates, 227
Oxidative stress. *See* Free radicals

Oxidative stress testing, 168–69
Oxygen
    and exercise, 425
    and free radical damage, 115–19

P
Pain control, TENS units, 381
Pancreas
    diet for care of, 233
    and digestive process, 29, 30–31
    glandular supplements, 232
    nutritional needs, 313–14
    pancreatic cancer, 574–75
    pancreatitis, 575–78
Pancreatic enzymes
    supplemental, 186, 205–206
    testing enzyme levels, 78
    types of, 30–31
Panos, Maesimund, 402, 414
Panreatin, 205–206, 546
    side effects, 206, 233–34
Pantothenic acid, 316
Papain, 354
Paracidin, 206
ParaGONE, 206
Para-Guard, 206
Para-Relief, 206
Parasite antibody panel, 144
Parasite elimination routine
    antibiotics, 202–203
    antiparasite formulas, 206
    continued therapy, 207–208
    die-off reaction, 204–205
    digestive enzymes, 205–206
    herbal therapy, 203–204, 206, 360–62,
        367–68
    mineral-based supplements, 206
    preparation for therapy, 202, 204
    supportive supplements, 207
Parasites, 20, 22–24
    and candida, 151
    diagnostic difficulties, 20, 23, 148–49,
        197, 200–201
    diagnostic tests, 150–51, 201
    helminths, 144
    illness caused by, 20, 150, 151
    new/emerging pathogens, 149, 198
    protozoa, 144
    risk of exposure, 147–48
    self-assessment quiz, 23
    signs of, 20, 22–24, 147, 194
    transmission of, 145–46, 193–94
    types of, 144, 195, 197–98
Parenteral nutrition, 337
Parex Intensive Care, 206
Pathogens
    candida, 21–22
    categories of, 252–54
    in GI tract, 16, 35, 127, 195
    parasites, 22–24
    protection against. *See* Digestive system
        and immunity
    See also Dysbiosis

Pau d'arco, 206, 366–67, 517
Peppermint, 354–55
Pepsin, 27
Peptides
    food allergy trigger, 77
    for inflammation, 305–306
    role of, 92, 399–400
    secretion of, 91, 92
    supplements, 243, 584
Pepto-Bismol, 206, 313, 534
Permavite, 242, 522
Pesticides, 218–21, 226–28
    avoidance strategy, 219, 220
    digestive symptoms, 77, 81
    and free radical formation, 122
    sources of, 218–19
    testing for exposure, 227, 228
    types of, 223, 227–28
Peyer's patches, 38, 41
Phosphatidyl choline, 61, 207, 249
Phosphorus, 406
Phyllanthus, 358
Pilates, 436–37
Pitta, 416–17
Plasma cells, function of, 39
Plautonol, 590
Plummer, Nigel, 46, 53
Podophyllum, 412
Polyps, colon cancer, 511, 512
Polyzyme, 242
Prednisone, 336, 569
Proactive patient, 503–507
    guidelines for, 505–507
Probioplex, 239
Probiotic Complex, 239
Probiotics, 47, 518, 529–30
Progesterone, 329–31
Protease, 30, 230
Proteozyme, 243
Proteus vulgaris, 362
Proton pump inhibitors, 582, 589
Protozoa, types of, 144
Protozyme, 233, 234, 242
Pruritus ani, 578–79
Pseudomonas aeruginosa, 362
Pseudowintera colorata, 367
Psyllium seed, 527
Pulsatilla, 406
Pulse test, 184
Putrefactive dysbiosis, 57
Pylorus, 313

Q
Qi, 384, 385, 387–88
Qigong, 428–31, 498
Quassia, 368
Quercitin, 61, 207, 242, 249, 542

R
Reflux. *See* Gastrointestinal reflux disease
Restaurant dining, 290
Rosenbaum, Michael, 35, 45, 71, 183, 247,
    278

Rossman, Martin, 96, 452
Rotation diet
    for food allergies, 185–86
    procedure for, 185–86

S

Saccharomyces boulardii, 207, 236
    benefits of, 237, 533
Salmonella, 195, 362
Salt, 284–85
    with sauna therapy, 258
    substitutes, 285
SAM (S-adenosyl-methionine), 524
Saputo, Len, 54, 61, 206, 469
Sauna therapy, 257–58
    nutrients used with, 257–58
Schizandra, 358, 365, 524, 570
Schizophrenia, and leaky gut, 69
Schuster's syndrome, 587
Scratch test, for food allergies, 187
Sea Cure, 190, 248, 303, 304, 306
Secretin, for pancreas testing, 140
Secretory immunoglobulin A (SIgA),
        32–33, 40–42, 44, 175
    measurement of, 171–73
Selenium, 124, 312
    deficiency, 312, 313
Self-care, 463–68
    healer within, 500–502
Shigella, 195
Short-chain fatty acids, 319–20, 534
Short gut syndrome, 337, 574
Shrader, W.A., Jr., 199, 370, 377
Sick building syndrome, 82–83, 223–24
Sigmoidoscopy, 512
Silica, 410
Silymarin, 250, 357, 524, 546, 570
Skin problems
    and food allergies, 158
    and leaky gut, 131
Skin testing, food allergy testing, 187
Sleep
    basic guidelines, 273–75
    Chinese medicine, 392
Slippery elm, 250, 303, 307, 356, 359, 529
Small intestine
    and digestive process, 30, 31–32
    nutritional needs, 314–19
    testing for inflammation, 173
Solvents, 220–21, 228–29
    testing for exposure, 228
Sore throat, treatment, 210
Spicebush, 367
Spontaneous remission, 500
Sprue, celiac disease, 519–22
Staphylococcus aureus, 362
Stevia, 284
Stine, Jerry, 13, 14, 200, 240, 242, 245
Stinging nettle, 250
Stomach
    and digestive process, 29–30
    nutritional needs, 312–13, 333–35
    viral diseases of, 210–11

Stomach acids
    functions of, 27, 29, 38
    testing levels of, 139–40, 231–32, 539
Stool analysis. *See* Comprehensive
        digestive stool analysis
Streptococcus thermophilus, 48
Stress
    Chinese medicine, 385–86
    and cortisol level, 174–75, 191
    destruction of microflora, 51, 58
    and digestion, 100–101
    and food allergies, 79
    and free radical formation, 120
    and immunity, 44, 60, 98
    positive use of, 101
    stress response, 98–99
    Types 1 and 2, 100
Stress management, 101–102, 191
    Chinese medicine, 398–99
    relaxation methods, 102, 103, 274,
        275–76
Strictures
    colon, 587
    esophageal stricture, 585–88
Sublingual antidote therapy, food
        allergies, 187–88
Sucralfate, 346
Sugar
    alternative sweeteners, 284
    cravings, 264, 295
    health problems related to, 263, 314
    supplements to curb cravings, 264–65
Sulfur, 410, 412, 413
Superoxide dismutase, 237, 590
Support system, 469–90
    basic guidelines, 477
    Circle of Life, 488–90
    healing relationships, 479–81
    online help, 476–77
    support groups, 476, 482–88

T

Tai chi, 429–30
Tannic acid, 206
Taurine, deficiency, 313
T cells (killer cells), 38, 39, 375–76
TENS units, 381
Therapy
    Ayurvedic medicine, 415–21
    bioelectromagnetic therapy, 379–83
    Chinese medicine, 384–401
    detoxification, 252–61
    exercise program, 272–73
    herbal, 349–69
    homeopathic remedies, 402–14
    lifestyle changes, 262–70
    mind/body. *See* Mind/body methods
    nutrition guidelines, 271–72
    repair phase, 240–45
    sleep in, 273–75
    steps in, 181–82, 250–51
    strengthening phase, 245–50
    See also specific illness/condition

Thioles, liver support, 113
Thrush, 311
Thymic Longevity Compound, 247
Thymus extract, 207, 247
Timmins, William, 170, 177
Tongue, and health status, 311
Tongue diagnosis, Chinese medicine, 389–90, 391
Toothpaste, toxic effects, 82
Touch, and healing, 473–74
Toxins
  bacterial. *See* Pathogens
  common sources of, 80–84, 215–23
  and destruction of microflora, 59, 89–90
  detoxification routine, 256–61
  diagnosis of exposure, 85–86, 224–29
  and digestive damage, 86–89, 91–95
  digestive symptoms, 84–85
  and free radical formation, 120, 121
  and heavy metals, 80
  sick building syndrome, 82–83, 223–24
  viral activation by, 90
Trace minerals, antioxidant, 124
Trans-fats, 322
Transit time, 58
Travel, and parasite infections, 147, 531
Tricycline, 206
Tumeric, 358, 359–360, 525

U
Ulcerative colitis, 555, 558
  treatment, 335, 359, 372
Ulcers, 588–590
  causes of, 334–335, 588–89
  with stricture, 586
  treatment, 356, 359, 589–90
UltraClear, 339, 534, 537
Ultra Dophilus, 239
Ultrasound, endoscopic, 137
Urso, 514, 545

V
Vata, 416–17
Vegetables
  in diet, 281
  juices, 207
  nutritional benefits, 281
Venereal warts, 212
Veratrum album, 406, 412
Verma Key, 206
Villi, 31, 32
Viral screens, 144

Viruses
  activation by toxins, 90
  of anal/perianal area, 212
  anti-viral herbs, 364–65
  and GI damage, 200
  of liver, 212
  of mouth, 209–10
  of small intestine, 211
  of stomach, 210–11
  types of, 144
Vitamin A, 190, 211, 314–16
  antioxidant, 124, 207
  and immune response, 42, 61, 78, 207, 248
Vitamin B complex, 249, 316–17
  deficiency, signs of, 311
Vitamin C, 317, 529
  antioxidant, 124
Vitamin D, 314, 317
Vitamin E, 123, 210
  anti-aging effect, 123
  antioxidant, 124, 207, 317–18
Vojdani, Aristo, 141, 144
Vomiting, treatment, 406–407
VRM 3 (wormseed), 206

W
Walking, 426–28
Water intake, 280, 313–14
  hot water, Chinese view, 394–95
Water supply
  minimizing toxins, 217–19
  toxins in, 80–81, 215–18
Water therapy, 276
Weight training, 432–34
Wheyplex, 239
White flour products, avoiding, 287
Wilson's disease, 568
Wine, red wine benefits, 289
Wobenzyme, 243
Wormseed, 368
Wound healing, 380–81

Y
Yellow dock root, 356–57, 529
Yoga, 419–20, 431–32
Yogurt-like foods, benefits of, 47–48, 50, 236, 533–34

Z
Zinc, 124, 190, 248, 534
  excess, 313